Initial Management of Acute Medical Patients

A Guide for Nurses and Healthcare Practitioners

Second Edition

Edited by

Ian Wood

MA, RN, DipN (Lond)
Lecturer
School of Nursing & Midwifery
Keele University
Keele
UK

Michelle Garner

MPhil, BSc (Hons), RN, DipN (Lond)
Senior Lecturer
Faculty of Health & Wellbeing
University of Cumbria
Carlisle
UK

WILEY-BLACKWELL

This edition first published 2012
© 2003 by Whurr Publishers
© 2012 by John Wiley & Sons, Ltd

Wiley-Blackwell is an imprint of John Wiley & Sons, formed by the merger
of Wiley's global Scientific, Technical and Medical business with Blackwell Publishing.

Registered Office
John Wiley & Sons, Ltd, The Atrium, Southern Gate, Chichester, West Sussex, PO19 8SQ, UK

Editorial Offices
9600 Garsington Road, Oxford, OX4 2DQ, UK
The Atrium, Southern Gate, Chichester, West Sussex, PO19 8SQ, UK
2121 State Avenue, Ames, Iowa 50014-8300, USA

For details of our global editorial offices, for customer services and for information about
how to apply for permission to reuse the copyright material in this book please see our website
at www.wiley.com/wiley-blackwell.

Library of Congress Cataloging-in-Publication Data

Initial management of acute medical patients : a guide for nurses and healthcare practitioners / edited
by Ian Wood, Michelle Garner. – 2nd ed.
      p. ; cm.
   Rev. ed. of: Medical assessment units / edited by Ian Wood and Michelle Rhodes. London : Whurr, 2003.
   Includes bibliographical references and index.
   ISBN 978-1-4443-3716-7 (pbk. : alk. paper)
I. Wood, Ian, 1962– II. Garner, Michelle. III. Medical assessment units. [DNLM:
1. Critical Care–methods. 2. Emergency Nursing–methods. 3. Acute Disease–nursing.
4. Nursing Assessment–methods. 5. Triage–methods. WY 154]
   616.02′8–dc23

                                              2011037445

A catalogue record for this book is available from the British Library.

Wiley also publishes its books in a variety of electronic formats. Some content that appears in print
may not be available in electronic books.

Set in 10/12.5 pt Sabon by SPi Publisher Services, Pondicherry, India
Printed and bound in Malaysia by Vivar Printing Sdn Bhd

1   2012

Contents

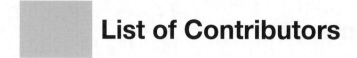

List of Contributors

Carole Donaldson
Staff Development Educator, Postgraduate Critical Care Nursing Program, Sir Charles Gairdner Hospital, Perth, Western Australia

Michelle Garner
Senior Lecturer, Faculty of Health & Wellbeing, University of Cumbria, Carlisle

Michael Gibbs
Lecturer, School of Nursing & Midwifery, Keele University, Keele

Ruth Harris
Consultant Gastroenterologist, Department of Gastroenterology, Countess of Chester NHS Foundation Trust, Chester

Susan Hope
Respiratory Nurse Specialist, Department of Respiratory Medicine, University Hospital of North Staffordshire NHS Trust, Stoke on Trent

Fiona Howell
Matron, Elderly Care Unit, University Hospital of North Staffordshire NHS Trust, Stoke on Trent

Scott Inglis
Senior Lecturer, Faculty of Health & Wellbeing, University of Cumbria, Carlisle

Jane Jervis
Medical Advanced Nurse Practitioner, University Hospital of North Staffordshire NHS Trust, Stoke on Trent and Institute for Life Course Studies, Keele University, Keele

Toni Jordan
Consultant Physician, University Hospital of North Staffordshire NHS Trust, Stoke on Trent

Judith Morgan
Consultant Nurse in Emergency Care, Local Accident Centre, Neath Port Talbot Hospital, Port Talbot

Louise Nelson
Principal Lecturer, Faculty of Health & Wellbeing, University of Cumbria, Carlisle

Sue Read
Reader in Learning Disability Nursing, School of Nursing & Midwifery, Keele University, Keele

Judi Thorley
Regional Lead, Learning Disability Health and Adult Safeguarding, NHS East Midlands

Terry Wardle
Consultant Gastroenterologist and General Physician, Countess of Chester NHS Foundation Trust, Chester

Ian Wood
Lecturer, School of Nursing & Midwifery, Keele University, Keele

Preface

Increasing demands on acute hospital resources, together with a reduction in the number of acute beds available, have placed greater emphasis on the need for rapid and effective assessment of patients in order to determine their need for hospital admission. The increased acuity of patients who are treated in hospital also means that they are at greater risk of deterioration than was previously the case. From a different perspective, it is equally important that those cared for in primary and intermediate care settings are assessed and managed in order to prevent their admission to acute hospital beds. In this context, it is vital that nurses and other healthcare practitioners caring for these patients are aware of how to assess and manage acutely ill patients.

This book provides an up-to-date guide for the initial assessment and management of patients with acute medical conditions. It presents a structured approach based on common presenting features and focuses on the first 24 hours of the patient's hospital stay. The book draws on a wide range of supporting evidence and also provides the reader with sources for further reading.

In writing this book, the authors have been able to draw on their experience as educators in the fields of acute and critical care and their clinical experiences as a charge nurse in emergency department nursing and a sister in acute cardiology, respectively.

Ian Wood
Michelle Garner

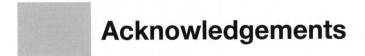

Acknowledgements

The Editors would like to thank the following people for their valuable contributions to the writing of this book:

- The contributors for their hard work in writing and revising their respective chapters
- Magenta Styles and her colleagues at Wiley-Blackwell for their support
- Our families (Sam, Steph and Alex [IW], and Andy and Matthew [MG]) for their support and patience

Introduction

Initial Management of Acute Medical Patients: A Guide for Nurses and Healthcare Practitioners builds on the success of the first edition in meeting the need for a nursing text which relates to the assessment and management of acutely ill medical patients. This second edition has been extensively updated and expanded to include greater focus on the recognition and management of those patients whose condition deteriorates while they are in hospital. The book focuses on the assessment and management of acutely ill medical patients during the first 24 hours of their care but will also appeal to primary and intermediate care professionals whose aim may be to prevent patients' admission to hospital.

Written predominantly *by* nurses *for* nurses, the book has been designed as a quick reference text for use in clinical practice. To act as a source of further reading, the book is extensively referenced throughout, thus increasing its appeal to nurses at all stages of their careers and to those who are undertaking further study.

Each chapter offers clear, concise and down-to-earth information based on a common presenting symptom and provides practical advice, supported by best evidence and the most up-to-date clinical guidelines. The reader is led, step by step, through the initial assessment and management of the patient. Text boxes identify the most common conditions associated with each presenting symptom. A detailed explanation of the causes, pathophysiology, presenting features, investigations and initial management is given for each condition. Text boxes also identify the less common conditions associated with each presenting symptom. The book does not provide information relating to the continuing management of the patient, nor to the less common conditions associated with each presenting symptom. However, sources of further reading are identified.

Notably, the book contains chapters relating to the principles of initial assessment, management of cardiac arrest, sudden death and vulnerable groups. The latter two chapters are deliberately placed early in the book in recognition of their importance in the provision and organisation of care for older people, those with mental health needs and those with learning disabilities.

Normal physiological values are detailed within the preliminary pages. Specific aims and a reference list are contained within each chapter. Text boxes are used to highlight key points from the text and the book is cross-referenced throughout.

Normal Clinical Values

1. Haematology

Haemoglobin	
Male	14.0–17.7 g/dL
Female	12.0–16.0 g/dL
White cell count	$4–11 \times 10^9$/litre
Basophils	$<0.01–0.1 \times 10^9$/litre
Eosinophils	$0.04–0.4 \times 10^9$/litre
Lymphocytes	$1.5–4.0 \times 10^9$/litre
Monocytes	$0.2–0.8 \times 10^9$/litre
Neutrophils	$2.0–7.5 \times 10^9$/litre
Platelet count	$150–400 \times 10^9$/litre
Mean corpuscular haemoglobin (MCH)	27–35 pg
MCH concentration (MCHC)	32–35 g/dL
Mean corpuscular volume (MCV)	80–96 fL
Packed cell volume (PCV)	
Male	0.42–0.53 litres/litre
Female	0.36–0.45 litres/litre
Erythrocyte sedimentation rate (ESR)	<20 mm in 1 hour

Coagulation studies

Activated partial thromboplastin time (aPTT)	25–35s
Usually recorded in relation to the laboratory control or reference level	
Partial thromboplastin time (PTTK)	24–31s
Prothrombin time	12–16s
International normalised ratio (INR)	1
Activated clotting time (ACT)	70–120s

2. Biochemistry

Amylase	< 220 U/litre
Bicarbonate	22–30 mmol/L
Bilirubin	<17 µmol/L (0.3–1.5 mg/dL)
Calcium	2.2–2.67 mmol/L (8.5–10.5 mg/dL)
Chloride	95–106 mmol/L
Cholesterol	3.5–6.5 mmol/L (ideal <5.2 mmol/L)
Creatinine	0.06–0.12 mmol/L (0.6–1.5 mg/dL)
C-reactive protein (CRP)	<10 mg/L
Creatine kinase (CK)	
Male	24–195 U/litre
Female	24–170 U/litre
CK-MB fraction	25 U/litre (0–5% of total CK)
Glucose (fasting)	4.5–6.0 mmol/L (70–110 mg/L)
Magnesium	0.7–1.1 mmol/L
Phosphate	0.8–1.5 mmol/L
Potassium	3.5–5.0 mmol/L
Sodium	135–146 mmol/L
Urea	2.5–6.7 mmol/L (8–25 mg/dL)

Arterial blood gases (ABGs)

PaO_2	10.0–13.3 kPa (75–100 mmHg)
$PaCO_2$	4.8–6.1 kPa (36–46 mmHg)
pH	7.35–7.45
Base excess	–2 to +2 mEq/L
Bicarbonate	24–28 mmol/L
Hydrogen ions (H^+)	35–45 nmol/L
SaO_2	95–98%

1 Initial Assessment of the Acute Medical Patient

Judith Morgan and Ian Wood

Aims

This chapter will:

- describe a systematic approach for the initial assessment and management of acute medical patients
- discuss the components of physical assessment, history-taking and prioritisation
- discuss the principles of documentation and discharge planning as part of the initial assessment process

---

Introduction

Accurate assessment and the ability to prioritise and manage patients' needs underpin safe and effective practice in acute care settings. If initial assessment is inadequate, the clinical risk for the patient increases. Assessment involves the gathering of information regarding the patient's current physiological and psychological status along with a history of the present and past medical events. On seeing the patient for the first time, the assessment process begins. An initial 'eyeball' of the patient will quickly identify whether they are alert and talking, their age, sex, general appearance, behaviour and demeanour. Alongside this process, relevant investigations to aid diagnosis should be initiated, and appropriate treatments and care commenced. Early and effective assessment and initiation of investigations are essential if prompt and accurate decisions regarding the patient's need for medical attention, hospital admission or transfer to a more appropriate care setting are to be made.

The assessment process should always be carried out systematically, and comprises the following components:

- systematic physical assessment (Airway, Breathing, Circulation, Disability, Exposure)
- history taking

Initial Management of Acute Medical Patients: A Guide for Nurses and Healthcare Practitioners, Second Edition. Edited by Ian Wood and Michelle Garner.

- prioritisation of needs
- documentation of findings
- discharge planning

Systematic physical assessment (ABCDE)

Using the systematic ABCDE approach helps in the identification of serious, life-threatening complaints or complications at the earliest opportunity and saves lives. The identification and management of *airway* problems before the assessment of breathing is crucial, as an unrecognised airway problem may be the cause of a patient's breathing difficulties. As the first physiological responses to illness normally occur in the respiratory system, and breathing has a direct impact on the circulatory system (i.e. the circulation is dependent on oxygen supply), it is crucial to identify and correct life-threatening *breathing* problems before making an assessment of circulatory function. Once the patient's *circulatory* status has been assessed and problems managed, an assessment of neurological *disability* can be made. This systematic approach to the initial assessment of all patients is completed by undressing the patient (*exposure*), thus ensuring that important clinical indicators are not missed. As a baseline for this assessment, Table 1.1 gives details of normal adult physiological values.

Airway

Assess the patency of the patient's airway. In most cases, this will be a formality as the patient will be alert and talking. However, those patients who are unconscious or semi-conscious may not be able to maintain a clear airway, particularly if they are positioned supine. Failure to clear the airway will lead to inadequate ventilation of the lungs and reduced oxygenation. Complete airway occlusion will quickly result in respiratory arrest which, without intervention, will proceed to a full cardiac arrest. The other patients who are at risk of airway compromise are those presenting with an allergic response where the lips and tongue can swell and, if not treated promptly, can lead to full airway obstruction.

Look at the patient's chest for signs of accessory muscle use that may indicate increased respiratory effort caused by airway obstruction. Look at their lips and oral mucosa for cyanosis, pallor (with dark skins this may be difficult to assess),

Table 1.1 Baseline physiological values for adults

Respiratory rate	12–20 per minute
Heart rate	
Normal	60–100 beats per minute
Bradycardia	< 60 beats per minute
Tachycardia	> 100 beats per minute
Blood pressure	
Systolic	> 90 mmHg
Oxygen saturation	
Normal	95–98%

swelling, dryness or cracking. Check whether the patient has false teeth and if they are well fitting. If false teeth are ill fitting, remove them as they can cause obstruction. Listen for noise in the airway. Inspiratory noise (stridor) can be indicative of upper airway obstruction. Expiratory noise (wheeze) can indicate lower respiratory problems caused by airway collapse on expiration, e.g. acute asthma. A swollen, dry or cracked tongue can be indicative of dehydration.

In the unconscious patient, look inside the mouth for saliva, frothy sputum which can be pink in colour (pulmonary oedema), blood-stained spit (pulmonary embolism, TB, lung trauma), blood, vomit or foreign bodies. If the patient vomits, use suction to help clear large amounts of material from the mouth and oropharynx and tilt the head of the bed down to reduce the likelihood of pulmonary aspiration. In airway management, nursing interventions include clearing of obstructions (e.g. foreign bodies, poorly fitting dentures, vomit and flaccid tongue), use of head-tilt/chin-lift manoeuvres, administration of suction, insertion of airway adjuncts (oropharyngeal or nasopharyngeal airways) and moving the patient into the recovery position. If using suction through airway adjuncts, suctioning for more than 15 seconds can deplete the lungs of oxygen, so great care should be taken. If, when checking the airway, there is an inability to open the mouth due to muscle spasm, then trismus is present and insertion of a nasopharyngeal airway may be required. Further assessment of the airway includes obtaining any history relating to possible causes of airway problems (e.g. does the patient have any allergies that may have caused an airway problem?).

Breathing

Inadequate breathing may be acute or chronic, continuous or intermittent, and can lead to inadequate ventilation of the lungs and subsequent respiratory failure. Initial assessment of breathing focuses on the identification of immediately or potentially life-threatening conditions (Box 1.1; see also Chapter 7 – Shortness of breath and Chapter 8 – Chest pain), an increase in respiration rate is the first sign of the patient's condition deteriorating (Moore & Woodhouse 2004).

While considering the presence of one or more of these conditions, look at the patient for central or peripheral cyanosis. Assessing the pattern and rate of respiration is of vital significance (Kennedy 2007) as the respiration rate has been found to be a key predictor of cardiac arrest or a critically ill patient requiring intensive care (Goldhill et al. 1999). Count the respiratory rate using a stethoscope and assess the depth and effort of breathing. Measure the oxygen saturations using a pulse oximeter. Look at the symmetry of the patient's chest movements. Assess the patient for use of accessory muscles and for retraction of the skin around the clavicles and ribs, indicating increased respiratory effort. Listen for sounds of stridor or wheeze on inspiration (upper respiratory infections), on expiration (bronchospasm) or biphasic (wheeze on inspiration and expiration – foreign body, laryngospasm or very severe asthma attack). Assess whether the patient can talk in complete, full sentences, short sentences, words only, or is unable to give an oral response. Check the patient's lung expansion by feeling the chest bilaterally. A more detailed assessment includes percussion and auscultation of the patient's chest. Percuss anteriorly and posteriorly in the upper, middle and lower areas bilaterally.

Box 1.1   Immediately life-threatening and potentially life-threatening conditions causing breathing problems

Immediately life-threatening conditions causing breathing problems:
Life-threatening asthma (defined by BTS & SIGN guidelines 2009)
Severe pulmonary oedema
Large pulmonary embolism
Cardiac arrhythmia
Cardiac tamponade
Tension pneumothorax

Potentially life-threatening conditions causing breathing problems:
Acute severe asthma (defined by BTS & SIGN guidelines 2009)
Acute exacerbation of COPD or respiratory failure
Chest infection
Myocardial infarction
Pulmonary oedema
Metabolic acidosis
Pulmonary embolism
Simple pneumothorax
Pleural effusion
Anaphylaxis

Resonance indicates presence of air while dullness indicates fluid underlying the area percussed. Auscultate the same areas, listening for the presence, type and quality of breath sounds as well as any additional sounds (Advanced Life Support Group 2010). Absent breath sounds (silent chest) may be caused by severe bronchospasm, bronchoconstriction and mucosal swelling. Such cases require immediate medical attention as this is normally is a sign that intubation is required. Remember to consider that the patient may be breathless or hot from simple physical activity. Likewise, if the patient is in pain their respiratory rate and depth may be increased. If appropriate, repeat the assessment at least 5 minutes after the patient has been resting (Kennedy 2007).

Ask the patient about any history of asthma, acute or chronic chest conditions or any deviation from their normal breathing pattern. In asthmatic patients, peak flow must be recorded to enable treatment according to the British Thoracic Society guidelines (BTS/SIGN 2009). Determine if the patient has taken medication (prescribed or not) before or after their breathing problem started. Make a note of the percentage of oxygen being given to the patient as this may be important if the patient has a chronic lung condition (e.g. chronic obstructive pulmonary disease) requiring lower percentages of oxygen to be given. Nursing interventions at this stage include positioning the patient upright or in the recovery position, as appropriate. Administer oxygen if required, according to BTS and SIGN (2009) guidelines. Patients with chronic pulmonary disorders will require careful monitoring if given oxygen. Where oxygen is to be administered for a prolonged period, a humidification device should be used to prevent drying of the patient's mucous membranes and secretions.

Monitor and record oxygen saturation levels using a pulse oximeter probe attached to a finger, toe, nose or earlobe. The blood requires 5 g/dL of haemoglobin to register a value (Chapin & Proehl 1999). Do not use with nails coloured with nail polish or henna as they can cause inaccurate readings. Pulse oximetry recordings can also be inaccurate if peripheral vasoconstriction is present or when carbon monoxide has been inhaled (Chapin & Proehl 1999). In patients with COPD, arterial oxygen content should be assessed by arterial blood gas analysis (with the inspired oxygen concentration also recorded) (National Institute for Health and Clinical Excellence 2010). Respiratory exhaustion could be indicative of the need for non-invasive or invasive mechanical ventilation (see Chapter 7 – Shortness of breath).

If the patient has an audible wheeze, is a known asthmatic or has an underlying chronic respiratory problem, measure their peak expiratory flow (PEF). To overcome problems with the patient's technique, ask them for three readings and record the highest. Compare this reading with what is normal for the patient. PEF is contra-indicated for patients who are haemodynamically unstable, have recently had eye surgery (Will 2009), haemoptysis, recent myocardial infarction or pulmonary embolism, aneurysms (thoracic, abdominal or cranial), or recent surgery to thorax or abdomen. If the patient is asthmatic, refer to the guidelines for the management of asthma (BTS/SIGN 2009) (see Chapter 7 – Shortness of breath).

Circulation

Circulatory problems may be primary or secondary. A primary problem involves the heart not pumping effectively (e.g. following a myocardial infarction; see Chapter 8 – Chest pain). A secondary problem involves a failure of the circulatory system (i.e. the arterial/venous system), for example, through severe blood loss. In essence, there is either 'pump' failure or 'pipe' failure. Both primary and secondary problems can lead to tissue hypoxia or 'shock' (see Box 1.2 and Chapter 5 – Shock). Circulatory problems can be assessed through several parameters (see Box 1.3).

Box 1.2   Potentially life-threatening circulatory problems

Hypovolaemia (see Chapter 5 – Shock)
Acute and severe left ventricular failure (see Chapter 7 – Shortness of breath)
Arrhythmias (see Chapter 4 – Cardiac arrest)
Pulmonary embolism (see Chapter 8 – Chest pain)
Myocardial infarction (see Chapter 8 – Chest pain)
Anaphylactic reaction (see Chapter 5 – Shock)
Sepsis (see Chapter 5 – Shock)
Cardiac tamponade (see Chapter 4 – Cardiac arrest)

Box 1.3   Parameters for assessing circulatory problems

Respiratory rate
Pulse site, rate, volume and regularity
Blood pressure
Skin colour, appearance, texture and turgor
Capillary refill
Urine output
Level of consciousness
Peripheral pulses
12-lead ECG

Respiratory rate

The rate and depth of respiration has already been noted when assessing the patient's breathing. However, it is important to remember that an increase in the respiratory rate is often the first physiological response to a reduction in circulating blood volume or heart failure.

Pulse site, rate, volume and regularity

Check the pulse manually as this enables the patient's pulse rate, volume and regularity to be assessed at the same time as feeling their skin temperature and texture. The site of which the pulse is palpable gives an indication of how critically ill the patient is; if the patient loses their peripheral pulses i.e. wrist / ankle it could indicate critical illness.

As other factors (e.g. emotional stress, pain, fitness or drugs) affect the heart rate, it is important that the heart rate alone is not used to assess cardiovascular state. As an example, a patient presenting with a heart rate of 80/min would not normally be associated with cardiovascular compromise. If this patient was a fit athlete, their heart can pump up to 6 times the normal volume with the consequence of having a bradycardic (Leski 2004) resting rate which can be as low as 40/min in this person; a rate of 80/min could be considered to be as a tachycardia. Similarly, patients taking beta-blockers (which slow the heart rate) may not develop a tachycardia. Great care must also be taken when assessing the older person as some have a limited response to catecholamine release (American College of Surgeons 1997) and do not develop a significant tachycardia even with substantial blood loss.

When palpating for a pulse or listening to the bleep on a cardiac monitor, the rhythm of the beat is detected. Any irregularity in pulse indicates that the patient potentially could have a mismatch between the cardiac heart beat and the pulse in the periphery, normally radial pulse. When this occurs an apex beat should be taken at the same time as a peripheral pulse and the difference noted. An irregularly irregular pulse may indicate atrial fibrillation which can be considered a peri-cardiac arrest arrhythmia requiring urgent or immediate management (Resuscitation Council (UK) 2010).

Blood pressure

Record the blood pressure. A systolic blood pressure of less than 90 mmHg (or 40 mmHg below baseline) should give immediate cause for alarm as it may indicate significant hypotension that warrants emergency intervention. Remember that patients taking beta-blocker medication may normally have a low systolic blood pressure. Pay attention to the pulse pressure (difference between the diastolic and systolic). This narrows as the diastolic pressure increases (peripheral venoconstriction causes an increase in peripheral vascular resistance) in order to increase the circulating volume by moving blood from the venous reservoir (Herbert & Sheppard 2005). The calculation of a mean arterial pressure (MAP) ($^1/_3$ pulse pressure added to the diastolic pressure) indicates the pressure that is driving the blood through the circulation. A normal MAP is considered to be between 70 and 105 mmHg (Morton et al. 2009) while a MAP less than 65 mmHg is an indicator of poor organ perfusion (Treacher 2009) such as can occur in dehydration, haemorrhage, or cardiac failure (Woodrow 2009). The blood pressure may need to be recorded in both arms as a difference of 10–15 mmHg could be indicative of a dissecting thoracic aortic aneurysm (American College of Surgeons 1988). Another indicator of blood volume is to assess for distension of the neck veins when the patient is laid flat. If no neck veins can be seen or they do not fill when the patient is positioned upright, dehydration may be present. Conversely, distended neck veins could be a sign of fluid overload, heart failure or an increase in thoracic pressure (e.g. tension pneumothorax). Care should be taken when handing over responsibility from one nurse to another, as one may record the diastolic as a muffling of heart sounds (fourth Korotkov sound) and the other may record it when the sound disappears (ffith Korotkov sound). An electronic sphygmomanometer records the average between the two sounds.

Skin colour, appearance, texture and turgor

Observe the patient for pallor (vasoconstriction, anaemia), flushing (pyrexia, carbon monoxide poisoning), cyanosis or a waxy appearance. The skin may feel cool and clammy due to vasoconstriction with no heat to evaporate insensible perspiration (Richards 2005) or hot and sweating due to vasodilation or pyrexia. Check skin turgor for signs of dehydration. Pinch some skin over the back of the hand or inner forearm, if the skin stays pinched for up to 30 seconds this indicates severe dehydration (Edwards 2005). Care should be taken in testing turgor in the older person as there is often an insidious loss of elasticity of their skin (Mentes 2006).

Capillary refill

Record a capillary refill test. Press a fingernail firmly for 5 seconds and, when the pressure is released, colour should return within 2 seconds. If the colour takes more than 2 seconds to restore then this is indicative of peripheral vasoconstriction and/or marked hypotension from circulatory deficit, i.e. bleeding or dehydration. This test can be inaccurate if the patient is cold or has a history of vessel disease such as atherosclerosis (Woodrow 2009).

Urine output

In critically ill patients, the placement of a urinary catheter may be necessary to assess hourly urine output as this is an accurate indicator of tissue perfusion. A trend for urine output of less than 0.5 mL/kg body weight per hour indicates inadequate renal perfusion. Exercise greater caution in using this as a measure in the older person, as their kidneys have a reduced ability to concentrate urine; approximately 30% of patients over 70 years have chronic renal disease with less than 50% function of normal glomerular filtration rate as compared with a young healthy adult (Robinson-Cohen et al. 2009). Good catheter care is important in reducing the likelihood of infection.

ECG recording

Any patient who is critically ill, has an irregular pulse, has a cardiovascular deficit or a history suggestive of a cardiac cause, should have a 12-lead electrocardiogram (ECG) recorded. This will establish the underlying heart rhythm and identify signs of an acute coronary syndrome (e.g. myocardial infarction or unstable angina (see Chapter 8 – Chest pain)). Continuously monitor the cardiac rhythm of critically ill patients and repeat 12-lead ECGs at any rhythm change and during chest pain.

Peripheral pulses

Check for the presence of pedal pulses (dorsalis pedis is found between the first and second metatarsals, and the posterior tibial is found posterior and just distal to the tip of the medial malleolus of the tibia) in patients with potential arterial or venous problems. Check for a history of sudden onset of pain and numbness in the affected limb. Observe the limbs for pallor and cyanosis and feel for coldness to touch.

Nursing interventions to manage circulatory problems include:

- The insertion of IV cannulae. Careful consideration should be given as to whether the patient requires an intravenous cannula; they are known to be a source of infection and reducing hospital-acquired infections is high on the priority list of *Saving 1000 Lives Campaign* (NHS Wales 2010).
- Collection of blood samples for:
  o urea and electrolytes
  o full blood count which includes haemoglobin, platelets and white cell count (possibly with differential)
  o blood glucose levels

     o   if hypovolaemia is suspected, request a group and cross-match or group and save, and consider if blood needs to be ordered.
- If hypovolaemic, administer IV fluids as prescribed via large-bore cannulae or, if severely affected, two large-bore cannulae and consider administering plasma expanders such as gelatine-based (Gelofusine®, Geloplasma®, Haemaccel®, Isoplex®, Volplex®), etherified starch (hetastarch, pentastarch, tetrastarch) or blood (see Chapter 5 – Shock).

Disability (neurological status)

Patients may have altered neurological status (consciousness level) for a variety of reasons (see Box 1.4).

A neurological assessment comprises three parts:

1   Use of a neurological assessment tool
2   Assessment of pupil reaction
3   Assessment of limb function

1.   Neurological assessment tool

Two tools can be used: the mnemonic AVPU and the Glasgow coma score (GCS). These give a clear indication of how obtunded the patient is and allow a quick assessment of the critically ill. AVPU is quick and easy to use and is ideal for initial assessments. The GCS (Table 1.2) is internationally accepted as the measurement of choice and should be used for assessment over longer periods. It does not always meet the needs of some patients who have a reduced consciousness level solely through drugs, alcohol or a metabolic cause when using a sedation score such as Ramsay sedation scale (Dawson et al. 2010) or solely the verbal component of the GCS may be of more benefit.

Box 1.4   Potential causes of altered consciousness

Hypoxia
Cerebrovascular accident (CVA) (see Chapter 6 – Altered consciousness)
Subarachnoid haemorrhage (see Chapter 6 – Altered consciousness)
Hypo- or hyperglycaemia (see Chapter 6 – Altered consciousness)
Transient ischaemic attack (TIA) (see Chapter 6 – Altered consciousness)
Drug overdose (see Chapter 6 – Altered consciousness)
Sepsis (see Chapter 5 – Shock)
Epileptic seizures (see Chapter 6 – Altered consciousness)
Meningitis (see Chapter 6 – Altered consciousness)
Head injury
Acidosis (respiratory and metabolic)
Alkalosis (respiratory and metabolic)
An unidentified reason

Table 1.2 Glasgow coma score (from Teasdale & Jennett 1974)

	Score	Description	Interpretation
Best eye response	4	Spontaneously	Eyes open without the need of a stimulus
	3	To speech	Eyes open to verbal stimulation (normal, raised or repeated)
	2	To pain	Eyes open to pain only
	1	None	No eye opening to verbal or painful stimulus
Best verbal response	5	Orientated	Knows: who they are, where they are and the month or year
	4	Confused	Incorrectly answers the above questions
	3	Inappropriate words	Responses given do not answer questions posed
	2	Incomprehensible sounds	Not able to formulate recognisable words
	1	None	No verbal response
Best motor response	6	Obeys commands	Follows and acts out commands and must undertake 2 out of 3
	5	Localises to pain	Purposeful movement to remove a painful stimulus – here supra-orbital pressure should be used as then one can see the patient localising to the pain as they lift their hand to push away the stimulus
	4	Withdrawing from pain or normal flexion	Flexes the arm at the elbow without wrist rotation in response to a painful stimulus
	3	Abnormal flexion to pain	Flexes arm at elbow with rotation of the wrist with resulting spastic posture in a response to a painful stimulus
	2	Extends to pain	Extends arm at elbow with inward rotation of the arm in response to a painful stimulus
	1	None	No motor response

There remains uncertainty about the choice of stimulus to use when assessing response to pain. Options for assessing central pain response include pressure on the supra-orbital bone and pinching the trapezium muscle (Waterhouse 2009). Sternal rubbing should be avoided (it often causes bruising) and so should application of pressure to the nail bed (it can lead to capillary damage and loss of the nail).

AVPU. The AVPU (**A**lert, responds to **V**oice, responds to **P**ain or **U**nresponsive) (ACS 1997) scale is self-explanatory. If the patient is conscious and able to talk regardless of whether they are confused or giving inappropriate answers to questions, they are considered to be 'alert'. If they are not talking but respond to 'voice' by opening their eyes or obeying commands, their consciousness level is obtunded. If they do not respond to voice but respond to a central 'pain' stimulus, their consciousness level is even further reduced. If they do not respond to pain, the patient is completely 'unresponsive'.

GCS.   The GCS (see Table 1.2) was developed to facilitate a common language between doctors in tertiary hospitals and neurosurgeons in specialist centres (Teasdale & Jennett 1974). The scale is designed to identify early deterioration in level of consciousness, to facilitate prompt intervention that reduces morbidity and mortality. The tool centres on the determination of three variables: best eye opening response, best verbal response and best motor response. Each area is assessed in turn and scored out of 15. A score of 15/15 considers the patient to be fully conscious. A score of less than 8/15 designates the patient as being in a coma.

Consider the following when using the using the GCS:

- When transferring accountability for care from one nurse to another, both nurses should undertake one set of neurological observations together, to ensure continuity and consistency of measurements.
- Best eye opening: If the patient has their eyes closed – for whatever reason, including sleep – and opens them at the commencement of the recording, they score 3.
- Best verbal response: To be assessed as orientated, the patient must know their name, that they are in hospital and either the month or the year. If they only answer two correctly, they are considered to be confused.
- Best motor response: To test for obeying commands, the patient should be asked to touch their nose, wriggle their toes and stick their tongue out. Two instructions must be successful to be assessed as obeying commands. Asking the patient just to squeeze fingers should be avoided as it cannot be ascertained if this was a reflex action. If this method is used, the command should be to squeeze and then let go.

Table 1.3 outlines a comparison between an AVPU assessment and respective scores using the GCS.

Table 1.3   Comparison between neurological scores

AVPU	Glasgow coma score
Alert	GCS 14/15
Responding to voice	GCS 8–13
Responding to pain	GCS 4–8
Unresponsive	GCS 3

2. Pupil reaction

Check pupil reactions using a bright light (not an ophthalmoscope) shone into each eye and record the size and reaction. While shining the light in one eye, check the other to confirm the presence of consensual reflexes. Altered pupil sizes (measured in millimetres) and reaction to light give some indication of underlying pathology. Pinpoint pupils may indicate the presence of opiates or a metabolic disorder, while dilated pupils may be present following seizures or the ingestion of some drugs (e.g. cocaine, amphetamines or tricyclic antidepressants). The size and reaction of the pupil may also indicate the site of damage in the brain. Consider the shape of the pupil, as one that is not round may indicate an underlying brain lesion (Shah 1999). Having unequal pupils without a reduced consciousness level is insignificant.

Pupil reaction is an essential component when undertaking a neurological assessment where there is potential for raised intracranial pressure. The pupil becomes fixed and dilated when significant pressure is placed on the third cranial (oculomotor) nerve that lies just above the tentorium. This is often unilateral. If this pressure continues, the brain will subsequently 'cone' whereby the uncal portion of the temporal lobe herniates through the foramen magnum in the base of the skull (Copstead-Kirkhorn & Banasik 2009).

3. Limb assessment

Assessment of the patient's best limb response will determine where specific brain injury has occurred. Limb response is assessed against normal power, mild weakness, severe weakness, flexion, extension and no response (see Table 1.4).

In a co-operative patient, normal power, mild or severe weakness can be confirmed by asking the patient to undertake some actions (e.g. touching their nose, lifting their arm or leg in the air). Take care when assessing the patient's arm weakness, because if the patient is asked to squeeze the nurse's fingers, one hand is usually dominant and has greater power. Assess patients with a reduced consciousness level by using a peripheral pain stimulus. Record subsequent limb movement. To confirm the presence of a mild arm weakness, lay the patient flat, ask them to close their eyes and hold their arms out in front of them. If one arm drifts, there is a mild weakness. Further assessment of neurological status includes

Table 1.4 Limb assessment of motor power (based on Shah 1999)

Normal power	Patient is able to match resistance applied by the observer to any joint movement
Mild weakness	Patient is able to move against resistance but is easily overcome
Severe weakness	Patient is able to move his or her limb but not against resistance
Flexion	Flexes the limb to painful peripheral stimulation
Extension	Extends the limb to painful peripheral stimulation
No response	No response

taking a history from the patient or relative regarding disorientation, confusion, fitting and loss of consciousness or head injury.

Exposure

It is not possible to complete a thorough assessment without undressing the patient. Inspect the patient's skin for integrity, colour, rashes, oedema and signs of possible abuse or self-harm. Take the opportunity to measure their blood glucose using a bedside glucometer, and record their temperature. Having exposed the patient, remember to keep them warm and preserve their dignity. Any suspicion of non-accidental injury in vulnerable patients should instigate an assessment with possible subsequent referral under adult safeguarding arrangements. In addition domestic abuse/violence assessments should be considered if there are unexplained signs of injury regardless of whether the patient is vulnerable or not. For patients who are experiencing domestic abuse it is imperative that the family unit should be considered, and if there are children at home then the safeguarding policy should be considered.

While exposing the patient, the patient's skin integrity should be examined and the presence of pressure ulcers noted. If no ulcers are present then a skin tolerance test should be undertaken to help determine if changes have started to occur. This should be accompanied by a pressure risk assessment using a formal tool such as Braden (Braden & Bergstrom 1987) or Waterlow (Griffiths & Jull 2010).

History taking

History is of paramount importance when assessing patients as approximately 90% of diagnoses are derived from the history alone (ACS 1997). When assessing a patient who is critically ill, the nurse must make a clinical decision as to when and how the history will be taken, the aim being to complete an accurate history as soon as possible. It is important to identify in chronological order the history of how each of the symptoms has developed and what, if any, events were related to them. Likewise, it is also important to determine how the patient feels about their illness and what aspect of their condition has led them to seek medical advice. The obvious presenting problem should not stop the nurse from questioning the patient further to satisfy themselves that this is indeed the most important complaint. On occasions, the presenting condition is not seen by the patient to be their main problem as other aspects of their physical state may cause them more concern. The 'news reporter's tool' may be a useful aide memoir when taking a patient's history (Box 1.5).

Details of the patient's family history of illness can be important as it may high-light the possibility of the patient developing the same condition. It may also allow the patient to express fears and anxieties regarding conditions suffered by their family, which they are concerned may also affect them. Similarly, gathering information about the patient's personal and social history helps to identify their employment status. This may be relevant if their work is associated with particular

---

Box 1.5   The news reporter's tool (Who? What? Where? When? Why? How?)

1 Who is the patient?
   ● Are they male or female?
   ● What is their age?
   ● What is their ethnicity and culture?
   ● Do they have any particular religious beliefs?
   ● How do they appear? Pale, cyanosed or do they have a mobility deficit?
   ● Are they appropriately dressed for the time of the year? Does their clothing depict a lack of care or poverty or are they unkempt? Is this related to their social circumstances (e.g. homelessness)?
2 What happened to cause them to seek assistance today?
   ● Has their condition changed?
   ● Is their condition acute or chronic?
   ● What is their presenting complaint?
3 Where did the problem start?
   ● Was it at home or work?
   ● What were they doing at the time?
   ● Where exactly is the problem?
   ● Does it affect their activities of daily living? If so, what is affected?
4 When did it start?
   ● How long have they had it?
   ● Was the onset sudden or slow?
   ● Was the onset insidious or overt?
   ● Has it happened before?
5 Why did this occur?
   ● Have they done anything different today that may have caused the problem?
   ● Are there any other symptoms in addition to the main problem?
6 How did this happen?
   ● Was the problem precipitated by anything?

---

physical or mental health risks. Consider also the patient's weekly alcohol intake, smoking habits and recreational drug use. Drug use is sometimes a difficult and sensitive subject to discuss and it is often much easier to approach the subject when asking about alcohol and smoking habits. In some hospitals every patient is assessed for alcohol problems; one test that is easy, quick and appropriate to use in initial assessment is the Paddington alcohol test (Touquet & Brown 2009).

An insight into a patient's social circumstance is important. Gather details of the patient's next of kin, who they live with, whether they are cared for or whether they themselves act as a carer to someone else. This information helps if the patient needs admission as provision can then be made for dependants. If the patient so wishes, relatives, friends and carers can be kept informed of their hospital admission. This information is also important in the discharge planning process. Social workers and other members of the healthcare team benefit from this information in planning the provision of services for the patient if they are discharged. In the context of contemporary issues relating to patient consent and in relevant cases,

Box 1.6   The AMPLE mnemonic

Allergies
- Does the patient have any? If so, what are they?
- Are they relevant to your plan of care?

Medications
- Does the patient currently take any medications?
- What medications have they previously taken?
- Are they prescribed, over the counter, herbal, illicit drugs or smoking?
- With what frequency and for how long have they been taking them?

Past medical history
- Is the present problem an exacerbation of a previously experienced condition (e.g. asthma)?
- Are there any underlying conditions that could complicate this presentation (e.g. diabetes mellitus, alcohol dependence, hypertension)?
- Is the patient at risk of pressure sore development?

Last ate
- Nutritional assessment
- Is the patient well nourished?
- What type of diet do they eat?
- Do they have any special dietary needs?
- Should they receive food or fluid by mouth?
- Are they likely to have vitamin or mineral deficiencies (e.g. alcoholism)?

Events/environment
- What events led the patient to come to you today?
- What is their home environment like?
- Are they able to return home safely?
- What social support do they receive?
- Does this require cancelling or rearranging?
- Do they care for anyone else?
- Who has come to hospital with them today?

discussion with the patient about their wishes regarding resuscitation and if they wish their family to be present should be considered.

Another mnemonic that may act as an aide memoir is AMPLE (ACS 1997) relating to allergies, medications, previous medical history, the patient's nutritional/dietary status and the events surrounding the presenting problem (Box 1.6).

An important component of any history relates to the type of any pain experienced by the patient in relation to their presenting problem. There are many pain assessment tools in use in general nursing; the quick and easy to remember PQRST mnemonic was developed by Rogers et al. (1989). This assesses what provokes the pain, its quality, whether it radiates, its site and severity and how long it has been present (Box 1.7). Remember that older people may be reluctant to acknowledge and disclose pain and may have their own descriptors (British Pain Society & British Geriatric Society 2007).

Box 1.7   The PQRST mnemonic

Provokes
- What provokes the pain?
- Does anything make it better or worse (e.g. positioning, heat or cold)?
- Is it present only on movement?

Pattern
- Continuous or intermittent?
- Insidious or sudden onset?

Quality
- Ask the patient to describe the pain.
- Is it stabbing, crushing, spasmodic or continuous?

Radiation
- Does the pain radiate anywhere?
- If so, where to? Remember not to ask leading questions.

Site/severity
- Where exactly is the pain?
- Is it localised?
- Can it be pinpointed?
- What is the severity? A pain scoring system may be used.
- Is the pain the same now as it was last time?
- Does it impair any bodily functions? If so, which ones?

Time/treatment
- How long has the pain been present?
- Has the patient taken any analgesia? If so, what and when?
- If they have taken analgesia, are they presenting a true picture of the severity and quality of their pain?

The use of the above mnemonics is not compulsory but they act as a guide to the history-taking process during which questions should be asked in a tactful and caring way. A nurse requires experience and expertise to obtain this information during the assessment process. Any assessment guide or tool should be designed specifically to help the nurse collect the information necessary to make an accurate and effective assessment. An acute problem has to be clearly differentiated from a chronic condition. This will aid the implementation of the correct plan of care for the patient's needs.

Infection control

During the assessment, the risk of infection to or from the patient should be considered. If the patient is at risk or potentially may be at risk then appropriate isolation measures should be instigated.

Prioritisation of patients' needs and referral

One option for effective referral is use of the SBAR tool (Situation, Background, Assessment, Recommendations). This is an easily remembered mnemonic that can be used to compose messages regarding urgent situations that require a colleague's immediate attention and action. It helps to clarify information that needs to be communicated between team members and can help to develop teamwork and foster a culture of patient safety (NHS Institute for Innovation and Improvement 2008).

The mnemonic consists of standardised prompt questions (Box 1.8) that ensure concise and focused information is shared. Furthermore, it enables assertive and effective communication and reduces repetition. It also helps clinicians to anticipate the information needed by their colleagues and encourages use of assessment skills. According to NHS III (2008), the SBAR tool prompts clinicians to formulate information with the right level of detail.

Box 1.8   SBAR communication tool

Situation
- Identify yourself and the site or unit you are calling from
- Identify the patient by name and the reason for your report
- Describe your concern

Background
- Give the patient's reason for admission
- Explain significant medical history

You then inform the consultant of the patient's background: admitting diagnosis, date of admission, prior procedures, current medications, allergies, pertinent laboratory results and other relevant diagnostic results. For this, you need to have collected information from the patient's chart, flow sheets and progress notes.

Assessment
- Vital signs
- Contraction pattern
- Clinical impressions, concerns

You need to think critically when informing the doctor of your assessment of the situation. This means that you have considered what might be the underlying reason for your patient's condition. Not only have you reviewed your findings from your assessment, you have also consolidated these with other objective indicators, such as laboratory results.

Recommendation
- Explain what you need: be specific about request and time frame
- Make suggestions
- Clarify expectations

Finally, what is your recommendation? That is, what would you like to happen by the end of the conversation with the physician? Any order that is given on the phone needs to be repeated back to ensure accuracy.

Source: NHS Institute for Innovation and Improvement (2008)

on

nt assessment, initial investigations and treatments, findings and ocumented. This serves the purpose of communicating details of members of the healthcare team and providing a written record of all activity relating to the patient. When documenting patient care, it is important to follow a structured approach to ensure that vital information is not omitted. This also ensures that all relevant information is available to be shared and used by the multidisciplinary team. The nurse should also undertake a final evaluation and document the findings before the patient is discharged from their care, irrespective of whether it is back into the community or to a ward. Box 1.9 outlines components of the documentation that should be included.

It is of the utmost importance that all information is documented accurately. Record the time using the 24-hour format to avoid the potential confusion from using am and pm. To be effective, documentation must be complete so that all information relating to the patient can be communicated without confusion to the members of the team.

Box 1.9   Components of documentation

- Demographic data (name, address, date of birth, next of kin, religion, occupation)
- Presenting complaint
- History of presenting complaint including pain scoring
- Previous medical history (PMH)
- Drug history
- Allergies
- Social history including dependents
- Examination
- Findings of airway, breathing, circulation, disability assessment including vital signs:
  o respiratory rate and depth
  o blood pressure
  o heart rate, regularity and pulse volume
  o temperature
  o oxygen saturation
  o Peak flow (PEFR)
  o AVPU/GCS
- Skin integrity and pressure risk assessment
- Nutritional assessment
- The patient's psychological state
- Details of investigations carried out:
  o blood glucose
  o ECG
  o laboratory tests (Hb, WCC, U&E)
  o X-rays
  o blood gas analysis
- Medical and nursing interventions and their effects
- Patient's current condition:
  o any changes in the patient's condition
  o plan of further care
- Date and time of entry
- Name and signature of the nurse completing the documentation

The Nursing and Midwifery Council (2005) identifies a number of important factors that affect accurate record keeping. These state that the entry should be made as soon as possible after the event, to maintain accuracy and to reflect the current condition of the patient. The records should be legible and written in such a way that they cannot be erased. Mistakes can occur as a result of illegible handwriting. Jargon and irrelevant speculation should not be included.

Historically, nursing and medical records have been maintained separately. A collaborative and integrated approach for doctors, nurses and other healthcare professionals in recording patient care and treatment has many benefits for the patient and staff. Integrated care pathways ensure that information is not duplicated needlessly. Each member of the team has access to all the information concerning the patient. This stops the patient being subjected to repetitive questioning and reduces the risk of relevant facts being omitted. Similarly, facts can be presented in a straightforward and comprehensive manner. Integrated care pathways can also be provided in the form of computerised records.

Recording of vital signs, GCS and other parameters should be made on an observation chart as this makes for easier identification of trends and readily demonstrates changes. This chart will accompany the patient on their journey to discharge. In areas that use 'track and trigger' early warning scoring systems (e.g. MEWS – see Table 1.5), a score should be calculated and action taken according

Table 1.5 Modified early warning score (MEWS)

	Scores						
	3	2	1	0	1	2	3
Heart rate (bpm)		<40	41–50	51–100	101–110	111–120	>120
Respiration rate (rpm)		<9		0–14	15–20	21–29	>30
Systolic BP (mmHg)	<70	71–80	81–100	101–199		>200	
Level of consciousness				Alert	Confused	Response to pain	Unconscious
Temperature (°C)		<35		35.1–37.8		>37.8	

Patients with a **low score of 1–2** on the MEWS: frequency of observations must be **4 hourly** as a minimum standard. If the patient is causing clinical concern at any time but not scoring on the MEWS, commence ABCDE and refer for appropriate advice (e.g. Outreach Team).

Patients with a **medium score of 3–6** on the MEWS: inform the nurse-in-charge and the Outreach Team (if available), commence ABCDE and initiate appropriate clinical interventions. Recheck observations and MEWS within 30 minutes.

Patients with a **high score of 7 or more** on the MEWS, or if it is anticipated at any time that the patient's condition will deteriorate quickly: **clinical emergency** – actions will be determined by local arrangements for initiating an appropriate emergency response.

to local guidelines. It should be recognised, however, that early warning systems may not be sufficiently sensitive to be able to prioritise patients' care needs prior to a diagnosis being made.

Discharge planning

It is essential that discharge planning is commenced during, or as soon as possible after, the initial assessment to avoid problems arising when the decision is finally made to discharge the patient home or to refer them elsewhere. Vulnerable patients (e.g. older adults, those with mental health needs or people with learning disabilities) may require multidisciplinary collaboration and consultation with the family or carers and GP.

The nurse should spend time with the patient's relatives or carers to discuss any concerns about how the patient and family will manage if the patient is discharged. Where appropriate, those involved in the patient's care before admission should be involved in planning their discharge.

Summary

This chapter has focused on the guiding principles involved in a systematic approach to the initial assessment of patients who may be referred to hospital because they are acutely ill or those who may become acutely ill while in hospital. It is imperative that all patients are assessed using the same approach, thereby ensuring that all life-threatening or potentially life-threatening conditions are identified and treated as promptly and effectively as possible. As nurses are the only 24-hour professional presence in most healthcare settings, it is vital that they are all familiar with this approach and use their knowledge and skills to ensure that patient care is optimised. It is also important to remember that the discharge process for many patients starts soon after their arrival. By using a team approach to the assessment of their patients, nurses can have a significant impact on a successful patient outcome.

References

Advanced Life Support Group (ALSG) (2010) *Acute Medical Emergencies: The Practical Approach* (2nd edition). Oxford: Wiley-Blackwell (BMJ Books).

American College of Surgeons (1988) Committee on Trauma. *Advanced Trauma Life Support for Doctors* (5th edition). Chicago: ACS.

American College of Surgeons (1997) Committee on Trauma. *Advanced Trauma Life Support for Doctors* (6th edition). Chicago: ACS.

Braden B & Bergstrom N (1987) A conceptual schema for the study of the etiology of pressure sores. *Rehabilitation Nursing*, 12, 8–12.

British Pain Society & British Geriatric Society (2007) *Guidance on Assessment of Pain in Older People*. www.bgs.org.uk/Publications/Publication%20Downloads/Sep2007PainAssessment.pdf (accessed 28 August 2011).

British Thoracic Society (2008) *BTS Guideline for Emergency Oxygen Use in Adult Patients*. London: BTS. www.brit-thoracic.org.uk/clinical-information/emergency-oxygen/emergency-oxygen-use-in-adult-patients.aspx (accessed 20 April 2011).

British Thoracic Society (BTS) & Scottish Intercollegiate Guidelines Network (SIGN) (2009) *British Guideline on the Management of Asthma*. www.sign.ac.uk/pdf/sign101.pdf (accessed: 27 January 2011).

Chapin J & Proehl J (1999) Pulse oximetry. In: Proehl J (ed.) *Emergency Nursing Procedures* (2nd edition). Philadelphia: WB Saunders.

Copstead-Kirkhorn L-E & Banasik J (2009) *Pathophysiology: Biological and Behavioral Perspectives* (4th edition). Philadelphia: Saunders.

Dawson R, Von Fintel N & Nairn S (2010) Sedation assessment using the Ramsay Scale. *Emergency Nurse*, 18(3), 18–20.

Edwards S (2005) Innate defences. In: Montague S, Watson R & Herbert R (eds) *Physiology for Nursing Practice* (3rd edition). London: Elsevier.

Goldhill D, Worthington L, Mulcahy A, Tarling M & Sumner M (1999) The patients at-risk team: identifying and managing seriously ill ward patients. *Anaethesia*, 54(9), 853–860.

Griffiths P & Jull A (2010) How good is the evidence for using risk assessment to prevent pressure ulcers? *Nursing Times*, 106(14), 10–13.

Herbert R & Sheppard M (2005) Cardiovascular function. In: Montague S, Watson R & Herbert R (eds) *Physiology for Nursing Practice* (3rd edition). London: Elsevier.

Kennedy S (2007) Detecting changes in the respiratory changes in ward patients. *Nursing Standard*, 21(49), 42–46.

Leski M (2004) Sudden cardiac death in athletes. *Southern Medical Journal*, 97(9), 861–862.

Mentes J (2006) Oral hydration in older adults. *American Journal of Nursing*, 106(6), 40–49.

Morton P, Reck K, Tucker T et al. (2009) Patient assessment: cardiovascular system. In Morton P & Fontaine D (eds) *Critical Care Nursing: A Holistic Approach* (9th edition). Philadelphia: Wolters Kluwer Health/Lippincott Williams & Wilkins.

National Institute for Health and Clinical Excellence (NICE) (2010) *Management of chronic obstructive pulmonary disease in adults in primary and secondary care*. London: NICE. http://guidance.nice.org.uk/CG101 (accessed 20 April 2011).

NHS Institute for Innovation and Improvement (2008) *SBAR tool (Situation, Background, Assessment, Recommendations)*. NHS III. www.institute.nhs.uk/quality_and_service_improvement_tools/quality_and_service_improvement_tools/sbar_-_situation_-_background_-_assessment_-_recommendation.html (accessed 14 September 2011).

NHS Wales (2010) *Saving 1000 Lives Plus: Reducing Health Care Associated Infections*. www.wales.nhs.uk/sites3/home.cfm?orgid=781 (accessed 20 April 2011).

Nursing and Midwifery Council (NMC) (2005) *Guidelines for Records and Record Keeping*. London: NMC.

Resuscitation Council (UK) (2010) *Resuscitation Guideline: Adult tachycardia with Pulse Algorithm*. Resuscitation Council (UK). www.resus.org.uk/pages/tachalgo.pdf (accessed 20 April 2011).

Richards A (2005) The autonomic nervous system. In: Montague S, Watson R & Herbert R (eds) *Physiology for Nursing Practice* (3rd edition). London: Elsevier.

Robinson-Cohen C, Katz R, Mozaffarian D et al. (2009) Physical activity and rapid decline in kidney function among older adults. *Archives of Internal Medicine*, 169(22), 2116–2123.

Rogers J, Osborn H & Pousada L (1989) *Emergency Nursing: A Practice Guide*. Baltimore: Williams & Wilkins.

Shah S (1999) Neurological assessment. *Nursing Standard*, 13(22), 49–56.

Teasdale G & Jennett B (1974) Assessment of coma and impaired consciousness. *Lancet*, (2), 81–84.

Touquet R & Brown A (2009) PAT (2009) Revisions to the Paddington alcohol test for early identification of alcohol misuse and brief advice to reduce emergency department re-attendance. *Alcohol and Alcoholism*, 44(3), 284–286.

Treacher D (2009) Acute heart failure. In Bersten A & Soni N (eds) *Oh's Intensive Care Manual* (6th edition). Edinburgh: Butterworth-Heinemann.

Waterhouse C (2009) The use of painful stimulus in relation to Glasgow Coma Scale observations. *British Journal of Neuroscience Nursing*, 5(5), 209–214.

Will T (2009) Peak expiratory flow measurement. In Proehl J, *Emergency Nursing Procedures* (4th edition). Missouri: Saunders Elsevier.

Woodrow P (2009) Haemodynamic assessment. In Moore T & Woodrow P (2009) *High Dependency Nursing Care Observation, Intervention and Support for Level 2 Patients* (2nd edition). London: Routledge.

2 Vulnerable Adults

Louise Nelson, Scott Inglis,
Fiona Howell, Michael Gibbs
and Judi Thorley

Aims

This chapter will:

- discuss the principles involved in assessing and managing the needs of the following groups of vulnerable adults who may be accessing services in acute care settings:
  - individuals with mental health needs
  - older adults
  - individuals with learning disabilities

Introduction

Early assessment and identification of abuse and neglect of vulnerable adults is vital for the protection of the individual and prevention of further abuse. This chapter highlights issues relating to three vulnerable groups of individuals in society: older adults, individuals with mental health needs and those with learning disabilities. The chapter is organised into three sections each devoted to one vulnerable group. The aim of each section is to offer a framework whereby the needs of these individuals can be assessed and treatment options developed. It is important to remember that individuals from vulnerable groups are as susceptible to 'medical' needs as other members of society. It should also be remembered that individuals with learning disabilities can have co-existing mental health needs. For the purposes of this chapter, a vulnerable adult is defined as a person aged 18 years or over:

> 'who is or may be in need of community care services by reason of mental or other disability, age or illness; and who is or may be unable to take care of him or herself, or unable to protect him or herself against significant harm or exploitation'.
> (Department of Health 2008, 49)

Initial Management of Acute Medical Patients: A Guide for Nurses and Healthcare Practitioners, Second Edition. Edited by Ian Wood and Michelle Garner.
© 2012 John Wiley & Sons, Ltd. Published 2012 by John Wiley & Sons, Ltd.

A: MEETING THE NEEDS OF PATIENTS WITH MENTAL HEALTH NEEDS
(Louise Nelson and Scott Inglis)

Aims

This section will:

- provide a structured approach to the assessment of patients with mental health needs
- describe the components of a combined physical and mental health assessment
- promote understanding of specific assessment strategies, including when and how to apply them in the acute clinical setting

Introduction

Most patients with mental health disorders first present to their general practitioners (GP) with physical complaints (for example, inability to sleep, vague aches and pains) as these frequently mask mental illnesses (Nash 2010). Similarly, patients may have co-existing physical and mental health needs (for example, poorly controlled diabetes or chronic pain which may lead to depression). This highlights the complex interplay between physical and psychological symptomology. At any given time, one in six of the UK population are experiencing mental health needs (Office for National Statistics 2000) and so it is self-evident that a significant proportion of patients within acute clinical settings may have concurrent mental health needs. Healthcare professionals may feel inadequately prepared to deal with issues perceived to be outside their scope of expertise and it is important, therefore, that nurses have a sound working knowledge of mental health issues so that patients' needs can be assessed and managed effectively (Nash 2010). It is part of each nurse's professional responsibility to deliver the best quality care in a non-judgemental manner (Nursing and Midwifery Council 2008).

Most common mental health disorders

The International Statistical Classification of Diseases (ICD) (WHO 2007) has defined 100 categories relating to mental health disorders. For ease of use, these are condensed into 10 divisions. The seven relating solely to adults are outlined in Table 2.1.

Within the acute settings, mental health disorders are usually described *in one of the following ways*.

Psychosis. This is a general term that refers to an individual's experience of pervasive mental changes characterised by delusions (fixed or false beliefs) and/or hallucinations (abnormal sensory perceptions). Patterns of symptoms can vary widely between individuals; however, psychosis is often characterised by a person

Table 2.1 ICD codes for mental health disorders (from WHO 2007)

ICD-10 code	Division	Categories include:
F00–F09	Organic – including symptomatic mental disorders	Dementia in Alzheimer's disease Vascular dementia Delirium not induced by alcohol/substances Brain disease/damage
F10–F19	Mental and behavioural disorders due to psychoactive substance abuse	Acute intoxication Dependence syndrome Withdrawal state Psychotic disorder
F20–F29	Schizophrenia, schizotypal and delusional disorders	Schizophrenia Persistent delusional disorders Acute and transient psychotic disorders Schizoaffective disorders
F30–F39	Mood (affective) disorders	Manic episodes Bipolar affective disorder Depressive episode Recurrent depressive disorder
F40–F49	Neurotic, stress related and somatoform disorders	Phobic anxiety disorders Obsessive–compulsive disorder Reaction to severe stress Hypochondriacal disorder
F50–F59	Behavioural syndromes associated with physiological disturbances and physical factors	Eating disorders Non-organic sleep disorders Sexual dysfunction Abuse of non-dependence-producing substances
F60–F69	Disorders of adult personality and behaviour	Personality disorders (borderline) Enduring personality change after catastrophic experience or psychiatric illness Habit and impulse disorders (e.g. gambling) Gender identity disorders

having disorganised thinking and behaviour, a flattened affect and unusual perceptual experiences (Tummey & Turner 2008). Psychosis can be present in a number of disorders and may include schizophrenia, psychotic depression, mania, toxic drug reaction, dementia and delirium. With the exception of delirium, hypothyroidism and dementia, there are no concrete physical tests to discern mental state. This definition can be further expanded by defining 'delusions' as 'false beliefs which are fixed and are not amenable to logic or explanation' and 'hallucinations' as 'false sensory perceptions that involve any of the five senses such as auditory hallucinations in schizophrenia' (Isaacs 2001).

Neurosis. Refers to disorders in which anxiety or emotional symptoms predominate (Townsend 2007). Neurotic disorders include anxiety, panic disorders and somatoform disorders (the latter being characterised by physical symptoms that mimic physical disease or injury for which there is no identifiable physical cause) (Davies & Craig 2009; Fontaine 2009).

Dementia and delirium.   Refer to disorders specifically affecting the architecture of the brain. These changes may occur for a number of reasons including specific diseases and cerebrovascular accidents (Morris & Morris 2010). Common dementias include Alzheimer's, Lewy body dementia, Korsakoff syndrome and as a result of transient ischaemic attacks. The symptoms of these commonly include memory loss, particularly short-term, mood and personality changes and communication difficulties. Symptoms of delirium may be mistaken for dementia as the presentation is very similar.

Admission to the acute clinical setting can be stressful for patients and carers alike and it is important that nurses recognise this to minimise stress. Everybody reacts to stress in a different way and those with mental health needs *may* feel vulnerable due to being cared for in an unfamiliar environment, particularly if the patient has some perceptual difficulties due to any of the aforementioned conditions.

Repeated visits to their GP and return visits to Emergency Departments by a patient with a mental health need could suggest that there may have been a failure to adequately address the patient's psychological needs. It could also be that the person's physical needs have been overlooked due to the stigma and discrimination of having a mental health label, or as previously mentioned inadequate mental health knowledge within the primary care system. Mental health provision in primary care settings is steadily improving with the advent of projects such as primary care mental health teams and also the publication of the document 'New Horizons' (DH 2010). The key to addressing the above issues in acute care settings is a combined physical and mental health assessment which can provide vital information to measure the patient's level of distress and define the treatment acuity that is essential for effective management. Assessment in this context aims to answer the questions in Box 2.1.

The assessment of patients with a mental health need has two components; the physical and assessment and the psychological assessment.

Box 2.1   Initial assessment of patient with possible mental health need

- Does the patient have any life-threatening or potentially life-threatening physical problems?
- Is the patient in distress?
- Are they able to co-operate with the assessment process?
- Is their behaviour likely to be unpredictable (e.g. noisy, aggressive, rude, disinhibited, abusive (Mavundla 2000)?
- Are they at risk because of mental distress or self-harm or are they likely to place others at risk (Atakan & Davies 1997)?
- Are they likely to abscond?
- Is there a supportive person with them?
- What level of supervision do they require?
- Are they likely to be a risk to others?

Physical assessment

Before physical symptoms can be attributed to a mental health need, an initial assessment of the patient's airway, breathing and circulation must be carried out to exclude an organic cause. In this way, any acute physical needs can be identified and treated. In addition to the assessment procedures discussed in Chapter 1 – Initial assessment, if a mental health need is suspected, consider adding the components of assessment in Box 2.2.

Many physical conditions may cause an alteration in normal behaviour patterns. The healthcare professional should be aware that a number of chronic illnesses could affect neurological or mental status. Table 2.2 outlines some of these conditions.

Box 2.2   Additional components of the initial assessment

Observations
- Head to toe observation for injury (signs of self-harm, needle or track marks)
- Neurological: Is the patient lethargic or alert? What is their pupil size and reactivity?
- Psychomotor activity: Do they have any tics or tremors, altered gait or agitated movements?
- Musculoskeletal: Is their co-ordination and movement altered?

Investigations
- Baseline blood work is required to rule out underlying physical causes (e.g. hypoglycaemia, electrolyte imbalance)

Patient records
- Past medical and psychiatric history
- Current medication (polypharmacy may cause interactions between medications)

Table 2.2 Physical conditions that may exhibit psychological symptoms (based on Good & Nelson 1986 and Molitor 1996)

Condition	Presenting features
Addison's disease	Withdrawal, apathy and depression
Hyperthyroidism	Hyperactivity (can mimic 'mania'), irritability
Hypoglycaemia	Personality changes
Lung cancer	Progressive dementia, anxiety or panic attacks
Phaeochromocytomas	Progressive dementia, anxiety or panic attacks
Vitamin B12 deficiency	Visual hallucinations, personality changes, dementia
Hypocalcaemia	Any psychiatric symptom
Alcohol withdrawal	Delirium, hallucinations, acute anxiety
Epilepsy	Repetitive behaviours, manic-like psychosis
Head injury/hypoxia	Altered consciousness level
Infection/constipation	Mental confusion

Psychological assessment

All patients should undergo an assessment of their mental health status even when there appear to be no apparent cognitive, behavioural or emotional needs. As a basis for the initial assessment of a patient's mental health status, consider factors relating to their presenting problem and insight, previous psychiatric history, environment, associated risk factors and the potential for violence and/or aggression.

Presenting problem and insight

The patient's answers to the following questions may help to give an indication of their current situation and their level of insight.

- What does the patient think is their main problem?
- What do they think caused it?
- What other needs does the patient have?
- Did the problems start recently or are they part of a chronic illness?
- Does the patient have a current physical illness that may be contributing to the problem?
- Has there been a recent trauma or head injury that could have contributed to the onset of symptoms?
- Is there anything that makes the problem worse or better? How is it affecting their daily lives?
- Does the patient think anything is wrong with them?
- What is their understanding of their present difficulty?
- Has the patient taken any illicit substance recently?

The patient should be encouraged to answer the questions in their own words, and may need encouragement to remain focused on the current need. When necessary and appropriate, information may be obtained from relatives, carers or friends. If this is the case, the source of the information must be recorded in the patient's notes.

Previous psychiatric history

The patient's previous psychiatric history can provide a valuable insight into their current situation. Details need to be confirmed for accuracy against previous medical records. Information to be collected should include:

- Previous psychiatric episodes/admissions?
- What were the patient's main problems?
- What therapy was given?

- Did they comply with therapy?
- Was the therapy effective?
- What was the mental state between episodes? (i.e. What was their level of recovery? Did any recovery take place with or without therapy?)

Environment

Essential details of the patient's background and social circumstances provide an invaluable context for their needs. Information already available through a patient's GP or hospital notes needs to be confirmed for accuracy. The information collected should include details regarding cohabitation, housing, employment, financial situation and any family history of mental health problems.

Risk factors

According to Harrison et al. (2010), Callaghan et al. (2009) and the Department of Health (2007a, 2009a), a detailed risk assessment is required for those patients who have expressed suicidal intentions, have a history of mood disorder, psychosis or substance abuse or a history of self-harm or violence. The assessment of risk associated with mental health problems is most often related to the danger that the patient presents to others. More commonly, and of equal importance, is the risk of harm to themselves and the risk of absconding prior to treatment. The history, assessment and the context of the present situation may reveal other features that are associated with risk of harm (Box 2.3).

Violence and aggression

In difficult situations (e.g. the unexpected admission to hospital, especially if the patient is in pain or confused, or experiences a feeling of being out of control), almost any patient (or their relatives/carers) may make threats or behave aggressively or violently. Although in most hospitals there is a policy of zero tolerance for violence and aggression, the need to take account of a patient's current condition is recognised, and not all will have an underlying mental health problem. No single assessment tool accurately predicts likelihood of violence; however, the strongest

---

Box 2.3   Factors associated with risk of harm

- Personal history of self-harm or violent behaviour
- Planning of a suicide attempt
- Recent stress or loss
- Considerable mood disturbances
- Substance misuse
- Chronic painful physical conditions

predictor of future behaviour is past behaviour (Callaghan et al. 2009). Norman and Ryrie (2009) have identified a number of risk factors which may enable the healthcare professional to predict a potentially violent situation. The risk factors include:

- gender and age (males aged 17–25)
- history of violent behaviour
- threats of violence (including depersonalising language and gestures)
- impaired psychological state (due to mental illness or substance/alcohol misuse)
- communication difficulties
- metabolic disorders (e.g. hypoxia, hypoglycaemia or delirium)

The above information can be collected as the basis of an initial assessment of a patient's mental health status. From this assessment, if a mental health need is suspected, the healthcare professional can use the following assessment tool to provide a more detailed mental health assessment (Seidel et al. 2010; Townsend 2007).

1   Appearance
2   Behaviour
3   Cognitive ability and communication
4   Disposition and emotional responses

1. *Appearance*

The patient's appearance can give an indication of their mental status; however, it is impossible to make generalisations in this respect. The following issues may be useful indicators:

- Clothing. Is the patient's clothing appropriate for the time of day, the weather and/or the time of year?
- Neglect. Are there obvious signs of self-neglect such as poor hygiene and body odour?
- Nutrition. Is the patient unusually thin or emaciated? Is there evidence of weight loss or gain? Recent weight loss may be indicative of physical illness or chronic anxiety.
- Body language. Assess the patient's posture. Is it tense? Are they slumped?
- Facial expression. Is the patient's expression suggestive of irritability or anxiety?
- Substance misuse. Is there any suggestion of drug, alcohol or substance misuse? Assess the patient's pupils. Are they dilated or pinpoint? Pupils become pinpoint with the use of opioids and dilated by alcohol.

2. *Behaviour*

This refers to the patient's observable activities and can include the following:

- Movements. Are there any unusual movements such as tremors, tics or ataxia?
- Psychomotor activity. Is the patient agitated? Are they pacing about the area? Patients with an elevated mood may be overactive and restless. Patients with a depressive illness may be slow in initiating movement and slow in performing that movement.

- Reaction. How does the patient respond to being assessed? Is the patient angry? Are they overfamiliar, fearful, tearful or guarded?

3. Cognitive ability and communication

Cognitive ability. The following aspects can give an indication of a patient's cognitive ability:

- Level of response. Is the patient alert, drowsy, responding to stimuli? Stupor (total immobility, no response to stimuli) can be a catatonic feature of schizophrenia or a feature of an organic disorder.
- Orientation. Is the patient orientated? Can they remember their name, where they are, what year it is?
- Memory and attention span. Can the patient remember three everyday items after 3 minutes?
- Judgement. Is the patient able to make accurate judgements about the situation? Are they able to give informed consent to treatment?
- Thought processes. Are they well-ordered, coherent and relevant? Is the patient preoccupied?
- Content. Is there flight of ideas? Is there poverty of thought? A patient with severe depression may complain of an inability to gather or express thoughts.
- Paranoia/delusions. Is the patient expressing hypochondriacal delusions of bodily disease which are rigidly maintained despite medical evidence to the contrary?
- Perceptual distortions. Has the patient any auditory hallucinations (described as voices that issue orders or make suggestions)? These are most common in psychotic disorders such as schizophrenia.

Communication. Aspects of verbal and non-verbal communication should be assessed along with the content of the conversation. Remember to consider language barriers and cultural influences when assessing communication.

- Speech. Is the verbal rate uninterruptible or is it slow? Is the volume loud or quiet? Is the quality of speech hesitant or slurred? Articulation difficulty can suggest a neurological disorder or the side effect of antipsychotic drugs.
- Content. Is the patient confused? Is the patient expressing unusual ideas, using inappropriate word substitutions? Are they expressing ideas of self-harm or harm to others? Do they feel in danger?
- Non-verbal. Is eye contact intense, staring or poor (if culturally appropriate)?

4. Disposition and emotional responses

This refers to the patient's mood, emotions and the atmosphere of the interview and includes the following:

- Mood. Subjectively, how does the patient perceive his or her own mood? Objectively, note the predominant mood during the assessment. Is it fluctuating?

Is it appropriate to the situation? Do the patient's perceptions and your own observations on mood correspond?

- Is the patient angry or agitated? Is the patient sad and despondent (depression) or euphoric and elated (bipolar disorder)? How does the patient feel about himself or herself? Is the patient feeling worthless or unreal (depersonalisation)? Is there an exaggerated sense of ability?

Using the above framework can help to build up a more detailed assessment of a patient's mental status. It is unlikely that any single patient will exhibit all of the above indicators.

Specific assessment tools

Assessment tools are a useful aid to identify a potential problem. Common tools include those for cognitive impairment, alcohol misuse and suicide. These should be used as indicated during the initial assessment:

Cognitive impairment

The mini mental state examination may be used to provide a numeric rating of cognitive ability (see Table 2.3); however this tool has a limited value outside of assessing potential dementias and can give a false reading if a patient has a learning disability. An alternative tool is the Addenbrookes Cognitive Evaluation Revised (ACE-R) (Mioshi et al. 2006) which gives a global picture of cognitive impairment. A score of 20 or less is indicative of confusion and/or impaired communication.

Alcohol or drug use

When assessing for potentially problematic alcohol or drug use, the CAGE-AID assessment tool can be used (Brown & Rounds 1995). In this approach, if the patient admits to being intoxicated or dependent this assessment tool can be applied. Consideration can only be given to signposting the patient to local drug and alcohol services.

- Have you ever felt you ought to Cut down on your drinking or drug use?
- Have people Annoyed you by criticising your drinking or drug use?
- Have you felt bad or Guilty about your drinking or drug use?
- Have you ever had a drink or used drugs first thing in the morning to steady your nerves or to get rid of a hangover (Eye-opener)?

Suicide

There are many assessment tools for assessing suicide risk. The 'preventing suicide toolkit' (National Patient Safety Agency 2009) supports the prevention of suicide

Table 2.3 The mini mental state examination (based on Wyatt et al. 2005 and Seidel et al. 2010)

Assess	Method	Score
Orientation for time	Day, date, month, season, year	1 point each
Orientation for place	Country, county, city/town, hospital, name of the ward/unit	1 point each
Learning of new information	Name three unrelated objects (clock, umbrella, carrot) Patient must remember all three objects	1 point each, at first attempt only
Attention and concentration	Spell 'world' backwards	1 point for each letter in the correct order
Short-term memory	'Tell me the three items that we named a few minutes ago'	1 point each
Language	Point to a pen and wristwatch and ask the patient to name them	2 points
	Repeat the phrase 'No ifs, ands or buts'	1 point
	Tell the patient to follow these instructions 'Take this piece of paper in your right hand, fold it in half and put it on the floor'	1 point for each part
	Read and obey: show the patient a piece of paper with the phrase 'Close your eyes' written on it and ask them to follow the instructions	1 point
	Ask the patient to write a short sentence	1 point, if it makes sense
	Ask the patient to copy a diagram (e.g. Two five-sided shapes that are intersecting)	1 point

strategy and is to be used in conjunction with local risk assessment tools and crisis services. Suicide risk factors include:

- age (younger age groups 19–34, and older age groups 85+)
- gender (males more likely than females)
- physical health (presence of chronic physical illness)
- psychological health (depression, psychosis, etc.)
- history of self-harm or previous suicide attempts
- social situation (lack of close, confiding relationships)
- high intent (have chosen method and means, and made plans)

It is important to differentiate between self-harm as a coping strategy and suicidal intent. Patients who self-harm may not necessarily be suicidal and should be treated with respect and dignity as they may be unable to cope with the strength of their distress in any other way. There is evidence that frequently patients perceive a punitive attitude from the treatment team (Norman & Ryrie 2009). In cases of self-harm, a full risk assessment and urgent referral to mental health services (e.g. crisis team) should be made.

Management of the patient with a mental health need

The medical and/or mental health diagnosis and stage of the illness will determine the selection of psychological, pharmacological or social options of management. Following the nursing assessment of both medical and mental health needs, an analysis is required to determine the priorities in the plan of care. The analysis may determine needs common to many disorders. The priorities for a plan of care are as follows (Polli & Lazear 2000):

- identify and treat life-threatening emergencies
- maintain airway, breathing, and circulation
- prevent complications
- maintain safety of the patient, other patients, relatives/carers and staff
- administer medications as prescribed and monitor effects
- provide a suitable ward environment

A nursing care plan for patients with specific mental health needs can be seen in Table 2.4.

Any attendance at hospital is filled with anxiety-provoking stimuli, and nurses can help reduce these by providing order and keeping the patient informed so that they can prepare themselves. Facilitating patient choice and including the patient in decisions when possible can increase their sense of being in control of the situation.

Nurses also need to manage risk, which encompasses the need for psychiatric referral, risk of self-harm or suicide, and/or risk of aggression/violence (Heslop et al. 2000). If a patient has been assessed as being at risk of harming themselves or others (an ongoing process), then appropriate measures must be employed to prevent them causing harm (see Table 2.5). Common Law allows reasonable restraint of such patients until appropriate medical/psychiatric personnel arrive, however, the initiation of restraint could escalate a situation and could result in injury to all parties and thus caution is to be advised. The emergency admission to hospital of a mentally ill patient is covered by the Mental Health Act in England and Wales (DH 2007b). If the Act is invoked, the correct documentation must be used and completed accurately. It is useful for acute care staff to familiarise themselves with the requirements of the Act and the relevant documentation before they are needed. Methods for managing the patient at risk are identified in Table 2.5.

Table 2.4 A nursing care plan based on the patient's mental health need (based on Polli & Lazear 2000 and Isaacs 2001)

Disorder	Clinical features	Nursing care
Anxiety	Not always sure what they are anxious about History of panic attacks Precipitating incident tachycardia, headache, hyperventilation, nausea, diarrhoea, chest tightness, hypertension Tremors, irritability, anger, pacing, restless, crying Expect the worst outcome Lack of concentration Difficulty sleeping	Acknowledge stress and anxiety Provide support by being available Discuss coping strategy for any physical tests to be performed Provide information on tests and keep patient up to date with the plan of care Encourage calm breathing and relaxation Nurse in quiet area of unit/ward if medical condition allows Consideration of anxiolytic medication
Dementia (including Alzheimer's disease)	Loss of memory in union with lack of concentration Confusion about time and place Signs of self-neglect Wanders aimlessly Reasoning slow and muddled Depressed, agitated and restless	Orientate patient to time, place and person at level of ability Reduce environmental stimuli Maintain safety Work with family in setting realistic goals Encourage to follow set routine of rest and activity
Suicidal behaviour	Previous history of chronic illness and/or mental health disorder Signs of depression Suicidal ideas Respiratory/cardiovascular status may be altered from drug ingestion Self-inflicted injuries Presence of risk factors	Encourage to talk about feelings Listen objectively and non-judgementally Provide safe environment in an observable area Specific treatment for any substance ingested Ensure patient is aware of care plan Orientate to unit/ward
Depression	History of depression A precipitating incident Quiet, withdrawn, tired Crying Insomnia, hypersomnia Loss of interest Feelings of worthlessness Possible brady-cardia Slowed gait and movements	Provide emotional support Discuss with patient possible cause(s) of depression Assess suicide risk Facilitate adequate nutrition Signpost to appropriate mental health services
Bipolar disease	Alternating mania and depression History of bipolar disease Hallucinations Agitation or withdrawal Flight of ideas or flat affect (mood) Delusions or thoughts of grandeur Not sleeping Over-activity or slowed movement	Orientate patient to ward and plan of care Minimise environmental stimulation Administer mood-stabilising medication as required Monitor nutritional intake, high calorie Promote rest periods if manic Advise patient on importance of taking prescribed medications
Psychosis	Delusions Hallucinations Paranoia Bizarre behaviour (e.g. inability to care for self) Pressure of thought Thought blocking Thoughts are being broadcast, being inserted or removed	Observe for early cues of agitation Orientate patient to time, place and person Reduce environmental stimuli Maintain calm, helpful approach Administer anti-psychotic medication as prescribed

Table 2.5 Management of the aggressive patient

Indications of risk	Nursing action	Monitoring
Extreme agitation, excited behaviour, pacing, shouting, violent gestures, slamming doors, threats, abusive language **indicate a high risk of violence** May be the result of the effects of excessive use of drugs or alcohol	**Always keep an exit clear** **Always have an escape route** Inform security personnel of potential for violence Ask them to attend the clinical area prior to attempting to deal with the situation Move other patients quietly Remove potential weapons (e.g. furniture, equipment) Ensure assistance is available from staff trained for such situations Talk calmly, be clear and non-threatening Allow space between self and patient If possible, try to find cause of outburst but avoid confrontation Use a sideways posture (reduce target) and keep hands open Contact crisis resolution/home treatment team	Security personnel to stay until situation under control Consider physical restraint only if absolutely necessary Monitor continually according to mental health assessment Offer drinks and food Respect space and dignity Ensure other staff are continually aware of situation
Expressing desire to harm self High suicide risk Tries to leave	Seek immediate assistance from available unit/ward staff trained for such situations Contact medical staff and mental health services Inform security and ask them to attend the unit Administer medications as prescribed (dependant on cause of symptoms) Nurse to be relieved regularly (at least every hour) Review level of observation regularly	One or two nurses to wait with the patient Consider physical restraint only if absolutely necessary Monitor at all times Restrict movement so that there is minimum opportunity to abscond by routes such as windows, fire exits
Frightened, impulsive, may not wait	Seek urgent medical or psychiatric assessment Keep patient informed of plan of care	Sit with patient Offer support and reassurance Monitor closely
Appears to be under the influence of drugs or alcohol but no physical compromise	Monitor clinical signs as indicated by substance Nurse in high observation area	Discreet observation Check regularly for deterioration in physical or mental state
Wandering (coping mechanism – boredom, hunger)	Check at regular intervals the whereabouts of the patient Keep patient informed of the unit/ward routine (e.g. meals, when they will be reviewed by doctor) At handover, the patients whereabouts must be confirmed	Discreet observation Check regularly for deterioration in mental status Do not forget nutritional needs
Patient absconds	Inform security personnel, medical staff and manager Contact GP and next of kin Contact the Police if patient is at high risk of harm to self or others	

Documentation

As a guide to future patient management an accurate and concise history of the current problem must be recorded. This should include:

- details of the presenting complaint, duration and intensity, psychiatric and physical assessments, include both positive and negative findings (Brown & Cadogan 2006)
- an estimate of the degree of urgency of treatment in terms of risk to patient and others
- source of information and relationship to patient
- full details of any behavioural problems encountered and any action taken
- risk assessment
- plan of care with treatment goals, medication prescribed and/or reason for referral to any other agency
- close communication between the acute clinical setting and the responsible mental health team
- evaluation of care given
- date and time of assessment and name of assessor

Referral options

An important minority of these vulnerable patients will require referral to a community mental health team or crisis resolution/home treatment team for an expert assessment of their mental health status, suicide risk or substance dependency. Based on this referral, a decision whether to admit or discharge will be made.

If the patient is discharged with a serious (e.g. chronic illness) but low-risk (of harm to self or others) mental health need, follow-up must include an outpatient's clinic appointment or GP referral. When any patient with a mental health disorder is discharged their GP and community care co-ordinator must be informed of their attendance and subsequent discharge. The role of the care co-ordinator is to monitor the patient's mental health in their home environment.

Discharge planning

Failure to ensure follow-up for a mental health disorder denies the patient an opportunity for effective treatment and can adversely affect the quality of life for both them and their family. This makes discharge planning vital for effective transfer of information and management of care. Before discharge, and being aware of the requirements of confidentiality, ensure that the patient (and their carers) is aware of their diagnosis and plan of care. Give instructions regarding prescribed medications, their side effects and where and when to get a follow-up prescription. Details of any support that has been arranged should be given in written form along with details of where to attend in case of a crisis. The date, time and location of outpatient appointments should also be written down. Finally, the patient should know who has been informed of their discharge (e.g. their GP and any community services that are involved in their care).

Summary

Among vulnerable groups of people who attend acute care settings, one of the most complex are those who present with a co-existing mental health need. This vulnerability can be compounded by the individual's own reluctance to acknowledge a mental health need. They may be feared by the public, may be vulnerable to assault and may be the victims rather than perpetrators of violence (Atakan & Davies 1997). Their health can be vulnerable as a result of their own behaviour; from the physical injuries of attempted suicide or self-neglect in cases of severe depression. These individuals can be vulnerable to a decline in their social circumstances, to social violence and to the use and abuse of alcohol and drugs (Mavundla 2000). This situation is often compounded on general hospital wards by the insecurity of nursing staff in their skills and knowledge of mental health issues. This leads to apprehension among nurses which is often generated by patients' invasive behaviours and aggression (Brinn 2000; Heslop et al. 2000). In these circumstances, care plans often focus on the physical elements of care as these are perceived as being more familiar and easier to achieve.

This section has aimed to provide a structure for the assessment of patients with mental health needs. By so doing, it is hoped that these patients will receive the individualised care that they require and that nurses will overcome their apprehensions in respect of this vulnerable group of people.

B: RECOGNISING AND REPORTING ACTUAL AND POTENTIAL ABUSE IN THE OLDER ADULT: A GUIDE FOR THE FIRST 24 HOURS OF ACUTE CARE PROVISION
Fiona Howell

Aims

This section will:

- explore the concept of abuse in relation to the older person
- provide a definition of abuse and the categories that are commonly known to exist in relation to the mistreatment of older people
- offer a framework for good practice in the identification and reporting of suspected cases of alleged abuse
- review the current legislation and professional practice guidance around the safeguarding of vulnerable adults

Introduction

Despite the recent development of procedures for the safeguarding of vulnerable adults, the abuse of older people is not a new concept, but one which has seen an ebb and flow of interest since the early 1970s. In 1995, Penhale and Kingston acknowledged the potential for elder abuse to become a societal concern in the same way that recognition of the abuse and neglect of children gained momentum in the mid-1970s, leading to legislative and practical responses across health and social care providers. Irrespective of the potential similarities to child abuse, the identification and management of 'elder' abuse presents the health worker with some significant challenges. Physical presentation, a lack of education and skills or ability of nurses to identify abuse, coupled with the frequent reluctance of the victim to disclose episodes of abuse, may have a significant impact on the care these patients receive and the ongoing support they require.

Over the last decade, there have been significant legislative changes relating to the protection of the vulnerable adult. These include the Mental Capacity Act (DH 2005) and its subsequent component, the Deprivation of Liberty Safeguards (DH 2009b), which both provide guidance on assessing vulnerable individuals' ability to make informed decisions. Preceding this, the Department of Health published 'No Secrets' (DH 2000) which provided comprehensive guidance for health and social organisations on how to work in partnership regarding the challenges of protecting vulnerable adults from abuse. Despite this increase in awareness, a review of 'No Secrets' (DH 2008a) identified that whilst good progress had been made in addressing the key issues surrounding the protection of vulnerable adults, there was the perception that the nursing profession continues to face challenges in relation to the recognition and reporting of abuse (Morgan 2009).

In situations where abuse is suspected, it is essential that clear local reporting mechanisms are in place and that these are rigorously adhered to. Health and Social Care organisations must provide evidence of working in partnership (DH 2000) in respect of safeguarding issues. They must have robust procedures for the identification, management and support of individuals experiencing or working with patients who have been exposed to abusive situations. Despite these recommendations, integrated systems appear to have been slow to develop (Morgan 2009).

Recognition of abuse

The World Health Organization (WHO) identifies elder abuse as a problem that exists in both developing and developed countries, yet it is believed to be under-reported globally. Data on prevalence exist only in developed countries – with ranges reported as being between 1 in 6 and 1 in 15 older adults experiencing abuse, although such low numbers may demonstrate the hidden nature of this phenomenon (WHO 2008). In the United Kingdom, the extent of mistreatment of older people is unknown, but it is believed to affect between 4 and 5% of older adults (O'Keeffe et al. 2007). In the UK, where three-quarters of all acute hospital beds are occupied by those over 65 years of age (DH 2001a), a fundamental understanding of the physiology of ageing is a useful starting point for all nurses working in these settings.

Changes in body systems occur as the individual ages and a physical reduction in functional reserve may result in an increase in those illnesses and physical characteristics associated with natural ageing. Without question, the complexity of the ageing process is such that during the initial assessment there may be few clear distinctions between the frailty of a naturally ageing body and those physical and psychological signs associated with abuse. For example, an infection of the urinary tract is a common condition that may require a period of hospitalisation for the older adult. Presenting with this condition in isolation is unlikely to raise concerns, but coupled with, for example, a presentation of general neglect, bruising around the perineum and/or unexplained genital bleeding, the nurse must be alert to the potential for sexual abuse to have occurred. Such suspicions should be documented and communicated effectively across the healthcare team. Similarly, whereas physical presentations such as multiple bruises or skin tears in a younger adult or child will automatically raise suspicion, particularly when associated with an implausible explanation, this is less likely in the case of older people as it is widely acknowledged that they undergo physical changes as part of the natural ageing process (Mattson-Porth 2005) and damage to the upper layers of the skin is a common occurrence. Poor recollection of the incident, memory problems or the presence of dementia will reduce the capacity of the older person to recall the origins of their injury, so it is vital that a detailed history is taken from those who accompany the individual. Severe bruising, lacerations and skin tears should not be taken as a definitive sign that abuse has occurred, but suspicions should be documented and consideration given to the plausibility of any explanation.

Categories of abuse

Throughout the last decade, efforts to categorise abuse have resulted in a variety of definitions. The most widely accepted definition originated from the charity, Action on Elder Abuse, and was adopted by WHO, which acknowledges the concept of abuse as being:

> a single, or repeated act, or lack of appropriate action, occurring within any relationship where there is an expectation of trust which causes harm or distress to an older person.
>
> (WHO 2008)

It is recognised that if suspicions are raised about the possibility of abuse having occurred, healthcare workers should be aware that more than one category of abuse may co-exist and more than one perpetrator may be involved. Categories of abuse are generally agreed to include physical, financial, sexual, intentional and unintentional neglect, emotional abuse and discriminatory practice (McGarry & Simpson 2008) (see Table 2.6). Baker and Heitkemper (2005) suggest that abuse can be a hidden problem, particularly in relation to reporting mechanisms and the unwillingness of the individual to disclose the breakdown of the relationship with their family or care-giver. Consequently, where abuse is suspected, it is not enough to focus solely on the older person experiencing the abuse. The complex interpersonal

Table 2.6   Categories of abuse with indicative signs (adapted from McGarry & Simpson 2008)

Type of abuse	Possible presenting features
Physical	Bruising, cuts, burns or fractures that are inconsistent with explanation given Bruising in various stages of healing and with unusual shaped patterns Cigarette burns or unexplained welts across aspects of the body Unexplained burns, especially on soles, palms and back, hot water immersion burns, rope burns, electric appliance or carpet burns Signs of medication misuse (over- or under-medication) Nervous or flinching behaviour Failure of carer to report injuries in a timely manner
Sexual	Unexplained bruising/bleeding and skin damage to the perianal region Torn, stained or bloody underclothing Sexually transmitted infections Unexplained urinary of faecal incontinence Bruises or finger marks around thighs and on arms
Emotional/psychological	Fearfulness and inability to maintain eye contact Reported emotional withdrawal Resignation/passivity and deference to care-givers Low self-esteem/self-depreciation Behaviour towards elder person by caregiver seen as aggressive, belittling or humiliating
Intentional or unintentional neglect	Clothing in poor condition – inappropriate for time of year or day Poor state of personal hygiene or malnourishment Existence of pressure damage to skin or untreated leg ulcers Delay in seeking timely medical treatment Wide discrepancy in general appearance between care-giver and cared for Care-giver frailty, poor cognition or poor health
Discrimination	Inappropriate choices given with little recognition of race or gender or functional ability Failure to recognise and support religious, cultural or spiritual needs Psychological or physical abuse on the basis of the descriptors above

relationships which often exist between the abused and the abuser may subvert attempts to provide subsequent support and assistance to the abused. According to the charity Action on Elder Abuse (2004), abuse is predominantly experienced within the individual's home, with a greater proportion of women reporting abusive environments than men. Male perpetrators tend more commonly to be family members; female perpetrators also include paid carers.

A framework for good practice

Recognising the signs of abuse and understanding the circumstances around the occasions of abuse is the starting point for a thorough assessment and holistic management plan.

There may be many manifestations of an abusive situation (Table 2.6) and separating those which raise suspicion from the natural ageing process or increasing frailty of the individual is a challenge for the most experienced of health workers (Meeks-Sjostrom 2004).

Undertaking a thorough assessment of the patient's physical and mental health along with a comprehensive history of events is vital, particularly where there is conflicting information between the patient and formal or informal care-giver. The Mental Capacity Act (DH 2005) provides clear guidance on the support that should be afforded to patients who may have a fluctuating mental capacity such as those with diagnosed or suspected dementia. Within the Mental Capacity Act, it is clear that all initial contacts with an individual start with the assumption that the patient has mental capacity.

Communication

Prior to any assessments, patients must be given the opportunity to provide consent and be fully informed of the process. Concerted efforts should be made to ensure adjuncts to communication are in place where appropriate, such as glasses, hearing aids and teeth. Without these, attempts to ascertain comprehensive information may be hampered and vital information may not be disclosed. The provision of sufficient time to undertake a comprehensive assessment is one of the greatest challenges for nurses in acute care settings as this is one of the most important factors when working with older people. It should be noted that, for the older person, a projected belief that the nurse is too busy to listen or take time with them will raise anxiety levels and significantly reduce effective communication between nurse and patient. This has the potential to lead to an inaccurate and insufficient account of the patient's circumstances.

Physical assessment

Physical assessments should entail a head-to-toe approach (starting with ABCDE priorities), particularly where there is a heightened suspicion of physical abuse having occurred. Unusual marks, blemishes and lacerations should be documented clearly and where necessary photographic evidence obtained through the adherence to strict local guidelines around such practice. A thorough understanding of the cause of any skin damage will help in ruling out abuse or enable the practitioner to build a comprehensive account of events that may have occurred.

Psychological assessment

Psychological assessments should be undertaken in a sympathetic and calm environment with the recognition that, for some older patients, an acute hospital may elicit feelings of fear and anxiety, particularly when guilt or shame relating to an abusive situation may exist. The use of an assessment tool such as the Abbreviated Mental Test (AMT) (Hodgkinson 1972) to ascertain short- and long-term recollection will provide a useful baseline for assessment. However, in the presence of a systemic infection, altered consciousness level or increasing anxiety, these may produce a misleading score and should be repeated on a frequent basis to monitor recovery to the patient's usual cognitive level.

Social assessment

Close consideration must be given to the patient's social circumstances, and a complete review of their individual abilities in relation to their activities of daily living, mobility and dietary intake should be undertaken within the first 24 hours of admission. This essential information will determine the level of support required during admission or as a part of the discharge process.

Documentation

In recognising that abuse may have occurred, documentation and the recording of events as relayed to the nurse is an essential component of any subsequent enquiry. Care should be taken not to lead the patient with questions about who perpetrated the possible abuse or what took place. They should be given gentle encouragement to talk and time allowed for the patient to reflect and consider the experiences. The resultant plan of care is a vital aspect of the overall management of the situation and should be developed in partnership with the individual and their family or care-giver. A multi-agency approach to future management should be considered and good communications established between those involved with ongoing care delivery, particularly if the patient is moved between wards, hospitals or community settings. Additionally, informal care-giver stress relating to a number of factors including dependency/financial pressures (Action on Elder Abuse 2004) has been highlighted as a risk factor associated with the potential for perpetrating abuse. For those patients living within institutional settings (such as nursing or residential accommodation), and where abuse is thought to have occurred, it is essential that a multidisciplinary approach is taken to safeguard and protect patients at risk. Nurses should have a good understanding of local policies and procedures in relation to safeguarding vulnerable adults and the reporting of potential abuse. Robust mechanisms must be in place at a local level to enable a full and thorough investigation. Additionally, the 'No Secrets' publication review (DH 2008a) recommended that hospital trusts should introduce an adult safeguarding post to ensure that a standardised and co-ordinated approach to abuse is in place (Morgan 2009), and that support and information is readily available to those in a position to report suspicions of abuse.

It should be remembered that patients who have the mental capacity to make informed decisions may and do refuse help and support, even if they have acknowledged that they are in an abusive situation. As an adult, these patients have the legal right to do so and supportive mechanisms such as referrals to their GP, community nurses and social care colleagues should be made in order to reduce the potential impact on discharge to their usual place of residence. The Nursing and Midwifery Council (NMC) makes it clear that nurses have a specific responsibility to safeguard the patients in their care, document accurately and communicate effectively with their colleagues relating to patients at risk (NMC 2008). Where patients have the capacity to do so, they should be supported to make informed decisions about their future care; the nurse should fully understand the risk of harm occurring and have a clear and comprehensive approach to documentation and following up areas of concern (NMC 2008). Since 2009, the 'Deprivation of Liberty Safeguards' (DoLS) has been part of the legal framework for the care of people lacking mental capacity (Jerram 2010). The DoLS exists as guidance for individuals seeking to prevent harm (or potential of harm) occurring to patients in any formal care setting. Its key elements ensure protective measures are in place for both the individual concerned and the organisation making the application. Consequently, this will ensure that those patients who lack capacity to make decisions have a voice in their care and those organisations making a DoLS application are able to protect an individual's human rights while regularly reviewing and monitoring the appropriateness of that application.

Summary

The mistreatment of older people presents significant challenges for those involved in the provision of care, both in recognising that an abusive situation has occurred and in relation to the most appropriate and timely management thereof. Despite a growing body of literature associated with this phenomenon, there are still no clear statistics which demonstrate the true scale of the problem within the UK although recent studies have demonstrated that between 4 and 5% of the UK older population may have experienced a form of abuse. The real extent of the problem, however, is believed to be much greater.

For nurses working in acute care settings, having and understanding clear policies and guidelines for action in the event of suspected abuse are vital if vulnerable adult patients are to be protected and supported through this significant event.

Clear assessment strategies and an ability to recognise subtle differences between the ageing body and the symptoms of abuse is a challenge. Nurses are at the forefront of managing the difficulties associated with the mistreatment of older people and as such are well placed to develop and sustain processes that support individuals at risk of abuse. Legislation has developed over the past decade which enables a standardised and anti-discriminatory approach to working with patients who lack the mental capacity to make informed decisions. With the increase in diagnosis of dementia within the older population, the Mental Capacity Act (DH 2005) and Deprivation of Liberty Safeguards (DH 2009b) have become a welcome addition to the supportive mechanisms which now exist for those individuals who are experiencing abusive situations now and in the future.

C: MEETING THE NEEDS OF INDIVIDUALS WITH LEARNING DISABILITIES
Michael Gibbs and Judi Thorley

Aims

This section will:

* provide a definition of learning disability
* facilitate an understanding of the development of contemporary policy relating to the health needs of people with learning disability
* equip the healthcare professional with an awareness of the skills, knowledge and understanding to assess, manage and deliver high quality care to people with learning disability
* consider the need to make reasonable adjustments as part of everyday healthcare practice
* describe how the healthcare professional undertaking acute assessment can optimise the patient experience and outcome through partnership with acute liaison nurses, health facilitators, family carers and the wider community nursing team

What is learning disability?

The current working definition as outlined by the Department of Health, and accepted nationally, is that learning disability is 'a significantly reduced ability to understand new or complex information and to learn new skills, with a reduced ability to cope independently, which started before adulthood with a lasting effect on development' (DH 2001b). From an international perspective, the term 'intellectual disability' is often used to identify the same group of people; indeed, the terms can be, and are, used interchangeably. In lay terms, these conditions mean that a person may experience many barriers when attempting to participate in everyday functions and activities that are often taken for granted, for example, making friends, having a job and coming into hospital. Learning disability is not a learning difficulty. In the UK Education Act of 1996, a learning difficulty is defined as 'a significantly greater difficulty in learning than the majority of persons of his (sic) age' (HMSO 1996). More recently, the government suggests that it includes people with mental health difficulties, autistic spectrum conditions, dyslexia, attention deficit hyperactivity disorder, physical, sensory and cognitive impairments, and other identified and non-identified difficulties in learning which may (or may not) have led to special educational needs interventions at school (Department for Education 2010). Learning disability is often confused with mental health needs; however, like the general population, people with learning disability can experience mental health issues, and mental health in itself is not a learning disability.

Fundamental principles

The foundations of any care, support and service delivered to people with learning disabilities sit in the values of independence, rights, choice and inclusion (DH 2001b). Significantly, this means allowing people with learning disabilities to be in control of their lives, to make choices and take decisions, and to be respected as members of society thus having equal access to healthcare and other mainstream services. These fundamental principles underpin the assertion that people with learning disabilities have the same right to services including healthcare provision. It is unacceptable to refuse or to offer inferior treatment to anyone because he or she has a learning disability (Lindsey 1998).

The UK government takes this philosophy further by suggesting that the NHS must be responsive to the needs of different groups and individuals within society. It states that discrimination on the grounds of age, gender, ethnicity, religion, disability or sexuality must be challenged. To achieve quality and equality in best practice, nursing staff (and all other healthcare professionals) need to be aware of the potential vulnerability of their patients and acknowledge their responsibility to make adjustments to ensure fair and equal experiences of care delivery.

The current political and professional focus on vulnerable people illustrates the point that to get things right for people with learning disability or older people or people with mental health needs merely requires nurses to work in a person-centred way with dignity, respect and understanding.

UK legislation through the Equalities Act directs all public services to ensure fair and equal access for all people (HMSO 2010). Equal access does not mean the same access; in fact, to achieve an equal experience of services people with learning disability may require 'reasonable adjustments' which are changes to the way in which services are delivered and planned to have the same fair and equal outcome or experience. In terms of healthcare provision, it is widely acknowledged that if you get it right for people with learning disability, you get it right for all (DH 2008b). The Michael Report (DH 2008b) emphasised the importance of providing holistic care for people with learning disability, who are acknowledged as one of the most vulnerable groups of people in society. Recently, the Health Service Ombudsman (2011) has presented to the UK Parliament a report which highlighted the failure of the NHS to treat older people with dignity, respect and value; these are the very same issues identified in the Michael Report in 2008. Emerson and Baines (2010) concluded that responding to the health inequalities faced by people with learning disabilities is a critically important issue and it is clear from the Ombudsman report that these inequalities exist for other vulnerable people. This reinforces the need for all healthcare staff to treat every person as an individual, thus achieving the core values of the NHS constitution (Health Service Ombudsman 2011).

For the registered nurse, this means actively listening to the person, their family and paid carers, and being flexible in supporting the individual by making reasonable adjustments. For example, over 30 years ago, it was recognised that 'pain is whatever the experiencing person says it is' (McCaffery & Beebe 1989, 7) but if the person doesn't use words to communicate then what should you do in order to understand what the person is experiencing and what they need? Reasonable adjustments can be made through the use of the person's own communication system, involving their carers, using a pen and paper to draw a picture, or by formalised tools such as the Disability Distress Assessment Tool (DisDAT) (Regnard et al. 2007). In 2010, Keele University, in partnership with key stakeholders including people with learning disability and family carers, produced a toolkit to support people with learning disability when accessing hospital care (Read 2010). This toolkit includes resources such as a Hospital Communication Book and the Traffic Light Assessment tool which can help to make reasonable adjustments when carrying out assessments and planning care. It is important to reiterate that it is the healthcare professional's responsibility to make these adjustments to ensure that the person has a safe and positive experience of healthcare.

Contemporary healthcare policy in learning disability

As previously stated by Emerson and Baines (2010), the health of people with learning disability is widely documented and demonstrates that this group of people within society are at higher risks of poor health and health inequalities than the general population. Much of the current debate surrounding these inequalities stem from a report in which healthcare providers were simply asked to 'Treat Me Right' (Mencap 2004). This report examined the healthcare experiences of people with learning disability. It reported both positive and negative issues and concluded that there were still problems when providing healthcare to people with learning disability. Two main issues identified were poor communication skills on the part of healthcare staff and their lack of understanding of the health needs of people with learning disability. The report made a number of recommendations, in particular, that all healthcare professionals should receive training and education regarding learning disability with the intention that they would be better able to meet the healthcare needs of people with a learning disability (Mencap 2004).

The awareness of the health needs and the way in which people with learning disability receive healthcare within acute care settings has gained significant scrutiny with the publication of a further report from Mencap. *Death by Indifference* (Mencap 2007) documented the experiences of six people with learning disabilities who died in NHS care. It is Mencap's view that these people would not have died if they had received the same standard of care provided to the general population. This report led to the establishment of an independent inquiry into access to healthcare for people with learning disability. The outcome of the inquiry, *Healthcare for All* (DH 2008b), called for major changes in the NHS. It found that people with learning disabilities experienced unequal treatment and that there was a lack of 'reasonable adjustments' being made by NHS services. The 10 recommendations made in the Healthcare for All inquiry, which included training for all healthcare staff, tracking and flagging of patients with learning disability, and ensuring reasonable adjustments to services and approaches, were accepted by the UK government. All 10 recommendations were incorporated into *Valuing People Now: A new three year strategy for people with learning disability*

(DH 2009c). The *Death by Indifference* report was investigated by the Parliamentary and Health Service Ombudsman and their report, *Six Lives* (HSO 2009), found that the basic human rights of the people who died had been infringed, and that on several occasions 'basic policy, standards and guidance were not observed, adjustments were not made and services were not coordinated'. Since the publication of *Six Lives* in 2009, there has been much work generated to prevent such occurrences happening again. The *Six Lives Progress Report* (DH 2010b) clearly demonstrates that the NHS is changing its working patterns, and experience of health services is improving for people with learning disability. However, there is still more to do, particularly when considering mental capacity and decision-making, and ensuring that mainstream staff receive awareness training about learning disability.

Using assessment skills to support a patient with learning disability

The skills required when assessing a person with learning disability are identical to those employed for any other person accessing your service, in that their immediate physiological and psychological needs are identified and treated as a priority. When a person with learning disability enters the hospital environment, they often experience a range of emotions. Research shows that many people with learning disability experience fear and anxiety and it is part of the nurse's role to alleviate these fears and anxieties. By making reasonable adjustments these fears and anxieties can be reduced or even overcome. For example, if possible, provide a separate waiting area, allow extra time for assessment/examination, use plain language with no jargon, and talk with the person and involve their carer as opposed to talking to the carer only. The often diverse and complex health needs of the person with learning disability mean that the assessment process is dynamic and a different approach to communication is therefore required. During the assessment, it is essential that you include the patient's carer(s), both as a source of effective communication with the patient and of information regarding the patient's previous medical and social history. Wood and Thorley (2010) highlighted the need for a flexible approach to assessment which draws on the family or paid carer's knowledge of how the person communicates.

Many nurses feel that they do not possess the necessary skills and knowledge of learning disability to deliver care to a high standard. It is evident that nurses and other healthcare professionals need to feel confident in caring for people with learning disability in order to effectively use their skills in delivering appropriate care (Glasby 2002). However, nurses already possess the key skills required to assess patients and this includes patients with learning disability. The challenge lies in realising that the nurse's existing skills as carer, communicator, observer, therapist, advocate and counsellor (Baldwin & Birchenall 1993; Jones 1999) apply to these patients. Confidence can be gained through an in-depth understanding of communication, through education and training and by accessing a range of resources.

Communication

Communication is a social activity that we all take part in from the day we are born. The way in which we communicate can vary widely, with verbal and non-verbal being the umbrella terms used to describe these methods. Communication is the process of exchanging ideas, thoughts and wishes that involves at least two people. This process involves sending and receiving information via symbols, words, signs, gestures and other actions (Peate 2006). Indeed, communication is vital in developing a therapeutic relationship with patients. For the person with a learning disability, your interpretation of the individual's non-verbal communication may be of paramount importance. Given that some people with learning disability give fewer non-verbal cues, it is often difficult to recognise that they are trying to convey a message. If these non-verbal cues are not recognised, the patient may reduce the number of cues even further, making communication even more difficult (Ferris-Taylor 1997). This interactive mode of communication, in which the interaction may not be verbal, is illustrated in case example 1.

Case example 1

Mary, a 46-year-old lady, was referred to the assessment unit by her GP. She had been complaining of chest pain for two days. On arrival, she looked well but was constantly hitting herself. When the nurse attempted to ask her questions, Mary started to shout and scream loudly and used increasing amounts of force to hit herself. This made it impossible for the nurse to make an assessment at this time.

Mary's response may not be a sign of self-injurious behaviour or of a physical threat to others, but may be this particular individual's way of communicating her fears of being in a strange and potentially threatening environment. You could attempt to reduce her anxieties and fears by moving her to a smaller and quieter area to be assessed. Another approach may be the use of simple conversation supplemented by the use of pictures, images or signs. Similarly, you may try demonstrating a blood pressure being taken on yourself or a carer before this procedure is carried out on the patient. Such an approach may help you to gain the patient's confidence and co-operation.

The approach to communication in this case example is time consuming, but it is important that the person with a learning disability has complete trust in you. Consequently, you may have to delay the completion of a physical assessment and any investigations until the individual is less anxious. Demonstration of procedures can assist with the development of trust. Despite the fact that admission areas operate on the principle of patients being rapidly assessed and treated, it is important for you to recognise that your priorities might need to be directed by the individual's needs rather than by nursing or medical procedures. This can be difficult in busy admission areas where patient throughput is high, treatments need to be delivered within specified time periods and nurses have multiple demands upon their time. To

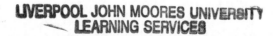

> **Box 2.4   Principles of communication with patients who have a learning disability**
>
> - Always introduce yourself and all appropriate others
> - Use language that the person is likely to understand
> - Avoid the use of jargon or abbreviations – these may cause confusion and increase the person's anxiety
> - Always re-direct the focus of the conversation to the individual concerned – 'ice-breaking' statements can assist with this process
> - Be aware of the importance of body language
> - Note the positioning of the patient, relatives and staff – if necessary change positions so that the nurse can observe the non-verbal cues clearly
> - Sitting at the same level and trying not to stand over the person creates a better therapeutic relationship
> - Assist the person to answer questions by giving them extra time to think
> - Be careful not to rush in with pre-determined answers
> - Make reasonable adjustments to how you communicate both with the patient with learning disability and their carer (where appropriate) by involving and listening
> - Make full use of any communication resource available

ensure effective communication and assist in patient assessment, a degree of lateral thinking may be required. In order to facilitate social interaction, the principles outlined in Box 2.4 can be applied.

To improve communication with patients with learning disability, you need to supplement your verbal communication skills with non-verbal tools such as sign language and pictures. The person with a learning disability may have a communication book, traffic light assessment or other such information tool that will help you to understand the individual's communication needs. Involving carers to help you to understand what is usual for the person and what certain gestures and movements mean is important. It will help you to feel more confident and the person with learning disability less anxious.

By using these principles, you can facilitate effective interaction and communication. Repeated and continually giving information and explanations can help to support this process. Using the example of taking a blood pressure, 'ice-breaking' statements that may be used include:

- 'Can I sit here while I take your blood pressure?'
- 'I would like to take your blood pressure with this machine. Do you want to hold it? This is what is does.'
- 'Let me show you on me first.'

These are simple ways of breaking down barriers and overcoming patients' fears. Be prepared to leave the patient for a short time. This enables the person to familiarise themselves with the situation and seek clarification from their carer. When you return, ask the patient if they have any questions. Continuing the blood pressure example, this could involve leaving the machine with the patient and their carer to allow them to inspect the equipment. You may return a short time later and ask; 'Are you okay now, shall we take your blood pressure?'

Remember that the patient should be the focus of your attention. With this in mind, always ask the patient what they want rather than asking their carer. Be aware, though, that you will also need to pay attention to verbal and non-verbal cues from the carer. It is very important to realise that your behaviour gives cues to the patient. Consequently, if you behave respectfully the patient is more likely to feel less anxious.

To ensure that people with learning disability have a fair and equal experience of services (DH 2008b), the Mencap Charter (2010) highlighted the value of learning disability nurses working within hospital settings and primary care. A good example of this is the acute liaison nurse role which facilitates not only care but also education and training. Case examples 2 and 3, both of which are from clinical practice, demonstrate the value of an acute liaison nurse for the person with learning disability, their carers and healthcare professionals. For the purposes of anonymity, pseudonyms have been used.

Case example 2

David was a 34-year-old gentleman with a mild learning disability and mental health problems in the form of anxiety and depression. He lived alone and managed his day-to-day life very well. David's mother had died three years previously and he had struggled to come to terms with his loss. David had a community nurse, social worker and consultant psychiatrist with whom he maintained contact when he was feeling well. When his depression was acute, David isolated himself, refused to attend appointments and declined input from professionals. As David had previously expressed suicidal thoughts, the acute liaison nurse discussed the situation with David, other professionals involved and emergency department colleagues. This discussion led to the tracking and flagging of David and his individual needs within the hospital system. In addition to support, David and hospital staff his community nurse helped him to maintain his traffic light assessment which described his current health status, important actions to take and contact details of community professionals. A review of David's community package was facilitated and a care plan agreed which incorporated additional community support in the form of respite care that could be triggered by hospital staff.

This case example illustrates how a well-planned system enabled early intervention that prevented David having to wait in what to him may have been a threatening and strange environment (the emergency department). It also shows how an admission to an acute psychiatric ward was prevented, thereby, removing the need for David to deal with what may have been a potentially difficult situation for him.

Both of these case examples illustrate how nurses can positively influence the care delivered to this potentially vulnerable group of patients by making reasonable adjustments and working in partnership with learning disability professionals, the person with learning disability and their carers. All nurses have a role in health promotion but nurses working in acute care areas are in an enviable position, in that they have the opportunity to assess the overall health and well-being of the patients in their care.

> **Case example 3**
>
> Adam was a 40-year-old gentleman with mild to moderate learning disabilities. He lived in a private community home for people with learning disabilities. Adam was admitted to the assessment unit with a suspected gastro-intestinal bleed and, from the unit, was admitted to a medical ward. When no source of bleeding was found, Adam was discharged home the following day. During his initial assessment, nursing staff became concerned about Adam's other health needs. He had previously been diagnosed as asthmatic but seemed to be poorly controlled. He was also obese and smoked at least 25 cigarettes per day. Consequently, the nurses referred Adam to the learning disability liaison nurse to follow up these health issues with him at home.

Summary

Nurses already possess many of the skills required to support and ensure high quality care for people with learning disability. The challenge lies in recognising the need to make reasonable adjustments and developing existing skills and putting these skills into practice. The following key messages are taken from the Hospital Toolkit (Read 2010) and provide simple pointers to help nurses to care for a patient with learning disability:

You should ALWAYS:

- actively listen to the patient using verbal and non-verbal communication skills
- involve the patient in all aspects of their care
- make reasonable adjustments in the way you work and to the care environment

You should THINK about:

- Does the patient understand their health needs?
- How can the patient's knowledge and experience help their care?
- Does the patient need someone to support them during procedures?

What you should NEVER do:

- Don't assume that the patient can't understand because of their learning disability
- Don't assume that everything is linked to the patient's learning disability
- Don't give the patient too much information all at once

In all aspects of the patient's care it is important to involve family, carers and others who know the person well. This particularly includes listening and hearing in order to help you meet the patient's needs by supporting them in offering choices and making decisions if they are able to. Should the patient lack capacity to make such decisions and choices then the nurse must act in the patient's best interests, as clearly identified in the Mental Capacity Act (HMSO 2005) to provide best quality of care in a timely, respectful manner. As identified in the Mencap *Getting it Right*

Charter (2010), there is a need for education and training to raise awareness of the needs of people with learning disability. The nurse's responsibility is to recognise the need for, and to make, reasonable adjustments and importantly to understand and apply the five core principles of the Mental Capacity Act (2005). Finally, as already stated, it is widely accepted that if you get things right for people with learning disability you get it right for everyone (DH 2008b).

References

Action on Elder Abuse (2004) *Hidden Voices: Older People's Experience of Abuse*. London: Action on Elder Abuse.

Atakan Z & Davies T (1997) ABC of mental health: Mental health emergencies. *BMJ*, 314(7096), 1740–1742.

Baker M & Heitkemper M (2005) The roles of nurses on interprofessional teams to combat elder abuse. *Nursing Outlook*, 53(5), 253–259.

Baldwin S & Birchenall M (1993) The nurse's role in caring for people with learning disabilities. *British Journal of Nursing*, 2(17), 850–855.

Brinn F (2000) Patients with mental illness: General nurses' attitudes and expectations. *Nursing Standard*, 14(27), 32–36.

Brown A & Cadogan M (2006) Emergency medicine. *Emergency & Acute Medicine: Diagnosis and Management* (5th edition). Melbourne: Hodder Arnold.

Brown R & Rounds L (1995) Conjoint screening questionnaires for alcohol and drug abuse. *Wisconsin Medical Journal*, 94, 135–140.

Callaghan P, Playle J & Cooper L (eds) (2009) *Mental Health Nursing Skills*. Oxford: Oxford University Press.

Davies T & Craig T (2009) *ABC of Mental Health* (2nd edition). Oxford: Wiley: Blackwell.

Department for Education (2010) *Supporting young people with learning difficulties to participate and progress: incorporating guidance on Learning Difficulty Assessments*. London: Department for Education.

Department of Health (2000) *No Secrets: Guidance on the developing and implementing multi-agency policies and procedures to protect vulnerable adults from abuse*. London: Department of Health.

Department of Health (2001a) *National Service Framework for Older People*. London: Department of Health.

Department of Health (2001b) *Valuing People: A new strategy for learning disability for the 21ˢᵗ century*. London: Department of Health.

Department of Health (2005) *Mental Capacity Act*. London: Department of Health.

Department of Health (2007a) *Best Practice in Managing Risk: Principles and Evidence for Best Practice in the Assessment and Management of Risk to Self and Others in Mental Health Services*. London: Department of Health.

Department of Health (2007b) *Mental Health Act*. London: Department of Health.

Department of Health (2008a) *Safeguarding Adults: A consultation on the review of the 'No Secrets' guidance*. London: Department of Health.

Department of Health (2008b) *Healthcare for all: Report of the Independent Inquiry into Access to Healthcare for People with Learning Disabilities (The Michael Report)*. London: Department of Health.

Department of Health (2009a) *Information sharing and mental health*. London: Department of Health.

Department of Health (2009b) *Mental Capacity Act Deprivation of Liberty Safeguards.* London: Department of Health.

Department of Health (2009c) *Valuing People Now: A new three-year strategy for people with learning disabilities.* London: Department of Health.

Department of Health (2010a) *New Horizons.* London: Department of Health.

Department of Health (2010b) *Six Lives Progress Report.* London: Department of Health.

Emerson E & Baines S (2010) *Health Inequalities and People with Learning Disabilities in the UK: Improving Health and Lives.* Stockton on Tees: Learning Disabilities Observatory.

Ferris-Taylor R (1997) Communication. In Gates B (ed.) *Learning Disabilities* (3rd edition). Edinburgh: Churchill Livingstone.

Fontaine K (2009) *Mental Health Nursing* (6th edition). Upper Saddle River, NJ: Pearson Education.

Glasby A-M (2002) Meeting the needs of people with learning disabilities in acute care. *British Journal of Nursing,* 11(21), 1389–1392.

Good W & Nelson J (1986) *Psychiatry Made Ridiculously Simple* (3rd edition). Miami: MedMaster Inc.

Harrison P, Geddes J & Sharpe M (2010) *Lecture Notes: Psychiatry* (10th edition). Oxford: Wiley-Blackwell.

Health Service Ombudsman (2009) *Six Lives: The provision of public services to people with learning disabilities* London: Parliamentary & Health Service Ombudsman.

Health Service Ombudsman (2011) *Care and Compassion.* London: Parliamentary & Health Service Ombudsman.

Heslop L, Eslom S & Parker N (2000) Improving continuity of care across psychiatric and emergency services: Combining patient data within a participatory action research framework. *Journal of Advanced Nursing,* 31(1), 135–143.

HMSO (1996) *Education Act 1996: Section 15ZA* (6) & (7). London: HMSO.

HMSO (2005) *Mental Capacity Act 2005.* London: HMSO.

HMSO (2010) *Equality Act 2010.* London: HMSO.

Hodgkinson HM (1972) Evaluation of a mental test score for assessment of mental impairment in the elderly. *Age and Ageing,* 1, 233–238.

Isaacs A (2001) *Mental Health and Psychiatric Nursing* (3rd edition). Philadelphia: Lippincott.

Jerram S (2010) Practice Question: Care of people who lack capacity. *Nursing Older People,* 22(6), 14.

Jones S (1999) Learning disability nursing: Holistic care at its best. *Nursing Standard,* 13(52), 61.

Lindsey M (1998) *Signposts for success in the commissioning and providing health services for people with learning disabilities.* London: Department of Health.

Mattson-Porth C (2005) *Pathophysiology: Concepts of Altered Health States* (7th edition). London: Lippincott Williams & Wilkins.

Mavundla T (2000) Professional nurses' perception of nursing mentally ill people in a general hospital setting. *Journal of Advanced Nursing,* 32(6), 1569–1578.

McCaffery M & Beebe A (1989) *Pain: Clinical Manual for Nursing Practice.* St Louis: C V Mosby.

McGarry J & Simpson C (2008) Identifying, reporting and preventing elder abuse in the practice setting. *Nursing Older People,* 21(1), 33–39.

Meeks-Sjostrom D (2004) A comparison of three measures of elder abuse. *Journal of Nursing Scholarship,* 36(3), 247–250.

Mencap (2004) *Treat Me Right* London: Mencap.

Mencap (2007) *Death By Indifference*. London: Mencap.

Mencap (2010) *Getting it Right Charter*. London: Mencap.

Mioshi E, Dawson K, Mitchell J, Arnold R & Hodges J (2006) The Addenbrookes Cognitive Examination Revised (ACE-R): A brief cognitive test battery for dementia screening. *International Journal of Geriatric Psychiatry*, 21, 1078–1085.

Molitor L (ed.) (1996) *Emergency Department Handbook*. Gaithersbury, MD: Aspen Publishers Inc.

Morgan A (2009) Health service struggling to integrate safeguarding policy. *Nursing Older People*, 21(8), 8–9.

Morris G & Morris J (2010) *The dementia care workbook*. Maidenhead, UK: Open University Press.

Nash M (2010) *Physical Health and Well-Being in Mental Health Nursing: Clinical Skills for Practice*. Maidenhead, UK: Open University Press.

National Patient Safety Agency (2009) *Preventing suicide: A toolkit for mental health services*. London: NPSA.

Norman I & Ryrie I (eds) (2009) *The Art and Science of Mental Health Nursing*. Maidenhead, UK: Open University Press.

Nursing and Midwifery Council (2008) *The Code: Standards of Conduct, Performance and Ethics for Nurses and Midwives*. London: NMC.

Office for National Statistics (2000) *Psychiatric Morbidity Among Adults Living in Private Households*. London: ONS.

O'Keeffe M, Hills A, Doyle M et al. (2007) *UK Study of Abuse and Neglect of Older People. Prevalence Survey Report*. London: National Centre for Social Research.

Peate I (2006) *Becoming a Nurse in the 21st Century*. Chichester, UK: John Wiley & Sons.

Penhale B & Kingston P (1995) Elder abuse: An overview of current and recent developments. *Health and Social Care in the Community*, 3(5), 311–320.

Polli G & Lazear (2000) Mental Health Emergencies. In: *Emergency Nurses Association: Emergency Nursing Core Curriculum*. Philadelphia: W B Saunders Company.

Read S (2010) *My next patient has a learning disability* (2nd edition). Staffordshire: Keele University. www.keele.ac.uk/nursingandmidwifery/mnphald/ (accessed: 14 April 2011).

Regnard C, Reynolds J, Watson B, Matthews D, Gibson L, & Clarke C (2007) Understanding distress in people with severe communication difficulties: Developing and assessing the Disability Distress Assessment Tool (DisDAT). *Journal of Intellectual Disability Research*, 51(4), 277–292.

Seidel H, Ball J, Dains J, Flynn J, Solomon B & Stewart R (2010) *Mosby's Guide to Physical Examination* (7th edition). Missouri: Mosby.

Townsend M (2007) *Essentials of Psychiatric Mental Health Nursing: Concepts of Care in Evidence-based Practice* (4th edition). Philadelphia: F A Davis Company.

Tummey R & Turner T (eds) (2008) *Critical Issues in Mental Health*. Basingstoke, UK: Palgrave.

Wood I & Thorley J (2010) 'He's not himself today': Assessment of acute physical health needs. *Learning Disability Practice*, 13(3), 12–17.

World Health Organization (2007) *ICD 10: International Statistical Classification of Diseases and Related Health Problems* (10th revision). Geneva: WHO. http://apps.who.int/classifications/apps/icd/icd10online (accessed 28 September 2010).

World Health Organization (2008) *A global response to elder abuse and neglect: building primary care capacity to deal with the problem worldwide: Main Report*. Geneva: WHO.

Wyatt J, Illingworth R, Clancy M, Monro P & Robertson C (2005) *Oxford Handbook of Accident and Emergency Medicine* (2nd edition). Oxford: Oxford University Press.

3 Sudden Death

Sue Read and Jane Jervis

Aims

This chapter will:

- consider the practical issues relating to the care and support of the relatives of acute medical patients who have died suddenly in the hospital context
- introduce ethical and legal issues encountered in clinical practice
- clarify the impact of both giving and receiving bad news and identify ideas for best practice
- discuss environmental factors to promote best practice
- identify the support needs of relatives bereaved by sudden death
- explore typical responses to bad news from a counselling and support perspective
- provide a rationale for informal and formal staff support systems
- examine the professional development needs for, and provision of, nursing and medical education and training in relation to sudden death
- provide a checklist as an indicator of best practice

Introduction

Death is indiscriminate and will touch each and every one of us as we progress through life. Death is always waiting around the corner, sometimes a regular companion as, for example, people with life-limiting conditions live with the prospect of an untimely death for many months or even years (Read, in press). But death can also be a sudden and unexpected visitor, when it arrives without warning or time to prepare for it, and may be perceived as untimely (Read, in press). It is worth remembering that even those who have been living with a non-curable illness for many years may be admitted as an emergency and die suddenly of a completely different and unrelated illness.

There are many modes of death, from the debilitatingly slow to the traumatically quick; and there are many factors that might affect the way that any surviving relatives may cope with their loss. Such factors include the mode of death; the circumstances around the death; the age of the person who has died; whether it was a public death; whether it involved violence; whether it was an

Initial Management of Acute Medical Patients: A Guide for Nurses and Healthcare Practitioners, Second Edition. Edited by Ian Wood and Michelle Garner.
© 2012 John Wiley & Sons, Ltd. Published 2012 by John Wiley & Sons, Ltd.

avoidable death and whether it was an expected death (Worden 2001; Machin 2009). While research identifies that home is the preferred place of death for the majority of people (Gott et al. 2004; Gomes & Higginson 2006), the majority of the population still die in institutionalised care, whether this be in a private nursing home, hospital or hospice (National Council for Palliative Care 2009). All of these factors may be multifaceted and accumulative, for example a young person who dies suddenly and traumatically in a road traffic accident may evoke many emotions and issues within the surviving family – largely because of the combination of age and nature of the death (both sudden and traumatic). Such sudden, tragic and untimely death may also evoke emotions among the professionals who fought to save them, and remain 'profoundly distressing, individually and socially' (Machin 2009, 27).

According to Wright (1991), no other event in one's life has the same impact as sudden death. For the individual who has experienced the sudden death of a close relative, that impact may be immeasurable; for those health professionals caring for such relatives the stress of continually being involved in such difficult and sensitive activities can be variable and complex. Healthcare professionals must remain mindful of the personal and professional challenges involved when dealing with such situations. As Wright (1991) reminds us, professionals 'must be aware of its [sudden death's] strength, enormity and complexity' in order for constructive help and professional support to be most effective.

Supporting the dying patient is often described as 'one of the most fulfilling yet challenging times' for the nurse (Jevon 2010, vii). In acute medical care areas, nurses are often faced with anxious patients who are referred for assessment, investigation and initial treatment. Relatives, who are often distressed because of the uncertain future of their loved ones and who are also uncomfortable in this unfamiliar environment, often accompany them. Such relatives will have to talk to complete strangers (nursing and medical staff) who maintain total autonomy over their loved ones. Largely, the nursing and medical staff will be meeting these people for the first time. They have to establish, in a very short period of time, communication channels in order to nurture trusting relationships with the patient and their relatives. These professionals have to be highly skilled communicators who are competent at dealing with the presenting physical problems while simultaneously addressing the interpersonal challenges posed by anxious relatives. Nurses in acute care areas are in a front-line position, faced with a plethora of medical conditions, and have to cope with a range of problems resulting from serious illness to death.

At a time of a sudden death in the acute medical area, the effects may be multiple, as nurses are supporting relatives and often each other. Dealing with death is often difficult and can affect us in three specific ways:

- making us painfully aware of our own losses
- making us aware of our potential losses
- making us aware of our own pending mortality

Worden (1991, 133–4)

Dealing with death involves addressing a whole range of issues from an environmental, physical, psychological and sociological perspective. Consequently, when considering sudden death within any acute care area, a whole range of factors need to be identified, considered and explored from a practical, emotional and psychological perspective. Such factors range from the ethical dilemmas often presented (for example, with witnessed resuscitation) to supporting the resultant bereaved family. A checklist is offered at the end of this chapter as a good practice resource when dealing with sudden death of acute medical patients.

Ethical and legal issues

Death, by the very nature of its diversity, is surrounded by social and cultural traditions and superstition. This contributes to the complex arena that is healthcare, in which many moral and ethical questions provide continuous debate. In the past, death could be defined as the absence of breathing and a heartbeat. However, advances in medical technology have caused great debate as to the modern definition of death (Stanley 1987; Gillon 1990; Chaloner 1996) and result in changing patterns of mortality and death rituals throughout the world (Seale 2000). Within critical care settings, advances (e.g. mechanical ventilation and drug therapies) have increased the complexity of ethical and philosophical questions surrounding the definition of death, as technology can now sustain the heart and lungs even when the brain can no longer perform these functions. Ultimately, this leads to such ethical dilemmas as withdrawal of treatment, brain death and organ donation.

As an acute medical nurse, the most common ethical dilemmas encountered relating to death and bereavement are those involving cardiopulmonary resuscitation (CPR). These tend to relate to resuscitation decisions (e.g. 'do not attempt resuscitation' – DNAR – orders and advance decisions to refuse treatment), but also include the patient's right to refuse life-saving treatment and relative-witnessed resuscitation (see Chapter 4 – Cardiac arrest).

CPR was originally introduced as a method to resuscitate the victim of a witnessed catastrophe or trauma such as drowning or electrocution (Page & Meerabeau 1996). Since this time, its use has increased so that, in recent times, anyone who has a cardiopulmonary arrest may receive CPR. It is important then to consider the first ethical question that arises: is it appropriate to give CPR in all cases of cardiopulmonary arrest? As one can see, it is possible to glimpse the moral and ethical minefield that surrounds CPR decisions from this one question alone.

All ethical decisions are guided by the four principles of beneficence, non-maleficence, justice and respect for patient autonomy. These principles are also the basis on which resuscitation decisions are made. The principle of beneficence relates to the need to take deliberate actions in order to do good and non-maleficence refers to a person's duty to do no harm. Respect for patient autonomy involves the acute medical nurse respecting the patient's right to make personal treatment decisions regardless of professional opinion. Justice 'implies a duty to spread benefits and risks equally within a society' and so CPR should be available to all who would benefit from it within the resources available (Resuscitation Council (UK)

2006, 147). The debates surrounding the four principles are complex. However, they are often linked together and when related to nursing practice can be applied to the Nursing and Midwifery Council (2008) *Code of Conduct* which provides a framework to assist the nurse to act in both a legal and ethical manner.

In modern healthcare, resource allocation is a frequent concern to both healthcare providers and society as a whole. As such it is argued that considerations related to the concept of justice support the limited use of CPR and intensive care to those who would benefit from it. Inherent to this argument is the concept that providing futile or inappropriate care to one patient could be delaying treatment to another who has a greater chance of survival (Hilberman et al. 1997; Mohr & Kettler 1997) or even harming the wider population (Niederman & Berger 2010). Therefore, the concept of justice can be in opposition to the ideas of patient autonomy.

> Autonomy is by far the most significant value which has been promoted by contemporary medical ethics. The concept which has dominated medical ethics more than any other over the final four decades of the twentieth century is that the individual should have control over his own body, should make his own decisions relating to his medical treatment and should not be hindered in his search for self-fulfilment.
>
> Mason & McCall-Smith (1999, 6)

Therefore, the principle of autonomy must take into account patients' rights when making resuscitation decisions. Although providing a guide to decision making, these rights can be the cause of even more ethical and moral questions since:

- having rights does not mean that one is bound to exercise them
- having rights does not mean that their exercise is unlimited
- negative rights are in general stronger than positive ones

Thompson et al. (1988, 133)

The statement that 'negative rights are in general stronger than positive ones' is relevant when discussing resuscitation decisions as it relates to the patient's right to refuse life-saving treatment. Take, for example, the patient who has taken a drug overdose. Although this is often thought of as an action taken by young people, suicide also occurs in the older population due to chronic illness or pain, social isolation or financial problems (Toulson 1996). In the UK, the highest suicide rate in the 1990s was in men aged 75 years and older. Although the rate in this group has now decreased and is the lowest level in the male categories, the highest suicide rate in women is in the group between 45 and 74 years of age (Office for National Statistics 2010). What then happens if these patients refuse treatment or do not want to be resuscitated? Should the age of the patient have any relevance in the actions of the healthcare team in this case? The right to refuse treatment is virtually absolute in law, and treating a patient against their will can technically be considered a criminal assault. In these circumstances, establishing the patient's mental capacity to make the decision is required. The Mental Capacity Act 2005 (England and Wales) and the Adults with Incapacity Act 2000 (Scotland) provide guidance for medical and nursing teams on how to ensure that mental capacity is assessed and what actions are required when capacity is not demonstrated and best interests decisions must be made. This also applies to other vulnerable members within society, such as people with learning disabilities or mental health problems (see Chapter 2 – Vulnerable groups) who may be refusing treatment for any type of health problem. The giving of non-consensual treatment to involuntary patients with mental health problems applies to treatment for the mental condition only and does not include any intervention for any other health problem.

Do not attempt resuscitation orders

One of the main ethical issues in society today is that of consent. Therefore, the questions of when to make resuscitation decisions and deciding who should make them is of ethical concern not only to patients, relatives, medical and nursing staff, but also to society as a whole. CPR is a highly invasive procedure which is not appropriate for all patients. As it has been found to be effective in only one in five patients (De Vos et al. 1999), it is important to consider whether each individual patient would benefit from this intervention.

The decision to resuscitate or not must not be considered as a 'black and white' question whereby resuscitation is seen as good, as it restores life, and the DNAR order is seen as bad, as it symbolises defeat through death. Using this idea, the principles of non-maleficence and beneficence could change this view to its opposite. For the terminally ill patient, refusal to consider a DNAR order may negate that patient's right to receive palliative care, even in acute settings such as Medical Assessment Units and Emergency Departments and 'palliative care is, ethically, a mandatory part of the care of the dying' (Gordon & Singer 1995). Forcing resuscitation on those who do not want it only achieves a prolonged death and often the exclusion of relatives at the end of life. 'The philosophical acceptance of dying combined with support for what valuable life remains have to be incorporated into clinical practice if unnecessary suffering at life's end is to be avoided' (Gordon & Singer 1995, p. 165). It is also important to remember that a DNAR order applies to CPR only and not to other resuscitative procedures such as intravenous fluids and non-invasive ventilation.

As an aid to good practice and uniformity throughout the NHS, guidelines for making decisions related to CPR are available in a Joint Statement from the British Medical Association, the Resuscitation Council (UK) and the Royal College of Nursing (BMA et al. 2007). In this paper, a number of factors are identified which should be addressed when making DNAR decisions. These include:

- *the likely clinical outcome*, including the likelihood of successfully re-starting the patient's heart and breathing for a sustained period, and the level of recovery that can realistically be expected after successful CPR
- *the patient's known or ascertainable wishes*, including information about previously expressed views, feelings, beliefs and values
- *the patient's human rights*, including the right to life and the right to be free from degrading treatment

- the likelihood of the patient experiencing *severe unmanageable pain or suffering*
- *the level of awareness the patient has* of their existence and surroundings

BMA et al. (2007)

These guidelines stress that it is best practice (where possible) to discuss resuscitation with the patient and/or their relatives and that any discussion should be documented clearly in the patient's notes and regularly updated in accordance with hospital policy. It is the responsibility of the most senior clinician in charge of a patient's care, in line with local policy, to make resuscitation decisions (BMA et al. 2007). In the acute medical area, this is likely to be the most senior medical doctor but in some areas, such as specialist palliative care areas, it could be a senior nurse. If there is an anticipated risk of cardiopulmonary arrest in a patient who has capacity, then the patient should be given the opportunity to discuss resuscitation and its risks and benefits as soon as is feasibly possible (BMA et al. 2007). Failure to involve the patient may contravene the principle of patient autonomy. Discussion with the patient is often not possible in the acute medical environment due to the nature of the patient's condition. Therefore, for the doctor to make a valid resuscitation decision, information from relatives is invaluable in gaining an insight into the patient's views and previous health status.

For those patients who lack capacity, resuscitation decisions should be agreed between the healthcare team and relevant relatives or representatives. It is a requirement of the Human Rights Act 1998, the Mental Capacity Act 2005 (England and Wales) and the Adults with Incapacity Act 2000 (Scotland) that those patients who lack capacity have decisions made in their best interests and that these decisions are made in collaboration with their relatives, friends, welfare attorney, court-appointed guardian or an independent mental capacity advocate (IMCA) (BMA et al. 2007). People with a mental health problem and/or a learning disability have the same rights as any other individual and, therefore, any resuscitation decision should be made in the same way as for any patient. This is the same as when dealing with the elderly, as an individual's age should not be the main factor in the decision for a DNAR order.

Effective interpersonal skills are required when discussing resuscitation decisions with relatives as a number of variables affect the family's decision. These include:

- functional role in the family
- emotional dependence
- family problem-solving style
- ethnicity and religion

Blatt (1999, 220)

These factors identify potential differences within families. For example, different religions hold different traditions about death and dying. Likewise, family dynamics can affect their ability to make a unified decision. Some may communicate their feelings in a non-blaming, open and flexible way while others may mistrust the healthcare team and be unable to express feelings without showing anger or distress (Blatt 1999). In order to gain an informed decision from relatives, information must be given in an honest and jargon-free way. There is evidence to suggest that both patients and relatives frequently overestimate the effectiveness of CPR (Mead & Turnbull 1995; Schonwetter et al. 1991).

Advanced decisions to refuse treatment

Advance decisions are written instructions from mentally competent patients to their family and healthcare professionals that detail their wishes in relation to future treatment if they become unable to express themselves. This could be a request not to receive CPR or other life-sustaining measures. Advance decisions refusing treatment are covered by the Mental Capacity Act 2005 in England and Wales. There is currently no statute covering refusal in Scotland and Northern Ireland. In England and Wales, an advance decision to refuse is considered valid and legally binding if:

- the patient was 18 years old or over and had capacity when the decision was made
- the decision is in writing, signed and witnessed
- it includes a statement that the advance decision is to apply even if the patient's life is at risk
- the advance decision has not been withdrawn
- the patient has not, since the advance decision was made, appointed a welfare attorney to make decisions about CPR on their behalf
- the patient has not done anything clearly inconsistent with its terms
- the circumstances that have arisen match those envisaged in the advance decision
                                                                    BMA et al. (2007)

Although the advance decision is legally binding on doctors, it remains a controversial subject for a number of reasons in various healthcare settings. First, there are questions relating to the interpretation and usage of terminology and language within the decision documentation. For those with life-limiting or progressive illnesses, such as motor neurone disease, guidance and templates have been developed which can aid the individual to provide clear documentation of their decisions about future treatment (Motor Neurone Disease Association 2009). Second, the decision document must be available to medical staff. Third, the authenticity of the decision must be ascertained. These issues are a particular problem in acute medical areas where the healthcare team is unlikely to know the patient and where there may often be no immediate access to their medical notes. As patients are admitted with a degree of urgency, the relatives may have forgotten the decision documentation in their hurry to get to the hospital.

End of life care

The importance of quality in end-of-life care has been widely recognised in recent years. Despite many deaths in acute medical areas relating to sudden, unexpected illness in previously well patients, others will be due to the final stages of chronic illnesses, such as heart failure and cancers. It is important, therefore, for the acute medical nurse to be aware of up-to-date palliative and end-of-life initiatives, such as the Liverpool Care Pathway for the Dying Patient (Ellershaw 2007). The National End of Life Care Programme provides guidance to practitioners in both primary and secondary care in improving care at the end of life. Examples include, 'Advance care planning: a guide for health and social care staff' (2007) which provides information about discussing and documenting preferences in care, and 'Care towards the end of life for people with dementia' (2010). Awareness of the issues and access to palliative care experts can enable the acute medical nurse to improve the quality of care provided, in addition to balancing the legal and ethical questions which may arise.

Critical thinking – Exercise one

These three short vignettes illustrate the potential ethical complexities involved in the acute medical environment. Discuss them with your colleagues.

Vignette 1

Mr Hicks, a 46-year-old with profound learning disabilities, has been admitted with pneumonia. On examination, his condition is critical. He is hypotensive, pyrexial and desaturates without 100% oxygen. Over the past five years, Mr Hicks has had recurrent admissions with pneumonia and on each admission he has required more aggressive treatment. The doctor thinks that admission to ITU or CPR in the event of cardiac arrest would not be appropriate due to his past history, futility of the interventions and the patient's quality of life. However, his family does want active treatment to be given.
Consider: How would your healthcare team approach this situation? Does your hospital policy provide adequate guidelines relating to these circumstances?

Vignette 2

Mrs Evans, aged 85, is referred following an overdose of diazepam and alcohol. She did leave a note and took steps not to be found. On arrival, she expresses the wish that she does not want to receive treatment and if she stops breathing she wants to be left to die.
Consider: What actions should the healthcare team take? Discuss whether Mrs Evans is competent to make this decision at this time using the Mental Capacity Act guidelines. Now reconsider this question as if Mrs Evans were 22 years old. Would her age affect the decisions made by your team?

Vignette 3

Mr Smith has a history of inoperable cancer of the prostate. He is admitted with an acute myocardial infarction. While in the department he has a VF arrest.
Consider: Would a DNAR order be appropriate in this case? Does Mr Smith currently have a good quality of life? Consider whether or not Mr Smith should be defibrillated. VF is a reversible rhythm. Would the age of the patient make a difference to your decision in this case? Would an advance decision to refuse treatment make a difference to your decision?

These examples are typical of the range of acutely ill medical patients presenting at any hospital in the UK. Ethical dilemmas relating to treatment and diagnosis in the acute medical areas have been identified. Once the professional team have explored various medical options, fully informing the patient and relatives and involving them in the future management of the presenting condition and ultimate decision-making is vital. Consequently, the manner of breaking such news is crucial to this process.

Breaking bad news

Buckman (1984, 288) describes bad news as 'any news that drastically and negatively alters the patient's view of his or her future'. Consequently, such news could emanate from a whole range of situations – from negative and positive test results, to failing exams, to hearing of enforced redundancy. Accepting this broad-based definition indicates that most nurses will be involved in the breaking of bad news on a regular basis and, as such, need to be aware of the factors that might enhance, rather than negate, effective communication. Historically, medical staff have been largely responsible for breaking bad news; however, contemporary practice suggest that this task should fall to the most appropriate person, and sometimes this may be an experienced nurse (Resuscitation Council (UK) 2006).

Death is among the most difficult of bad news to receive, largely because of its negative impact, permanence and irreversibility. Where acutely ill medical patients are assessed and treated, bad news might involve the giving of test results; receiving a diagnosis or prognosis; undergoing surgery or other invasive procedures; implementing the Liverpool Care Pathway (Ellershaw 2007); the acknowledgement and sharing of uncertainty related to undetermined illness; sudden death or the impending death of a patient.

Spall & Callis (1997) suggest that healthcare professionals may break news badly because they have not been adequately trained or prepared. Some nurses may lack self-awareness; fail to appreciate their role and the importance of effective communication (both verbal and non-verbal skills); be unaware of their own feelings of self-consciousness; and remain anxious about issues of mortality and reactions from relatives. Clinical areas are extremely busy places, and they may not have observed good examples of this process in the clinical practice setting. According to Buckman (1992), individuals may dread breaking bad news due to a whole range of professional and personal factors.

Social factors: where, in our society, great emphasis is placed upon health, wealth and youth. Anything that detracts from these values is likely to be frowned upon. Consequently severe ill health, and the practical, emotional and financial losses that often accompany injury or illness may affect the individual and their family most significantly.

Patient factors: such as the stigma associated with certain phrases or conditions (e.g. cancer). Some patients might grudgingly accept a diagnosis of a 'tumour' but become distraught at the confirmation of 'cancer'. Some illnesses that may be self-inflicted (e.g. drug or substance abuse), often carry social stigma that surviving relatives may have difficulty accepting or coping with.

Professional factors: These include:

- fear of causing pain
- sympathetic pain
- fear of being blamed
- fear of the untaught
- fear of eliciting a response
- fear of admitting what we don't know
- fear of expressing our emotions
- personal fears

Some of these identified fears may be contrary to the perceived role of healthcare professionals (e.g. causing pain, being blamed, and admitting that one does not know all the answers to indeterminable questions) and hence, may affect individual skill performance. Some fears may result purely from lack of training and perceived expertise. However, Kaye (1995) advocates that effectively breaking bad news is important to both professionals and patients in order to:

- maintain trust between patients and professionals
- reduce uncertainty
- allow appropriate adjustment (practical and emotional) so that the patient can make informed decisions
- prevent a conspiracy of silence which may destroy family communication and prevent mutual support

Kaye (1995, 3)

Breaking bad news is an unenviable task that many nurses and doctors would avoid, given the chance. However, it cannot be avoided. Breaking bad news effectively can promote patient autonomy, avoid collusive relationships and maintain open, honest and professional relationships and as such is an important aspect of the healthcare professional's repertoire of skills. Specific objectives of breaking bad news are presented in Box 3.1. Effective communication is the key to delivering news in a caring, clear, sensitive and accurate way that does not add to, or detract from, the heavy burden of the content.

Box 3.1   Key objectives of breaking bad news

- Gather information
- Relay information at an appropriate pace
- Provide support for the recipient
- Develop a future strategy or management plan

Source: Jevon (2010, 157)

Breaking bad news for the first time can be fraught with anxiety for any nurse as they may be unsure as to how the relative or patient may respond. All professionals should be given the opportunity to explore the potential challenges associated with breaking bad news in a safe, multidisciplinary and supportive environment and to explore the need for effective communication within this sensitive context.

A framework for effective communication

Many authors have explored breaking bad news from a process perspective and offer frameworks or models that guide professional practice (Buckman 1992, 2005; Kaye 1995; Spall & Callis 1997). Such models may be seen as practice guidelines by which professionals can gather cues or reference points to aid the bad news process. Although rather dated, an easy to use, easy to remember and effective framework provided by Buckman (1992) comprises six steps:

Step one: Getting started.

- Getting the physical context right. (Where should the news be broken? Who should be there? How does the professional begin?)

Step two: Finding out how much the patient/relative knows (language and knowledge).

Step three: Finding out how much the patient/relative wants to know.

Step four: Sharing the information (aligning and educating).

- Decide on your agenda (diagnosis, treatment)
- Start from the patient's/relatives' starting point (aligning)
- Educating:
  - o   give information in small chunks
  - o   use plain English not medical jargon
  - o   check reception frequently and clarify
  - o   reinforce the information frequently and clarify
  - o   check your level (Are you staying with the patient/relative?)
  - o   listen for their agenda
  - o   try to blend your agenda with theirs

Step five: Responding to the patient's/relatives' feelings (acknowledging and identifying their reactions).

Step six: Planning and follow through.

- organising
- making professional contact and following through

Buckman (1992)

Such a simple, yet realistic, framework can help the healthcare professional to deliver the news in a systematic and meaningful way. Some professionals may dislike the use of a framework in this context for fear of such an important personal process becoming mechanical. In the authors' experience, people are unique individuals who deal with any confronting challenges in individual and unique ways and would be unlikely to become processed by the use of guidelines. Such guidelines should be perceived as a professional tool that can act as meaningful guidance for those who need it. Professionals must also remain aware of the different perspectives of illness from a patient and/or relative versus the professional viewpoint. For example, news about a condition that may, to professionals, seem relatively common and easy to overcome and treat might feel overwhelming to the patient and relatives who have little experience of such conditions.

Guidelines are available (British Association for Accident and Emergency Medicine in conjunction with the RCN 1995; Department of Health 2005) which offer indicators of ways in which practice might be improved. There are a number of examples of how guidelines have been used in practice to improve the service provided (Wilkins & Dalby 2000; Williams et al. 2000), for example, when considering the environment in which difficult news is given. Breaking bad news in a corridor with little privacy or in the midst of distracting and busy activities is not recommended but may be unavoidable. The work compiled by BAAEM and RCN (1995) offers many salient recommendations that could be usefully translated into acute care areas. The environment is important and rooms designed for relatives must offer accessibility yet privacy and comfort, without creating a sense of foreboding or isolation. Informal terms (e.g. sitting room) help to humanise these facilities and such rooms should be designed to seat a minimum of eight people comfortably. Toilet facilities should be close by and the room should be bright and well lit. In addition to comfortable chairs, a table, tissues, a direct line telephone, wash-basin and toiletries, toys and books for children should be available (BAAEM & RCN 1995). Issues regarding the environment are incorporated within the checklist at the end of this chapter.

Responding to bad news

The principles of giving bad news remain the same across differing contexts; however, following an unexpected death, Jevon (2010) reminds us of two important additional points for consideration (see Box 3.2). When giving someone news that they do not want to hear, nurses should be prepared for a whole range of responses. Wright (1991) identified nine emotional responses often exhibited by people receiving news of a sudden death. These nine emotions are identified in descending order of difficulty for nurses in Box 3.3.

Withdrawal is identified as being the most difficult response to deal with by healthcare staff since it renders them impotent and unable to offer practical help. Sitting next to someone who has physically, emotionally and psychologically

---

Box 3.2   Important points to consider when breaking news of a sudden death

1   Following an unsuccessful resuscitation attempt, ensure that the deceased is present-able (e.g. check clothing for blood, wash their hands, and so on) (Resuscitation Council (UK) 2006)
2   Remain perfectly frank from the outset, using unambiguous terms such as death and dying. Avoid ambiguous language (Resuscitation Council (UK) 2006)

Source: Jevon (2010, 171)

Box 3.3   Possible emotions displayed by people receiving bad news

- Withdrawal
- Denial
- Anger
- Isolation
- Bargaining
- Inappropriate responses
- Guilt
- Crying, sobbing and weeping
- Acceptance

Source: Wright (1992, 88)

Box 3.4   Essential communication skills within the bad news context

- Active listening
- Questioning (open and closed)
- Answering questions
- Clarifying and reiterating
- Responding appropriately to patient and relatives emotions

Source: after Jevon (2010, 158)

---

withdrawn is extremely difficult and the nurse needs a wealth of patience and understanding to sit and 'be with' the person at this difficult time.

Acceptance, crying and weeping are probably the easiest to cope with because many professionals anticipate such a response. *Anger* is a natural response, and professionals need to hear this anger, acknowledge it, help the person to focus and reflect their understanding of such anger back to them in a clear and comprehensive way. Wright's work (1991) could help to prepare nurses to anticipate reactions from relatives and illustrates where support may be needed most from a bereavement perspective. It also serves to indicate development needs of the professionals involved. Essential communication skills within the bad new context are presented in Box 3.4.

Support for relatives

In human society, the loss of one who is dearly loved brings great emotional pain and grief. Some suggest that this pain has significance for the species – that it serves the function of binding the social group, the group essential for survival.

Raphael (1984, 3)

Trying to appreciate or understand how another person feels can be difficult, and exploring the recipient's understanding and acceptance of any bad news delivered, and validating the person's feelings in response to this, can promote support at this difficult time (Buckman 2005). Back et al. (2003) advocate that the two most important elements to breaking bad news is the professional's willingness to discuss dying and their sensitivities to the inherent difficulties around this topic and these conversations.

Bereavement is described as the loss of a significant other person in one's life, which typically triggers a reaction we call grief which is manifest in a set of behaviours we call mourning (Stroebe et al. 1993). While the patient's needs are seen to end at death, the needs of associated family members are just beginning (Warren 1997) and nurses need to be alert to these needs in order to respond effectively. For those people for whom loss is imminent, Hampe (1975) and Breu and Bacup (1978) identify the needs of a relative anticipating loss (Box 3.5).

Wright (1993) identified that relatives who have been suddenly bereaved want clear and concise messages and information about the death; welcome confirmation and affirmation about the circumstances; value the opportunity to ask questions and discuss major issues; need opportunities to spend time with the deceased; and, finally, welcome a further chance to clarify the circumstances surrounding the death before they leave the hospital. Such attention may be time consuming for nurses but may help relatives both in the initial coming to terms with the enormity of the loss and in the long-term accommodation of their loss (Dubin & Sarnoff 1986). Offering choices to bereaved relatives at this time may help them to begin to accept the death of their loved one. Such choices might involve offering bereaved

---

Box 3.5   The needs of relatives anticipating loss

- Be with the dying person
- Be helpful to the dying person
- Be assured that the dying person is comfortable
- Be kept informed of the dying person's condition
- Know of the impending death
- Experience and express emotions
- Comfort and support family members
- Be accepted, supported and comforted by healthcare professional
- Be relieved of anxiety

Source: Hampe (1975) and Breu & Bacup (1978)

relatives the opportunity to participate in performing the last rites; the choice to see the deceased and to be with them in private surroundings; the choice about which other relatives should be informed about the death; the choice to instruct others (or participate themselves) in the differing cultural and spiritual rituals surrounding death (Neuberger 1987; Lothian Racial Equality Council 1992; Green 1993). Of course, being able to respond positively to such choices is important and systems need to be in place to ensure that this happens. For example, if relatives are offered access to the mortuary to view their loved one, this option must be available before the information is given to the bereaved relatives.

Nurses need to listen and to hear the concerns of both the patient (if sufficiently aware) and the family (Intensive Care Society 1997) and to involve them as much as possible (and as much as they wish to be involved) in the care of and decision-making for the patient. Medical staff and nurses may play a major role in these initial stages of grief as they often 'become trusted confidantes (who) provide a tangible link with the dead person, and talking over the death with those who knew what happened helps to make the loss real' (Parkes et al. 1996, 132).

Death never occurs in a vacuum but within a social context and this context may be indicative of how well the bereaved deal with the death of their loved one in the future (Read, 2008). While every death is unique and everyone grieves in their own unique way, certain circumstances may affect the way that the individual responds to their loss. The ICS *Guidelines for Bereavement Care in Intensive Care Units* (Intensive Care Society 1997) have identified several factors, which potentially indicate a high risk of intense bereavement reaction:

- unexpected loss – if the patient is less than 65 years of age, with no history of serious or chronic disease and no previous life-threatening illness
- sudden loss – the relative has had no preparation for the death
- the relative perceives their family as unsupportive
- the bereavement is traumatic
- the relationship between the deceased and the relative is ambivalent – often manifesting as anger, dependency or guilt
- the relative has life crisis other than bereavement e.g. financial

Intensive Care Society (1997, 9)

Sudden death issues in acute care areas run through many of the above indicators (for example, unexpected, sudden and sometimes traumatic death) and may affect how the relatives react to their loss. Bereaved people respond to their loss in many different and unique ways, often from an emotional, physical, behavioural and psychological perspective. Worden (1991) identified typical responses to grief (Table 3.1).

Knowledge of these reactions will enable the nurse to anticipate possible responses from bereaved relatives and develop potential support strategies in a proactive and thoughtful way. In the acute care setting, it would be helpful if nurses attend at least a basic, preferably multidisciplinary, bereavement course, during which personal and professional responses to grief can be explored in a constructive

Table 3.1 Typical grief responses (Worden 2001)

Emotional	Physical	Behavioural	Psychological
Sadness	Hollowness in the stomach	Sleep disturbance	Disbelief
Anger	Tightness in the chest	Appetite disturbance	Confusion
Guilt	Tightness in the throat	Absent-mindedness	Preoccupation
Self-reproach	Oversensitivity to noise	Social withdrawal	Sense of presence
Anxiety	A sense of depersonalisation	Dreaming	Hallucinations
Loneliness	Breathlessness	Searching	
Fatigue	Muscle weakness	Crying	
Helplessness	Lack of energy	Sighing	
Shock	Dry mouth	Restless over-activity	
Yearning		Visiting old haunts	
Relief			
Numbness			

way. Bereavement follow-up support is also important and acute care areas must have formal guidelines regarding professional responsibilities in relation to:

- written information offered regarding local or national counselling and/or support groups
- communicating with the patient's GP
- liaising with the local coroner and the mortuary
- accessing an interpreter as appropriate
- involving independent mental capacity advocates (IMCAs)
- supporting a range of vulnerable groups (such as people with a learning disability, children, and different ethnic populations)

Dealing with death regularly may be particularly draining, and one must not forget the effect that this may have on healthcare professionals and the ongoing support needs of those involved.

Support for staff

Saines's (1997) phenomenological study identified the following four chronological themes of nurses' experiences of sudden death:

- encountering (e.g. suddenness, unacceptability, individuality)
- facing (e.g. related to self, physical reality, emotional reality)

- dealing with (e.g. witnessed resuscitation, professional competence, grief reactions, advocacy, emotional labour, cultural, religious, legal and gender issues, control and conflicts)
- reflecting upon sudden death (e.g. emotional release, support, time element, conclusion, experience)

Hence, involvement in a sudden death incident is likely to evoke many feelings, thoughts and emotions for the nurses involved. Acknowledging the personal and professional difficulties in dealing with sudden death by encouraging and providing regular access to peer support, professional counselling agencies and the constructive provision of critical incident debriefing (Wright 1989) is crucial. A critical incident is described by Wright (1993, 189) as 'any situation, faced by emergency personnel, that causes them to experience unusually strong emotional reactions. These feelings have the potential to interfere with their ability to function at the time or later'. Despite controversy over the use of critical incident debriefing over the years, it is still widely used in the workplace (Regel 2007) but clearly should be introduced by those experienced in the field in order to prevent the possibility of causing harm. Clinical supervision will play an active, useful role, but more immediate measures that can be called upon at short notice should also be routinely available. Such mechanisms enable professionals to constructively reflect on practice from a technical, practical, social, political and economic and self perspective (Clarke et al. 1996), thus supporting and promoting the development of professional expertise.

In recognition of its importance, some services (for example, Gloucestershire Royal NHS Trust 1997) have created written documentation regarding bereavement debriefing after a sudden death. Such guidelines are invaluable to both healthcare professionals and the relatives with whom they are in contact. Indeed, the ICS (1997) recommend that all intensive care units should have a written policy for bereavement care. It is also recommended, in the provision of follow-up bereavement services, that staff should have access to bereavement training, opportunities to participate in critical incident analysis and case reviews, and that staff support systems should be in place (ICS 1997; DH 2005). These recommendations can be applicable to any acute medical or critical care area, given that staff often deal with sudden death and its aftermath. *Help is at Hand*, a DH resource (2010), is an excellent guide for people bereaved by suicide or other sudden traumatic death, which may help professionals to appreciate the complexities around this type of loss.

Professional development needs

The BAEEM and RCN (1995) identify the need for appropriately trained staff 'to provide optimum care for the deceased person and their relatives'. The continuing professional development needs of the acute medical nurse in respect of sudden death have been highlighted throughout this chapter. Such areas to be addressed include ethical and legal awareness, giving and receiving psychological support (both personally and professionally), communication and counselling skills, dealing with difficult news and bereavement. Not all acute medical nurses will have specialist skills in all of these areas but the nursing team needs to be aware of the actual and desirable skill mix of those involved in order to identify skill deficits. Similarly, all individuals need to be aware of their own personal development needs and how these could be met by academic or skills-based education.

Practice development

To identify the skills, environmental features and practical issues associated with sudden death in the acute medical area, a checklist has been developed based on the issues raised within this chapter. This checklist (Critical thinking – Exercise two) is not intended to be a prescription for what every acute medical area needs to address but it does identify a number of realistic issues that should be considered when dealing with sudden death. The checklist consists of five sections, incorporating 61 indicators, which might be used to:

- highlight issues for discussion by the acute medical team
- measure existing baseline resources and act as an indicator of future developments
- help identify professional training and development issues

The checklist is offered as a practical guide and may be photocopied for professional use. It has been based upon other existing checklists (BAEEM & RCN 1995; Gloucestershire NHS Trust 1995; ICS 1997). Readers are guided to these documents for additional information.

Summary

This chapter has considered the practical issues often associated with the care and support of patients and relatives involved in sudden death situations in the acute care environment from a nursing perspective. Personal and professional challenges have been identified through the sensitive exploration of breaking difficult news from both the giver and receiver perspective, and the clarification and analysis of ethical issues in practice is provided through case-related vignettes. The importance of providing an appropriate environment has been highlighted and suggestions for the development of professional guidelines have been introduced. In acknowledgement of the identified and resultant support and developmental needs of both clinicians and families, a checklist has been introduced to audit current practice and to identify future developments required in the acute care setting from a sudden death perspective. While such checklists and guidelines are an aid to promoting good practice, professionals need to be mindful of the uniqueness of every situation involving death and that the need for individual and sensitive professional responses is crucial at this difficult time. Unless nurses can overcome their discomfort when talking about death and dying to patients and their families, then they can never truly offer them the support they deserve (and, indeed, need) at the time they need it the most (Read, in press).

Critical thinking – Exercise two

Dealing with sudden death – a checklist for positive practice

Tick the appropriate indicators if they are currently available within the acute care setting.

1.   Environmental factors:
1.1   Is the clinical area clearly signposted?   ☐
1.2   Is the name of the relatives' room/sitting room informal and friendly?   ☐
1.3   Is the sitting room within earshot of the main treatment area?   ☐
1.4   Is the relatives' room easily accessible for disabled and non-disabled people?   ☐
1.5   Does the relatives' room offer comfort and privacy?   ☐
1.6   Does the relatives' room seat eight people comfortably
        (if not, is there potential for temporary extension)?   ☐
1.7   Can relatives easily access toilet facilities?   ☐
1.8   Does the relatives' room contain basic necessities
        (chairs, tables, tissues, telephone, wash-basin and toiletries?   ☐
1.9   Does the sitting room have a window? If so, are there blinds fitted?   ☐
1.10   Is the relatives' room child friendly (books and toys)?   ☐
1.11   Are there concrete methods (e.g. books, photographs) to support
        individuals who may have cognitive difficulties in understanding the
        complexities of death (for example, children, people with learning
        disabilities, and elderly, confused or people with dementia)?   ☐
1.12   Is there a visiting room where relatives can view their deceased?   ☐
1.13   Is the visiting room en-suite with the sitting room?   ☐
1.14   Do the relatives have to walk through public areas to view the deceased?   ☐
1.15   Is there anything further that could be done to the sitting room,
        that would provide more comfort, privacy and dignity?   ☐

2.   Psychological support:
2.1   How many of the staff team have attended counselling courses?   ☐
2.2   Is there a formal staff support system in place?   ☐
2.3   Do team members have access to confidential counselling?   ☐
2.4   Is there critical incident debriefing system operating?   ☐
2.5   Are members of the team actively encouraged to talk about death?   ☐
2.6   Do the staff wear uniforms which are easily identifiable to the general public?   ☐
2.7   Is a named nurse allocated to the relatives for the duration of time
        that they are in the clinical area?   ☐
2.8   Is there an up-to-date bereavement package available for bereaved relatives?   ☐
2.9   Is there a bereavement follow-up service in operation?   ☐
2.10   Is there a nominated person to lead the bereavement developments
        within the staff team?   ☐
2.11   Does the staff team have good relations with appropriate bereavement
        services, outside agencies (e.g. the local Coroner's Court,
        medical illustration)?   ☐
2.12   Are there any members of the staff team who are identified as being
        specialist in the area of bereavement?   ☐

2.13 Are relatives given the choice of seeing the deceased/witnessing
      resuscitation/performing the last offices with their loved ones?   ☐
2.14 Are their guidelines regarding multi-cultural aspects of death?   ☐
2.15 Is there an up-to-date directory of religious leaders within the local area? ☐
2.16 Can the staff team contact spiritual leaders of different denominations
      throughout the twenty-four hour period?   ☐
2.17 Are the staff team aware of the different cultures and associated
      rituals in your geographical area?   ☐
2.18 Is there appropriate literature (e.g. information on the
      Coroner's Court, death notification and registration, funeral directors)
      available to bereaved relatives?   ☐
2.19 Are members of the staff team adequately equipped to deal with
      initial contact with relatives, preparing relatives for news of the death,
      breaking bad news and answering difficult questions?   ☐
2.20 Can the team arrange for deceased patients to be viewed in the mortuary
      throughout the 24-hour period by relatives who may have to travel
      long distances?   ☐

3.   Policy and procedures:
3.1   Does the hospital have a policy on resuscitation?   ☐
3.2   Does the hospital or clinical area have a policy on care of the
      bereaved and breaking bad news?   ☐
3.3   Is there guidance on requests for organ donation?   ☐
3.4   Does the resuscitation policy contain clear guidelines regarding
      DNAR orders and Advance Decisions to refuse treatment?   ☐
3.5   Who ensures that the patient's computer records are updated following death? ☐
3.6   Who informs the patient's GP?   ☐
3.7   What happens to the belongings of the deceased patient?   ☐
3.8   What is the policy for contacting relatives if the patient is unaccompanied? ☐
3.9   What are the team expected to do if they are unable to contact any next of kin? ☐

4.   Professional development:
4.1   Are there opportunities for multi-disciplinary training?   ☐
4.2   How many of the team have attended multidisciplinary sessions to
      explore issues such as ethics and breaking bad news?   ☐
4.3   How many of the staff team have attended multidisciplinary
      sessions to explore bereavement and loss?   ☐
4.4   How many of the team have attended multi-disciplinary opportunities   ☐
4.5   to explore sudden death?   ☐
4.6   Is research actively encouraged?   ☐
4.7   Have any of the team had work published in reputable journals?   ☐
4.8   Is there a personal review system in place?   ☐
4.9   Are there regular team meetings?   ☐
4.10 How many of the staff team are familiar with the multicultural
      dimensions of death and dying?   ☐
4.11 Are there training opportunities for all members of the team?   ☐
4.12 Are members of the team adequately prepared for asking
      difficult questions (such as organ donation)?   ☐

5.   Service development:
5.1   Are there regular reviews of the service?   ☐
5.2   Are there regular reviews of skill mix?   ☐
5.3   Is a feedback system from the patients, relatives and staff in operation? ☐
5.4   Is there a formal feedback system incorporating the results of such reviews? ☐
5.5   Is there an audit of how sudden death is managed?   ☐
5.6   Are checklists available in the clinical area to guide positive,
      consistent practice?   ☐

References

Back AL, Arnold RM & Tulsky JA (2003) Teaching communication skills to medical oncology fellows. *Journal of Clinical Oncology*, 21, 2433–2436.

Blatt L (1999) Working with families in reaching end-of-life decisions. *Clinical Nurse Specialist*, 13(5), 219–223.

Breu C & Bacup K (1978) Helping the spouses of critically ill patients. *American Journal of Nursing*, (78), 51–53.

British Association for Accident and Emergency Medicine & the Royal College of Nursing (1995) *Bereavement Care in A&E Departments: Report of the working Group*. London: BAAEM/RCN.

British Medical Association, the Resuscitation Council (UK) & the Royal College of Nursing (2007) *Decisions Relating to Cardiopulmonary Resuscitation: A Joint Statement*. London: Resuscitation Council (UK).

Buckman R (1984) Breaking bad news: Why is it so difficult? *BMJ*, (297), 1597–1599.

Buckman R (1992) *How to Break Bad News: A Guide for Health Care Professionals*. London: Papermac.

Buckman R (2005). Breaking bad news: the S-P-I-K-E-S strategy. *Community Oncology*, 2(2), 138–142.

Chaloner C (1996) The final frontier. *Nursing Times*, 92(33), 26–29.

Clarke B, James C & Kelly J (1996) Reflective practice: Reviewing the issues and refocusing the debate. *International Journal of Nursing Studies*, 33(2), 171–180.

Department of Health (2005) *When a Patient Dies*. London: Department of Health.

Department of Health (2010) *Help is at Hand: a resource for people bereaved by suicide and other sudden, traumatic death*. London: DH. http://webarchive.nationalarchives.gov.uk/+/www.dh.gov.uk/en/Publicationsandstatistics/Publications/PublicationsPolicyAnd Guidance/DH_087031 (accessed 10 April 2011).

De Vos R, Koster R, De Haan R, Oosting H, Van Der Wouw P & Lampe-Schoenmaeckers A (1999) In-hospital cardiopulmonary resuscitation: Prearrest morbidity and outcome. *Archives of International Medicine*, (159), 845–850.

Dubin W & Sarnoff J (1986) Sudden and unexpected death: Interventions with the survivors. *Annals of Emergency Medicine*, 15(1), 54–57.

Ellershaw J (2007) Care of the dying: What a difference an LCP makes! *Palliative Medicine*, 21, 365–368.

Gillon R (1990) Death. *Journal of Medical Ethics*, (16), 3–4.

Gloucestershire Royal NHS Trust (1997) *Bereavement Debriefing Service Following a Sudden Death*. Gloucester: Gloucestershire Royal NHS Trust.

Gomes B & Higginson I (2006) Factors influencing death at home in terminally ill patients with cancer: Systematic review. *BMJ*, 332(7540), 515–521.

Gordon M & Singer P (1995) Decisions and care at the end of life. *Lancet*, (346), 163–166.

Gott M, Seymour J, Bellamy G, Clark D & Ahmedzai S (2004) Older people's views about home as a place of care at the end of life. *Palliative Medicine*, 18(5), 460–467.

Green J (1993) *Death with Dignity (volume II)*. London: Nursing Times Publications.

Hampe S (1975) Needs of grieving spouse in a hospital setting. *Nursing Research*, (24), 113–120.

Hilberman M, Kutner J, Parsons D & Murphy D (1997) Marginally effective medical care: Ethical analysis of issues in cardiopulmonary resuscitation (CPR). *Journal of Medical Ethics*, 23, 61–367.

Intensive Care Society (1997) *Guidelines for Bereavement Care in Intensive Care Units*. London: Intensive Care Society of the United Kingdom.

Jevon P (ed.) (2010) *Care of the Dying and Deceased Patient: A practical guide for nurses*. Chichester, UK: Wiley-Blackwell.

Kaye P (1995) *Breaking Bad News: A ten-step approach*. Northampton: EPL Publications.

Lothian Racial Equality Council (1992) *Religions and Cultures: A guide to patients' beliefs and customs for health service staff*. Edinburgh: Lothian Racial Equality Council.

Machin L (2009). *Working with Loss and Grief: A New Model for Practitioners*. London: Sage.

Mason J & McCall-Smith R (1999) *Law and Medical Ethics* (5th edition). London: Butterworths.

Mead G & Turnbull C (1995) Cardiopulmonary resuscitation in the elderly: Patients' and relatives' views. *Journal of Medical Ethics*, (21), 39–44.

Mohr M & Kettler D (1997) Ethical aspects of resuscitation. *British Journal of Anaesthesia*, 79, 253–259.

Motor Neurone Disease Association (2009) *Advance Decision to Refuse Treatment Information Pack*. Motor Neurone Disease Association.

National Council for Palliative Care (2009) *End of Life Care Manifesto for 2010*. London: National Council for Palliative Care.

National End of Life Care Programme (2007) *Advance Care Planning: A Guide for Health and Social Care Staff*. www.endoflifecareforadults.nhs.uk (accessed 10 April 2011).

National End of Life Care Programme (2010) *Care Towards the End of Life for People with Dementia: An Online Resource Guide*. www.endoflifecareforadults.nhs.uk (accessed 10 April 2011).

Neuberger J (1987) *Caring for Dying People of Different Faiths*. Lisa Sainsbury Foundation series. London: Austin Cornish.

Niederman M & Berger J (2010) The delivery of futile care is harmful to other patients. *Critical Care Medicine*, 38(10 supp).

Nursing and Midwifery Council (2008) *The Code: Standards of Conduct, Performance and Ethics for Nurses and Midwives*. London: Nursing and Midwifery Council.

Office for National Statistics (2010) *Suicides*. www.statistics.gov.uk (accessed 10 April 2011).

Page S & Meerabeau L (1996) Nurses' accounts of cardiopulmonary resuscitation. *Journal of Advanced Nursing*, (24), 317–325.

Parkes C, Relf M & Couldrick A (1996) *Counselling in Terminal Care and Bereavement*. Leicester: British Psychological Society.

Read S (2008) Loss, bereavement, counselling and support: An intellectual disability perspective. *Grief Matters: Australian Journal of Grief and Bereavement*, 11(2), 54–59.

Read S (in press) End of life care. In H Atherton & D Crickmore (eds) *Learning Disabilities: Towards Inclusion*. Edinburgh: Elsevier.

Raphael B (1984) *The Anatomy of Bereavement: A Handbook for the Caring Professions*. London: Routledge.

Regel S (2007) Post-trauma support in the workplace: The current status and practice of critical incident stress management (CISM) and psychological debriefing (PD) within organisations in the UK. *Occupational Medicine (London)*, 57(6), 411–416.

Resuscitation Council (UK) (2006) *Advanced Life Support* (5th edition). London: Resuscitation Council (UK).

Saines J (1997) Phenomenon of sudden death: Part 1. *Accident & Emergency Nursing*, (5), 164–171.

Schonwetter R, Teasdale T, Taffet G, Robinson B & Luchi R (1991) Educating the elderly: Cardiopulmonary resuscitation decisions before and after Intervention. *Journal of the American Geriatric Society*, (39), 372–377.

Seale C (2000) Changing patterns of death and dying. *Social Science and Medicine*, 51, 917–930.

Spall B & Callis S (1997) *Loss, Bereavement and Grief: A Guide to Effective Caring.* Cheltenham, UK: Stanley Thornes Ltd.

Stanley J (1987) More fiddling with the definition of death? *Journal of Medical Ethics*, (13), 21–22.

Stroebe M, Stroebe W & Hansson R (eds) (1993) *Handbook of Bereavement.* Cambridge: Cambridge University Press.

Thompson I, Melia K & Boyd K (1988) *Nursing Ethics* (2nd edition). Edinburgh: Churchill Livingstone.

Toulson S (1996) The right to die: The dilemma for A&E nurses. *Professional Nurse*, 11(7), 35–436.

Warren N (1997) Bereavement care in critical care settings. *Critical Care Nursing Quarterly*, 20(2), 42–47.

Wilkins K & Dalby L (2000) A bereavement service in a critical care unit. *Nursing Times*, 96(45), 38.

Williams A, O'Brien D, Laughton, K & Jelinek G (2000) Improving services to bereaved relatives in the emergency department: Making healthcare more human. *Medical Journal of Australia*, 173, 480–483.

Worden J (2001) *Grief and Grief Therapy: A Handbook for Mental Health Practitioners* (3rd edition). London: Routledge.

Worden W (1991) *Grief Counselling and Grief Therapy: A Handbook for the Mental Health Practitioner* (2nd edition). London: Routledge.

Wright B (1989) Critical incidents. *Nursing Times*, 85(19), 34–36.

Wright B (1991) *Sudden Death: Intervention Skills for the Caring Professions.* London: Churchill Livingstone.

Wright B (1993) *Caring in Crisis: A Handbook of Intervention Skills.* Edinburgh: Churchill Livingstone.

Further reading

Department of Health (2010) *Help is at Hand: A resource for people bereaved by suicide and other sudden, traumatic death.* London: DH. http://webarchive.nationalarchives.gov.uk/+/www.dh.gov.uk/en/Publicationsandstatistics/Publications/PublicationsPolicyAnd Guidance/DH_087031 (accessed 10 April 2011).

General Medical Council (2010) *Treatment and Care Towards the End of Life: Good Practice in Decision Making.* London: General Medical Council.

Hannon L & Clift J (2010) *General Hospital Care for People with Learning Disabilities.* London: Wiley-Blackwell.

Joint Working Party between the National Council for Hospice and Specialist Palliative Care Services and the Ethics Committee of the Association for Palliative Medicine of Great Britain and Ireland (1997) *Ethical Decision Making in Palliative Care: Cardiopulmonary Resuscitation (CPR) for People who are Terminally Ill.*

Adults with Incapacity (Scotland) Act 2000

Scottish Executive. *Adults with Incapacity (Scotland) Act 2000.* www.legislation.gov.uk/asp/2000/4/contents (accessed 10 January 2011).

Carers Scotland: the voice of carers. www.carersscotland.org/Policyandpractice/KeylegislationandpolicyAdultswithIncapacityAct2000 (accessed 10 April 2011).

Mental Capacity Act 2005 England and Wales

Department for Constitutional Affairs (2007) *Mental Capacity Act 2005 Code of Practice.* London: Stationery Office.

Carers Direct. www.nhs.uk/CarersDirect/moneyandlegal/legal/Pages/MentalCapacityAct.aspx (accessed 10 April 2011).

4 Cardiac Arrest

Carole Donaldson

Aims

This chapter will:

- outline the importance of early recognition of the deteriorating patient
- describe a systematic approach for the assessment, treatment and post-resuscitative care in peri-arrest and cardiac arrest scenarios
- discuss the role of the nurse in cardiac arrest management
- discuss issues relating to witnessed resuscitation

The chapter is based on the Resuscitation Council (UK)'s guidelines for adult advanced life support (RCUK 2010a).

Introduction

Rates of survival and complete physiological recovery following in-hospital cardiac arrest are poor in all adult age groups, with fewer than 20% of patients surviving to discharge (Peberdy et al. 2003). Observable physiological and clinical abnormalities often precede cardiac arrest in the majority of hospitalised patients (Peberdy et al. 2007). There is evidence, however, that these warning signs are not always identified or acted upon appropriately (Kause et al. 2004; Australian Commission on Safety and Quality in Healthcare 2009). Therefore, it is incumbent that nursing staff recognise early signs of deterioration in their patients and take appropriate and timely actions to rescue the patient and prevent further deterioration to cardiac arrest. Each hospital should provide training for nursing staff to recognise patients at risk of a serious adverse event or cardiac arrest (RCUK 2008).

Although the National Institute for Health and Clinical Excellence (NICE) identified in 2007 the need to audit all cardiac arrests in the United Kingdom to determine causes and outcomes, it is only in the last year that collection of data

Initial Management of Acute Medical Patients: A Guide for Nurses and Healthcare Practitioners, Second Edition. Edited by Ian Wood and Michelle Garner.
© 2012 John Wiley & Sons, Ltd. Published 2012 by John Wiley & Sons, Ltd.

regarding in-hospital arrests has been commenced by the Intensive Care National Audit and Research Centre. Organisations informed by this data can implement policies and training to change future practices.

Effective management of a cardiac arrest requires rapid recognition, confirmation and response from an efficient and well-organised team. For the arrested patient to be given the best chance of survival, the optimum time from recognition of a shockable rhythm to the initiation of the first shock is 3 minutes (RCUK 2010); this is intended to improve the overall survival rate from in-hospital cardiac arrest to discharge. This championed the implementation of a compulsory education and training initiative by the RCUK in 2000 for nurse-led courses in cardiac defibrillation and immediate and advanced life support, aimed at improving survival to discharge (Spearpoint et al. 2009).

Early warning signs of deteriorating patients

Nurses working in acute care areas will recognise that many patients in their care are deemed high-acuity patients with multiple co-morbidities who, therefore, have a higher potential to deteriorate to cardiac arrest. From a meta-analysis of cardiac arrest studies, DeVita et al. (2006) identified that most in-hospital cardiac arrests are preceded by vital signs lying outside accepted normal ranges in 84% of patients in the 8 hours preceding cardiac arrest. Although nurses often intuitively recognise deterioration in their patients' condition, an understanding of 'early warning' scoring systems (for example, see Table 4.1) is fundamental in alerting either medical emergency, rapid response or outreach teams for a timely review of the patient in order to prevent the occurrence of cardiac arrest. Several studies highlight the impact that higher registered nurse staffing numbers make in the prevention of cardiac arrest scenarios and lower rates of failure-to-rescue (Aiken et al. 2002; Needleman et al. 2002; Tourangeau et al. 2006).

It is important to remember that no single sign or symptom is an indicative precursor to cardiac arrest. The patient must be assessed accurately and holistically to enable their clinical needs to be prioritised. However, several studies show that a higher early warning score (EWS) is associated with worse outcomes (Goldhill et al. 2005; Paterson & McLeod 2006; Smith et al. 2008). In the UK, USA and parts of Australia, there is a move away from the EWS to 'track and trigger' systems using single parameter multi-layered models (National Patient Safety Agency 2007; Lighthall et al. 2009) that enable nurses to escalate concerns regarding their patients' condition to a variety of appropriately skilled healthcare professionals for prompt review and implementation of management plans to prevent or reduce adverse clinical incidences.

It is imperative that nurses are competent in the use of EWS or 'track and trigger' systems and in the recognition and management of cardiac arrest. The Resuscitation Council (UK) (2010b) advocate that all hospital staff should undergo regular resuscitation training to a level compatible with their expected clinical responsibilities. This has been supported with the implementation of

Table 4.1 Modified early warning score (MEWS)

	Scores						
	3	2	1	0	1	2	3
Heart rate (bpm)		<40	41–50	51–100	101–110	111–120	>120
Respiration rate (rpm)		<9		0–14	15–20	21–29	>30
Systolic BP (mmHg)	<70	71–80	81–100	101–199		>200	
Level of consciousness				Alert	Confused	Response to pain	Unconscious
Temperature (°C)		<35		35.1–37.8		>37.8	

Patients with a **low score of 1–2** on the MEWS: frequency of observations must be **4 hourly** as a minimum standard. If the patient is causing clinical concern at any time but not scoring on the MEWS, commence ABCDE and refer for appropriate advice (e.g. Outreach Team).

Patients with a **medium score of 3–6** on the MEWS: inform the nurse-in-charge and the Outreach Team (if available), commence ABCDE and initiate appropriate clinical interventions. Recheck observations and MEWS within 30 minutes.

Patients with a **high score of 7 or more** on the MEWS, or if it is anticipated at any time that the patient's condition will deteriorate quickly: **clinical emergency** – actions will be determined by local arrangements for initiating an appropriate emergency response.

simple hospital life support training and immediate and advanced life support courses aimed at multidisciplinary teams.

Peri-arrest arrhythmias

Cardiac arrhythmias are relatively common in the peri-arrest period and are potentially fatal. They may also follow successful resuscitation and are well-recognised complications of myocardial infarction and other common conditions such as hypoxia (see Chapter 7 – Shortness of breath and Chapter 8 – Chest pain). It is advantageous to patient outcomes for nurses working in acute care areas to be able to recognise peri-arrest arrhythmias such as bradycardias and atrioventricular blocks, and broad and narrow complex tachycardias. Early recognition of these potentially life-threatening arrhythmias will facilitate timely and effective medical intervention to improve the patient's chances of returning to an adequately perfusing rhythm. Early detection of peri-arrest arrhythmias can only occur if the patient is haemodynamically monitored (non-invasive blood pressure, oxygen saturation and continuous cardiac monitoring).

The assessment of all arrhythmias is two-fold, first to accurately analyse the rhythm and second to determine if the patient is symptomatic of the rhythm.

Having made this assessment, there are then essentially two management strategies available, either electrical or pharmacological therapies depending upon the severity of the patient's symptoms.

Treatment of symptomatic arrhythmias

An ABCDE assessment (see Chapter 1 – Initial assessment) of your patient will identify if they are symptomatic of the arrhythmia and if they are stable or unstable. A patient is defined as 'symptomatic' when there is clinical evidence of shortness of breath and increased work of breathing, low cardiac output, leading to pallor, diaphoresis, hypotension, chest pain/myocardial ischaemia and/or impaired consciousness' (RCUK 2010a). The general principle before commencing treatment is to administer supplementary oxygen, monitor the patient through leads via a cardiac monitor/ defibrillation pads, ensure a defibrillator is close at hand, and secure intravenous (IV) access to allow for rapid advanced life support (ALS) management. In order to gain a true appreciation of the rhythm, record a 12-lead electrocardiograph (ECG) and correct deranged electrolytes or other reversible causes if the patient's condition allows (RCUK 2010c).

The treatment of unstable tachycardia

Having assessed the patient using the ABCDE model for adverse features such as shock, syncope, myocardial ischaemia and heart failure, a decision of stable versus unstable will have been established. If the patient has been assessed as unstable then a synchronised DC shock is advised (RCUK 2010c) (Figure 4.1). This can be repeated to a maximum of three shocks if required. Cardioversion will require the intervention of specialist help as the patient will require a general anaesthetic or conscious sedation, administered by a competent clinician, usually but not always an anaesthetist, who will also maintain a patent airway. Ensure that the patient has both three-lead monitoring through the defibrillator and defibrillator pads applied and select synchronised mode on the defibrillator. Defibrillator pads can be applied in the normal anterolateral or anterior-posterior position. A synchronised DC shock (cardioversion) can only be administered using the defibrillator in manual mode by a healthcare professional trained in the technique. The synchronised mode ensures that the counter-shock is not delivered during the repolarisation phase of the cardiac cycle ('T' wave) as this could induce ventricular fibrillation (VF). As the defibrillator is set to synchronise, there will be a delay from the discharge of the electrical current from the machine to the delivery of the shock. Synchronised shocks should commence at 120–150 J biphasic (200 J monophasic) for broad complex tachycardia or atrial fibrillation, increased in increments as indicated by a senior medical clinician if the initial synchronised cardioversion fails, and 70–120 J biphasic (100 J monophasic) for regular narrow complex tachycardias and atrial flutter that can often be terminated by lower energies (RCUK 2010c).

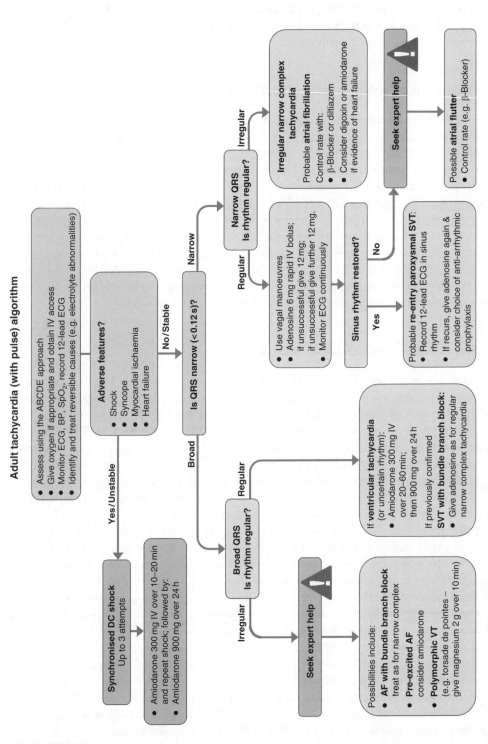

Figure 4.1 Tachycardia algorithm. Reproduced with the kind permission of the Resuscitation Council (UK).

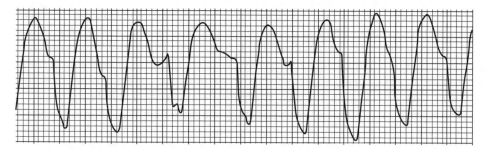

Figure 4.2 Broad complex ventricular tachycardia.

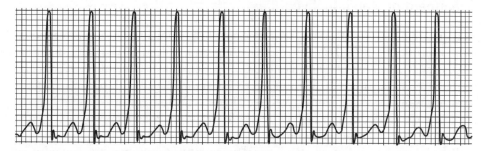

Figure 4.3 Narrow complex ventricular tachycardia.

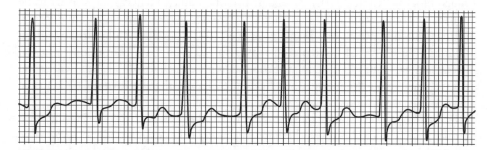

Figure 4.4 Atrial fibrillation.

A broad complex tachycardia (Figure 4.2) can either arise in the ventricles below the bifurcation of the bundle of His or may be a supraventricular tachycardia (SVT) conducted aberrantly. The rhythm characteristically has wide QRS complexes, no discernable P waves and a ventricular rate > 140 beats per minute.

Narrow complex or supraventricular tachycardia (Figure 4.3) is characterised by the presence of narrow, usually regular QRS complexes, with a ventricular rate often exceeding 200 bpm. The presence of P waves is difficult to determine due to the fast rate.

Atrial fibrillation (Figure 4.4) is characterised by disorganised electrical activity in the atria with irregular rate and morphology of P waves and narrow irregular ventricular QRS complexes.

In conjunction with synchronised cardioversion the use of intravenous amiodarone 300 mg diluted in 20 mL of 5% dextrose may be given into a peripheral vein in an emergency over 10–20 minutes (RCUK 2010c). Amiodarone 900 mg maximum dose in a 24-hour period may also be given via a continuous infusion into a central vein. The RCUK (2010c) also advocate the use of adenosine 6 mg for the unstable patient with narrow complex tachycardia while preparations are being made for synchronised cardioversion. However, they caution that the administration of adenosine should not delay the delivery of synchronised DC shocks.

Treatment of stable tachycardias

If there are no adverse features, seek specialist help from a healthcare professional who is proficient in analysing cardiac rhythms and 12-lead ECGs, while initiating the general management principles previously mentioned. Generally symptomatic stable patients who present with tachycardias are managed with pharmacological treatments and or vagal manoeuvres (see Figure 4.1). Analysis of a 12-lead ECG to calculate the QRS duration will determine narrow or broad complex tachycardia and subsequent management options.

Broad complex tachycardias are usually ventricular in origin, but may also be caused by supraventricular rhythms with aberrant conduction, such as bundle branch blocks (RCUK 2010c). A regular broad complex tachycardia is likely to be ventricular tachycardia (VT) and should be treated with intravenous amiodarone 300 mg diluted in 20 mL of 5% dextrose over 10–20 minutes. Amiodarone 900 mg maximum dose in a 24 hour period may also be given via a continuous infusion into a central vein. If a regular broad complex tachycardia is known to be supraventricular in origin with bundle branch block, then intravenous adenosine 6 mg can be administered.

Irregular broad complex tachycardia is most likely to be atrial fibrillation with bundle branch block; however, there may be many other causes and it is imperative that the 12-lead ECG is analysed by a specialist in order for the correct management to be implemented. Management may include intravenous amiodarone and adenosine in the doses previously mentioned for broad complex tachycardia. Intravenous magnesium 2 g over 10 minutes may also be administered in the presence of digoxin toxicity or hypomagnesaemia.

Several arrhythmias fall under the umbrella of regular narrow complex tachycardias; however, sinus tachycardia is not defined as an arrhythmia (Delecretaz 2006). Initially vagal manoeuvres such as carotid sinus massage or the Valsalva manoeuvre (forced expiration against a closed glottis) should be attempted. These manoeuvres stimulate the vagus nerve and induce a reflex that will slow the heart rate; they should only be attempted by a trained healthcare professional. Constant cardiac monitoring and preferably a 12-lead ECG recording during each manoeuvre are advised. This also applies to the administration of adenosine.

Adenosine is administered when vagal manoeuvres fail to terminate the arrhythmia. The patient must be informed of its potential for short-acting but alarming side effects, in particular, chest pain, momentary difficulty in breathing, nausea and hot flushing. Intravenous adenosine 6 mg should be administered rapidly into as large a vein as possible. If this is unsuccessful in terminating the arrhythmia, a further two doses of 12 mg may be administered intravenously. If adenosine is contra-indicated (such as in patients who suffer from Wolff-Parkinson-White syndrome and patients who are taking theophylline-related medications) or there is suspicion that the arrhythmia is atrial flutter, a calcium- channel blocker such as verapamil 2.5–5 mg may be administered intravenously over 2 minutes.

Irregular narrow complex tachycardia is most probably atrial fibrillation and expert help regarding further management must be sought early. When the patient is stable, treatment options are based on rate and rhythm control. If the duration of atrial fibrillation is less than 48 hours then rhythm control with a variety of pharmacological preparations is usually the management strategy. Heart failure should be carefully assessed for prior to administration of flecainide, as this drug is contra-indicated in these circumstances. Consultation with a clinical expert should be sought prior to the use of pharmacological agents when there is pre-existing ischaemic heart disease or a prolonged QT interval (RCUK 2010c).

The longer the patient remains in atrial fibrillation the great the likelihood of atrial thrombus developing (as blood collects in the fibrillating atria and is prone to clotting). If the patient has been in atrial fibrillation for > 48 hours then the patient should not be treated with electrical or pharmacological cardioversion until they have been anticoagulated for at least 3 weeks or trans-oesophageal echocardiography has shown the absence of any atrial thrombus (RCUK 2010c). If the patient's condition will not allow this, then intravenous bolus injection of unfractionated heparin followed by a continuous infusion can be administered until the activated partial thromboplastin time (APTT) sits at 1.5–2.0 times the reference control value. Further advice regarding the continuation of anticoagulation therapy should be sought from specialist clinicians.

When controlling the rate of atrial fibrillation the usual drug of choice is a beta-blocker; however, verapamil and diltiazem may also be used when beta-blockade is contraindicated.

Treatment of symptomatic bradycardia

In patients with poor cardiac function, ventricular rates of < 60 bpm may compromise the patient's circulating volume, leading to adverse signs (Figure 4.5). These include signs of shock (hypotension, diaphoresis and pallor), myocardial ischemia (chest pain, ECG changes), syncope and heart failure. A potential cause of the bradycardia must be explored. This includes recording of a 12-lead ECG to determine the rhythm, and treating electrolyte abnormalities. Calcium channel and beta-blocker overdose may also be a cause of symptomatic bradycardia; administration of glucagon is advocated as adjunctive treatment in these circumstances. The true mechanism of how glucagon works in these circumstances is still not fully known. However, it is believed that glucagon bypasses the beta-adrenergic receptor sites and thereby enhances myocardial contractility, increases heart rate and improves atrioventricular conduction (Shepherd & Pharm 2006).

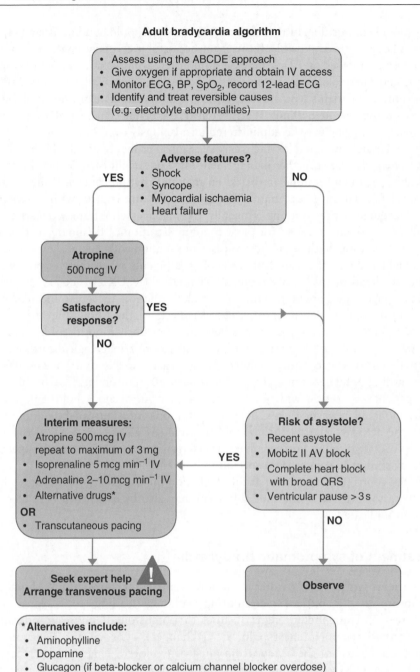

Adult bradycardia algorithm

- Assess using the ABCDE approach
- Give oxygen if appropriate and obtain IV access
- Monitor ECG, BP, SpO_2, record 12-lead ECG
- Identify and treat reversible causes
  (e.g. electrolyte abnormalities)

Adverse features?
- Shock
- Syncope
- Myocardial ischaemia
- Heart failure

YES   NO

Atropine
500 mcg IV

Satisfactory response?   YES

NO

Interim measures:
- Atropine 500 mcg IV
  repeat to maximum of 3 mg
- Isoprenaline 5 mcg min⁻¹ IV
- Adrenaline 2–10 mcg min⁻¹ IV
- Alternative drugs*

OR
- Transcutaneous pacing

YES

Risk of asystole?
- Recent asystole
- Mobitz II AV block
- Complete heart block
  with broad QRS
- Ventricular pause > 3 s

NO

**Seek expert help
Arrange transvenous pacing**   !

Observe

* Alternatives include:
- Aminophylline
- Dopamine
- Glucagon (if beta-blocker or calcium channel blocker overdose)
- Glycopyrrolate can be used instead of atropine

Figure 4.5   Bradycardia algorithm. Reproduced with the kind permission of the Resuscitation Council (UK).

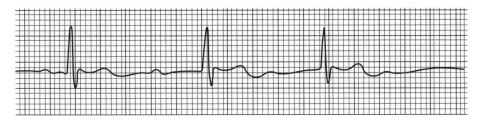

Figure 4.6   Heart block (Mobitz type 1/Wenckebach).

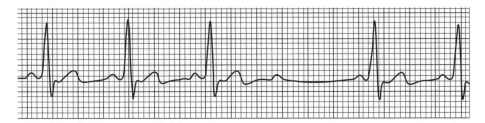

Figure 4.7   Heart block (Mobitz type 2).

A systematic patient assessment is required using the ABCD approach, acting upon any adverse findings during the assessment. As with the management of tachyarrhythmias, general principles of management apply. Ensure the patient has intravenous access, supplementary oxygen and continual monitoring of vital signs, oxygen saturations and cardiac rhythm. If time allows, record a 12-lead ECG to gain a better appreciation of the rhythm, which will assist with further management strategies. Rhythms normally associated with symptomatic bradycardia are Mobitz type 1 and 2 second-degree atrioventricular blocks, complete heart block (third-degree atrioventricular block) and sinus bradycardia.

Second-degree heart block, Mobitz type 1 (or Wenckebach phenomenon) (Figure 4.6), is characterised by a progressive prolongation of the PR interval until there is a pause where the atrioventricular node completely blocks the impulse reaching the ventricles and there is absence of a QRST complex. The next complex after this pause appears normal and the whole process starts again.

Second-degree heart block, Mobitz type 2 (Figure 4.7), is characterised by a normal PQRST complex and usually a normal PR interval. However not every P wave (atrial activity) is conducted to the ventricles to produce a QRS complex. This arrhythmia can be either a 2:1 or 3:1 block. In Figure 4.7 every other P wave fails to generate a QRS complex; this is therefore a 2:1 block.

Complete (third-degree) heart block (Figure 4.8) presents with complete dissociation between atrial and ventricular activity and usually with broad QRS complexes.

Initial management of the patient exhibiting adverse signs is with pharmacological preparations, with pacing being reserved for patients who have high risk factors for developing asystole or who are unresponsive to these interventions

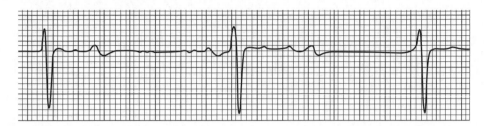

Figure 4.8 Complete heart block.

(RCUK 2010c). The treatment of symptomatic bradyarrhythmias requires the intravenous administration of atropine 500 μg to block the restraining effects of the vagus nerve, and therefore increase the ventricular rate. Repeat doses of atropine may be given every 3–5 minutes to a maximum dose of 3 mg (see Figure 4.5). Atropine should be carefully considered and used cautiously with post-infarction patients as the increased heart rate may exacerbate ischaemia and increase the size of the infarct (RCUK 2010c). Other drugs, such as isoprenaline and adrenaline, can be considered but require consultation with clinical experts. Aminophylline, dopamine and glycopyrrolate may also be considered as alternatives to atropine under the guidance of expert clinicians. Consider urgent referral to the cardiology team as transvenous cardiac pacing may be necessary if pharmacological interventions fail or are inappropriate.

Non-invasive transcutaneous pacing (external pacing) should only be used as a temporary measure. Before commencing external cardiac pacing, ensure that the chest is dry and free from combustible substances (such as GTN patches). In some circumstances, the chest hair may need to be clipped (not shaved) in order to provide a good contact with the two pacing pads. Pacing is usually delivered from a multifunction pacing-defibrillator system. If the system is limited to pacing only, place the pads in the anterior-posterior positions, so that they do not interfere with the positioning of defibrillation pads. If the patient is conscious they may require analgesia and/or light sedation as the procedure is often uncomfortable. The patient must be continually monitored via 3–5 lead ECG and vital signs monitoring throughout the process. Once the defibrillator pads are in position, the pacing mode must be selected. The nurse should set the beats per minute as directed by an appropriately trained colleague and then gradually increase the mA until a ventricular complex is seen after every pacing spike.

The nurse caring for the patient must confirm that both mechanical and electrical capture has occurred. Electrical capture is confirmed by the presence of QRS complexes after each pacing spike. The nurse should note the mA required for electrical capture to occur and then increase this by 10 mA to ensure electrical capture is not lost, thereby creating an electrical buffer. A palpable pulse (at the set rate) confirms that pacing is producing a cardiac output, or mechanical capture. Continuous monitoring of vital signs must be conducted to ensure that the intervention has had the desired effect. A 12-lead ECG pre- and post-procedure will be required.

In many UK hospitals, patients in need of transcutaneous pacing will require transfer to a critical care area such as a coronary care unit for further monitoring and management.

Patients with no adverse affects of the bradyarrhythmia should be assessed for the presence of atrioventricular blocks and the risk of the development of asystole. This requires the recording and analysis of a 12-lead ECG and monitoring of vital signs to determine ongoing management.

Assessment and management of cardiac arrest

Assessment

The confirmation of cardiac arrest is based on clinical assessment. The patient presents as unresponsive with the absence of normal respirations and no major pulse. Patients who are undergoing cardiac monitoring must have the absence of respirations and pulse confirmed (or absent signs of life, including swallowing or movement) rather than simply relying on what is displayed on the monitor. Remember to 'treat the patient and not the monitor'. Other clinical signs may also be present such as diaphoresis and skin mottling but their presence should not detract from the initial assessment of the patient's airway, breathing and circulation. Upon finding a patient collapsed, adopt the following sequence of assessment and management (Figure 4.9):

ABC initial assessment

Check responsiveness

Ensure it is safe for you to approach the patient as they may have collapsed in the bathroom or an area where access is difficult. Shake the patient gently by the shoulders and shout their name or a command such as 'open your eyes'. If the patient responds then they are obviously not in cardiac arrest. If the patient is unresponsive, sound the emergency bell and shout for help. Lie the patient flat and remove the bedhead if present. When help arrives, the second person should collect the defibrillator and resuscitation trolley, while the first person continues with assessment of the patient. Subsequent responders should call the resuscitation team on an identified emergency number (NPSA 2004) before returning to assist with the resuscitation.

Airway

Gently extend the patient's head slightly, look inside their mouth and clear any obstructions with the use of suction. When the mouth is clear, open the airway with a head tilt and chin lift, or jaw thrust if the other manoeuvres are contra-indicated (e.g. spinal precautions). These manoeuvres open the airway by removing the tongue from the posterior pharynx. If available, size and insert an oropharyngeal or nasopharyngeal airway. Do not delay further assessment to do this.

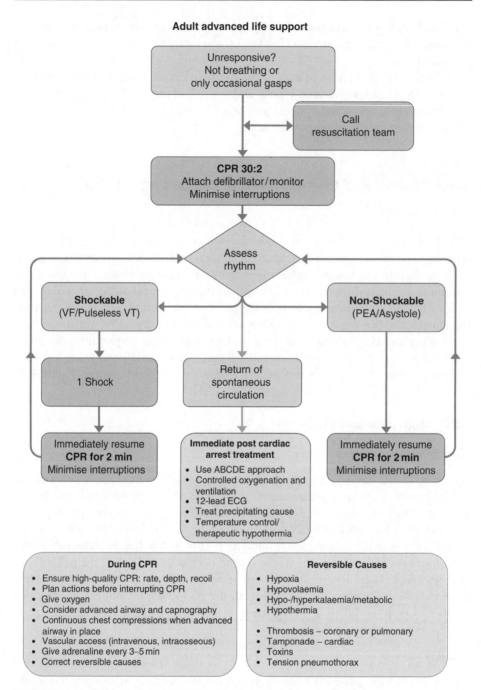

Figure 4.9 Cardiac arrest ALS algorithm. Reproduced with the kind permission of the Resuscitation Council (UK).

Breathing and circulation (signs of life)

Check for signs of respiratory effort for no longer than 10 seconds using the 'look, listen, feel' technique. Get close to the patient's mouth, listen and feel for breathing and look at their chest for signs of movement. Simultaneously palpate the carotid pulse if trained to do so. If no breathing is present or only occasional gasps are detected and there are no signs of life or a carotid pulse, commence chest compressions at a rate of 100 compressions per minute at a depth of at least 5 cm (European Resuscitation Council 2010) combined with ventilations at a ratio of 30:2.

The person performing compressions should locate the lower third of the sternum and place the heel of one hand in this area while interlocking the fingers of the other hand. Many research studies emphasise better patient outcomes with the implementation of early, uninterrupted effective chest compressions (RCUK 2010b). To ensure that this is achieved, team leaders are now encouraged to rotate team members performing cardiac compression every 2 minutes, even though they may not feel fatigued, and also to minimise time spent 'off the chest' by planning actions prior to ceasing compressions. It is important to remember that, even when chest compressions are delivered optimally, only 30% of the normal cerebral perfusion is achieved (Abella et al. 2005; Sutton et al. 2009).

Combine chest compressions with two ventilations using a bag-valve-mask device with reservoir (e.g. Ambu® bag) connected to oxygen with a flow rate of 15 L/min. Apply just enough pressure to the bag until a rise of the chest is seen. This usually equates to a tidal volume between 700 and 1000 mL. Any further pressure could lead to gastric insufflation with the consequent risk of regurgitation (vomiting) and aspiration with an unprotected airway. If the patient does vomit, tilt the bed head down and use suction. The airway adjunct will need replacing if occluded.

Defibrillation

If the semi-automated external defibrillator (SAED) is already attached to the patient then stop compressions momentarily and press 'analyse' if using in semi-automated mode, or manually analyse the rhythm if trained to do so. If the defibrillator is not attached and switched on, cardiac compressions should be continued while the second rescuer attaches the defibrillator pads and prepares to analyse the rhythm.

When placing hands-free pads onto the chest, place one pad to the right of the sternum just below the patient's right clavicle in the mid-clavicular line; place the second pad vertically over the patient's lower left ribs in the mid-anterior axillary line (centre of the pad in the V6 position). Pads should be rolled onto the chest to prevent air pockets forming, thereby ensuring a good contact with the skin. Pads should never be placed over breast tissue or body jewellery. The polarity of the paddles is unimportant (Weaver et al. 1993) although they are usually labelled 'sternum' and 'apex'. For safety reasons, the chest should be clear of GTN patches, fluids, vomit, free-flow oxygen and any other combustible material, before delivering a shock. Cardiac compressions should not be stopped while pads are being applied to the chest. The person applying the pads should work around the team member performing compressions. Figure 4.9 outlines the ALS algorithm based on UKRC guidelines.

Most nurses working in ward environments will be trained to use the defibrillator in SAED mode only. This mode does not require the nurse to analyse the rhythm and make decisions regarding the management of the rhythm, as the defibrillator analyses the rhythm and then advises if a shock is required. However, in high dependency and critical care areas, some nurses are trained in ALS techniques and will operate the defibrillator in manual mode as they are trained in the identification of arrhythmias.

During rhythm analysis the healthcare professional performing chest compressions is required to stop while the defibrillator analyses the rhythm and then automatically advises if a shock is required. Most defibrillators will then automatically charge to a pre-set joule setting. It is very difficult to return to implementing chest compressions during this time when the defibrillator is in SAED mode. However, when the defibrillator is used in manual mode and a healthcare professional is responsible for analysing the rhythm and confirming that a shock should be delivered, a team member must immediately recommence chest compressions while the defibrillator is charging. To reduce the pre-shock time off the chest, the European Resuscitation Council (ERC 2010) advocates that analysis should take no longer than 5 seconds. To limit the time off the chest further, some critical care environments are advocating that the defibrillator is automatically charged at the 2-minute analysis point while compressions are still being performed. An ALS provider will then ask for compressions to cease while the defibrillator is fully charged and will quickly analyse the rhythm. If a shockable rhythm is confirmed, the DC shock will be delivered. If a non-shockable rhythm is confirmed, the charge will be dumped and CPR re-initiated. The team leader should communicate clearly that ONLY the person performing the chest compressions is in contact with the patient while the defibrillator is charging. All other team members must stand clear and oxygen devices must be removed from the immediate vicinity of the patient. When the defibrillator has reached the selected joule setting, and the operator is ready to deliver the shock, the person operating the defibrillator must clearly tell the individual performing chest compressions to 'stand clear' and, when safe to do so, deliver the shock (RCUK 2010b).

Performing chest compressions while the defibrillator is charging is a huge paradigm shift and is underpinned by studies that have shown that relatively short interruptions in chest compressions to deliver rescue breaths and perform rhythm analysis are associated with reduced survival rates and reduce the chances of converting ventricular fibrillation (VF) to another rhythm (Berg et al. 2001; Eftestol et al. 2002). The ERC (2010) emphasise that the safety of the rescuer is paramount and the risk of harm in these circumstances is very small, particularly when wearing gloves.

In 25% of all adults in hospital cardiac arrest, the primary rhythm is VF/VT (Meaney et al. 2010). It must be remembered that a pulse can accompany VT and it is, therefore, imperative to determine the absence of a pulse before proceeding with the ALS algorithm (see Figure 4.9). The definitive treatment for both pulseless VT and VF is direct current (DC) counter-shock. The ALS guidelines (RCUK 2010b) recommend that, for uniformity, the first biphasic shock should be at least 150 J; however, if the first shock is unsuccessful at reverting the VF/VT, it is worth attempting subsequent shocks at higher joule settings. Conversely, a fixed-dose biphasic protocol has demonstrated good success rates (Hess et al. 2008). For nurses using defibrillators in SAED mode, the defibrillator will automatically set to a default joule setting, usually between 150 and 200 J and will not allow changes to this unless manual mode is selected. The team member operating the defibrillator is responsible for its safe use. A loud 'stand clear' should be announced and a visual check made to ensure that no-one (including the operator themselves) is touching the patient and no equipment is in contact with the patient prior to delivering a shock.

After the first shock is delivered, immediately carry out cardiopulmonary resuscitation (CPR) for 2 minutes, remembering that compressions are performed before ventilations. There is no need to analyse the rhythm or check for a pulse after delivering a shock, as studies indicate that there is a period of myocardial stunning before the heart converts to a perfusing rhythm (Deakin & Ambler 2006; Sandronic et al. 2008). During the 2 minutes of CPR, the team should attempt to gain intravenous access in order to administer drugs and fluids.

There is a reduced emphasis on securing the airway with an endotracheal tube (ETT) in the ALS guidelines (RCUK 2010b) as this necessitates halting cardiac compressions and time off the chest. Tracheal intubation should only be attempted by a skilled practitioner. An alternative to this method of airway management is the laryngeal mask airway (LMA). Once the airway is secured with either an LMA or ETT then cardiac compressions can be performed continuously without stopping for ventilations. Wherever possible, ensure capnography is attached to the ETT/LMA to monitor the tube's placement and provide an early indication of return of spontaneous circulation (ROSC) (RCUK 2010b). The team leader should also be considering potentially reversible causes for the cardiac arrest (see Box 4.1). The team should be informed of any actions required for treating these potential causes after the 2 minutes of CPR in order to minimise time off the chest when compressions are not taking place.

After 2 minutes of CPR, the rhythm must be analysed again using the same sequence of actions as previously outlined. If the patient remains in a shockable

---

Box 4.1   Potentially reversible causes of pulseless electrical activity

- Hypoxia
- Hypovolaemia
- Hypothermia
- Hypo/hyperkalaemia/ metabolic

- Thrombus: pulmonary or coronary
- Tension pneumothorax
- Toxins
- Tamponade, cardiac

rhythm, repeat the actions as above, delivering a second DC shock and then recommence CPR immediately.

During the 2 minutes of CPR, secure intravenous access (if not already achieved) and administer intravenous adrenaline (epinephrine) 1 mg/10 mL, or a 1:10,000 solution after the third shock and then every 3–5 minutes or during alternate cycles of CPR. In some areas, pre-prepared syringes or autojets are available as 1 mg of adrenaline diluted in 10 mL of normal saline (1:10,000 solution). Adrenaline is thought to improve both cerebral and myocardial perfusion by increasing coronary blood flow, which has been shown to improve the amplitude and waveform of VF and, in so doing, improves the chance of successful defibrillation (Achleitner et al. 2001). The administration of adrenaline should be followed by a 20 mL saline flush to expedite its entry into the circulation prior to administration of amiodarone 300 mg diluted in 20 mL 5% dextrose. This is given intravenously after the third shock and should also be followed by a 20 mL flush of saline.

If intravenous access cannot be obtained then administration of adrenaline by intraosseous (IO) route is the second option. The administration of any drug via the tracheal tube is no longer advocated (RCUK 2010). The insertion of central lines is not recommended during CPR as the risks associated with their insertion can be life-threatening and they require a substantial amount of time without cardiac compressions. If the patient remains in a shockable rhythm, repeat the actions above and administer epinephrine every 3–5 minutes.

If the patient is in asystole, pulseless electrical activity (PEA) or the defibrillator states that 'no shock is advised' then continue along the right arm of the ALS algorithm (Figure 4.9) by commencing CPR for 2 minutes after checking the absence of a major pulse. If there is any doubt as to whether the rhythm is fine VF or asystole, treat as asystole by immediately commencing CPR as this may improve the amplitude and frequency of the fine VF and improve the chances of successful defibrillation (Eftestol et al. 2004; RCUK 2005). If adrenaline has already been administered in the shockable side of the algorithm then withhold the next administration for 3–5 minutes. The use of atropine is no longer recommended in the routine management of asystole and PEA (RCUK 2010b). If the patient remains in a non-shockable rhythm, continue with CPR for another 2 minutes before reassessing. Only check a major pulse if there is a regular rhythm on the monitor that is compatible with a cardiac output, or if the patient shows signs of life. If the patient's initial rhythm is non-shockable then epinephrine may be administered as soon as intravenous access is secured.

Where PEA is the primary rhythm, the detection and treatment of potentially reversible causes becomes relatively more important. PEA is recognised by the presence on a monitor of a rhythm that would normally be compatible with a cardiac output but the carotid pulse is absent and the patient is lifeless. It is relatively common for the team to linger too long trying to diagnose the rhythm instead of recognising quickly that there is no cardiac output despite QRS complexes being present. There are broadly eight potentially reversible causes of PEA listed by the RCUK (2010b) and, for ease of recollection, these are known as 4Hs and 4Ts (see Box 4.1).

Potentially reversible causes of cardiac arrest

Hypoxia

This is a common cause of cardiac arrhythmias and subsequent cardiac arrest. Always assume its presence, even with evidence of normal arterial blood gas results. The best treatment is effective airway management with ventilatory support and high percentages of supplementary oxygen. The ALS algorithm highlights the use of buffers (for example, sodium bicarbonate); however, their role is still uncertain and only advocated when blood pH is < 7.1 (RCUK 2005).

Hypovolaemia

Blood/fluid loss leads to under-perfusion of vital organs with resultant hypoxia and loss of haemodynamic stability. A high index of suspicion for hypovolaemia should be given to any patient presenting with a recent history of surgery, haemorrhage, trauma, dehydration, sepsis or heat-related illnesses. Treatment is to replace volume with either a crystalloid (such as 1 L of 0.9% saline) or colloid (such as Haemaccel® or Gelofusine®) solution to restore adequate cardiac refilling and output. Ideally blood products should be administered if active bleeding is thought to be the cause of the arrest.

Hyper/hypokalaemia/metabolic

Cardiac arrest due to electrolyte abnormalities is uncommon except in the case of hypo- or hyperkalaemia. Renal failure is a common cause of hyperkalaemia, while dehydration and long-term use of diuretics may cause hypokalaemia. Obtain blood samples for electrolyte analysis and assess previous electrolyte results. Correcting any imbalance is based upon the severity of the problem. A blood gas analysis can also provide a fast potassium result if necessary. Ensure that a bedside blood glucose analysis is performed to exclude hypo- or hyperglycaemia.

Hypothermia

Hypothermia inhibits the movement of electrolytes across cell membranes and, therefore, affects the polarity of myocardial cells. Patients rarely present with hypothermia as a primary condition. However, there is a risk that patients who have returned from prolonged surgical procedures, are intoxicated, elderly or present in a collapsed state could be hypothermic (core temperature < 35 °C). The hypothermic heart may have a reduced response to pacemaker stimulation, defibrillation and cardioactive drugs. The latter may accumulate to toxic levels. Consequently, modification and prolongation of the ALS resuscitation may be required until the core temperature rises above 35 °C. Active rewarming with heaters and warmed intravenous fluids are the treatments of choice in ward areas. Other specialist critical care areas may attempt more invasive treatments.

Tension pneumothorax

This is a rare cause of PEA and is usually diagnosed with a high index of suspicion due to the patient's presenting problem before cardiac arrest. Once the patient's airway has been secured with an endotracheal tube, diagnosis may become easier as there will be increased resistance to ventilation and absence of air entry either unilaterally or bilaterally as the tension (pressure) within the thoracic cavity increases. Tension pneumothorax should always be considered in the young asthmatic patient who is in PEA. Immediate treatment is with needle decompression (i.e. placing a large-bore needle or cannula in the second intercostal space, mid-clavicular line on the affected side or bilaterally if indicated). This should be followed by the insertion of a chest drain if the resuscitation is successful.

Toxins

Toxic substances are the second most common cause of cardiac arrest in 18- to 35-year-olds (International Liaison Committee on Resuscitation 1997). In a ward environment, always check the medication chart to ascertain what may have been administered to the patient that could have precipitated the PEA arrest. The basic principles of restoring circulation and oxygenation apply here along with the identification of the toxic substance (e.g. opiate drugs, illegal substances) and the prevention of further absorption. The antidote to opiate medications, naloxone, may be given intramuscularly and intravenously if overdose is suspected. As the half-life of naloxone is relatively short, an intramuscular dose is given to ensure that therapeutic levels are maintained when the intravenous dose loses its effectiveness. Consult your local poisons unit for advice regarding antidotes for other drugs.

Thromboembolic

Usually caused by a large coronary or pulmonary embolus or cerebrovascular accident. Treatment is limited and the prognosis is poor. The use of anticoagulants or thrombolytic agents in this situation requires further research and may be administered in certain circumstances after consultation with expert clinicians.

Tamponade

Cardiac tamponade can occur with as little as 10 mL of fluid occupying the pericardial space. This leads to malfunctioning of the heart's pump action. The most common cause of acute tamponade in a ward environment is rupture of the ventricular free wall following acute myocardial infarction (Nolan et al. 1999). Cardiac tamponade is usually diagnosed by Beck's triad of symptoms. In usual circumstances, the three symptoms of muffled heart sounds, distended neck veins and hypotension are indicative of cardiac tamponade, but in the cardiac arrest situation they are not present.

As tamponade is so difficult to diagnose and treat, it is usually considered last in the potentially reversible causes of cardiac arrest. The exception to this is when chest trauma or cardiothoracic surgery is involved. Successful resuscitation in these circumstances usually requires a sternotomy. Treatment with thoracocentesis (needle aspiration) requires a confident approach, skill and accuracy (usually with use of ultrasound) that is almost impossible when CPR is in progress.

The nurse's role in the management of a cardiac arrest

Traditionally, nurses are the first healthcare providers to find a patient collapsed, confirm cardiac arrest and commence CPR. The advent of multidisciplinary ALS courses and the introduction of SAED have led to standardised approaches to cardiac arrest management in which nurses and doctors make equal contributions to improving patient outcomes. The emphasis when managing the patient in cardiac arrest is a co-ordinated team approach with an identifiable team leader. Prior to the arrival of the emergency/resuscitation team, an appropriately experienced nurse must assume the role of team leader in order to co-ordinate multiple activities in an efficient and time-critical sequence (Friedman & Berger 2004). Delegation of appropriate tasks to other healthcare professionals enables the team leader to gain a 'big picture' view of the resuscitation attempt, thereby identifying necessary interventions and co-ordinating activities. The team leader must communicate with the team calmly and effectively. This will allow for a cohesive and co-ordinated management approach. There is an abundance of literature surrounding crisis resource management that can be applied to cardiac arrest management (Cooper & Wakelam 1999; Gaba 2000; Friedman & Berger 2004; Salas et al. 2005).

Nurses are ideally placed to initiate the first link in the hospital 'chain of survival' whereby defibrillator pads are immediately attached to the patient upon recognition of cardiac arrest to assess for a rhythm. Studies conducted by Soar and McKay (1998) and Spearpoint et al. (2000) indicate that the majority of in-hospital survivors of cardiac arrest were in VF and had early defibrillation carried out by nursing staff. This is of paramount importance as the chances of successful defibrillation decline by around 5% with each minute that passes.

Defibrillation is arguably the most important enhanced role for nursing staff if they are to increase the chances of survival of the arrested patient. There are, however, issues associated with the use of manual defibrillators, in that the operator requires skill in cardiac rhythm interpretation. Unless practised on a regular basis, the skill in recognising cardiac rhythms may decline (Soar & McKay 1998). The use of SAED is advocated for healthcare professionals who deal infrequently with cardiac arrests as the operator requires no rhythm interpretation skills and the system uses the safer 'hands-off' approach.

The advent of resuscitation training officers in acute care facilities means that many nurses are now routinely taught how to size and insert oropharyngeal and nasopharyngeal airway adjuncts as well as performing simple airway management techniques (e.g. head tilt, chin lift). Knowledge of intubation equipment and how to assist with the procedure also play an important part in seamless cardiac arrest management. Many hospital-based nurses working in acute areas are trained to perform cannulation and to collect blood samples. Consequently, many have more expertise in this respect than their junior doctor colleagues. Cannulation should ideally be performed in the pre-arrest phase of the patient's care when superficial veins are more likely to be visible or palpable.

As well as being in a position to lead cardiac arrest situations until the emergency response team arrives, nurses are also required to maintain continuity of care. This continuity comprises drawing up of the correct drugs for administration at the appropriate time in the algorithm. The nurse responsible for the drugs can prompt the team leader when the next dose is due and maintain a record of the times and doses of the various drugs that have been administered along with the number of shocks delivered and the completion of the data collection tool. Nurses are also familiar with their ward surroundings and can obtain supplementary equipment required throughout the arrest.

Nursing staff provide the conduit between the arrest team and the patient's relatives. A nurse should be allocated to liaise with the family and to keep them informed as to their relative's progress. Similarly, important information can be gathered from relatives with regard to the patient's previous medical history and medications if they are a new admission to the ward. This liaison role continues in the post-resuscitation phase. Even though the family have no legal right to decide to terminate further medical intervention (RCUK 2001), their views should be sought and considered by the team as to the best way to further manage their loved one's condition. Consideration should also be given to facilitating the family presence during the resuscitation attempt.

Post-resuscitation care

If the outcome of the resuscitation is successful, a full ABCDE assessment is required and post-resuscitative care decisions need to be made. Documentation of the events and core data elements of the resuscitation should be recorded, usually on an Utstein-type chart. These data inform the hospital's Resuscitation Committee of the incidence of cardiac arrest along with 29 core data elements that can assist with improving the resuscitation process (Jacobs et al. 2004). Much of this data can be used nationally to inform research projects and ultimately to improve practice and patient outcome.

Patients who have been successfully resuscitated require ongoing cardiac monitoring for post-arrest arrhythmias, recording of their vital signs and additional documentation of preceding events. The patient's oxygen saturation levels should also be monitored to prevent potential harm from hyperoxaemia after return of spontaneous circulation (ROSC). The ERC (2010) recommend that saturation of arterial blood (SaO_2) should not exceed 94–98% via pulse oximetry monitoring in order to prevent this.

Specific knowledge of indications, contra-indications and dosages of medications used to support the patient's cardiac function is required. Nursing staff may perform post-resuscitation procedures such as recording an ECG, taking venous and arterial blood samples and ordering a chest X-ray. The patient may have a urinary catheter inserted to measure urine output and may require insertion of central venous and arterial lines. Nursing staff also play a pivotal role in the co-ordination of ongoing care by providing safe preparation and transfer to an intensive care unit, coronary care unit or another specialist facility.

Should the resuscitation attempt be unsuccessful, a nurse (and if necessary, a doctor) should inform the family as soon as possible. All the literature pertaining to 'breaking bad news' advocates a direct approach, using accurate wording that cannot be misinterpreted (Buckmann 1992; Kaye 1995). The environment in which relatives are told of the death of a loved one must have all the resources at hand to provide for their needs. The nurse liaising with the family should provide written as well as verbal information to the relatives regarding hospital procedures for post mortem, registration of death and the provision of support groups or bereavement liaison officers. Each family member is unique in the way that they react to distressing news and the nurse delivering this news should be prepared for this (see Chapter 3 – Sudden death). The nurse should be prepared to provide the family with details of treatments that have been given as this will help them to gain a more complete understanding of the events leading to their relative's death. Ideally, relatives should have been approached regarding their wishes to witness the resuscitation if they are in the clinical area at the time of the arrest, this will assist with the grieving process (Royal College of Nursing 2002).

Witnessed resuscitation

An important but controversial consideration during the resuscitation process is whether relatives should be offered the opportunity to witness the resuscitation taking place. This emotive subject has been discussed with increasing frequency over the past 12 years in nursing and medical literature (Tsai 2002). Professional organisations such as the American Association of Critical Care Nurses (2004), the Royal College of Nursing (2002) and the Resuscitation Council (UK) (1996) all advocate witnessed resuscitation in certain circumstances. Historically, the question of witnessed resuscitation has centred on emergency departments and intensive care units. Traditionally, relatives have been excluded when resuscitation involves adults but, with the increased coverage of these events by the media and TV dramatisations, relatives are more aware of what to expect. Several studies have found that relatives overwhelmingly report a desire to be present during end-of-life emergency treatments (Meyers et al. 2000; Grice et al. 2003; Kidby 2003; Mazer et al. 2006). Walker (1999) suggests that recognition of a relative's right to witness resuscitation is dependent upon healthcare professionals' willingness to promote the principles of respect and autonomy.

The literature shows that there is a difference of opinion between the public and healthcare professionals in this matter. Healthcare professionals believe the goal is to save human life and that the presence of relatives may be disruptive during resuscitation attempts (Duran et al. 2007; Mian et al. 2007; Twibell et al. 2008). From the family's perspective, the time that they have with their loved one during the resuscitation process may be the last contact before that individual's death. Meyers et al. (2000) and Twibell et al. (2008) suggest that witnessed resuscitation assists with the grieving process and many relatives believe it to be a positive experience. Findings of these studies suggest that the relatives be given the opportunity to touch and speak to their loved one and to ensure that they are not 'alone' in death. Similarly, the family's presence enables the medical team to view the patient as part of a loving family and less as a clinical challenge. However, despite the literature suggesting the benefits of providing the option of family presence during resuscitation, there are arguments against this. Medical and nursing opinions vary considerably but the main concerns expressed by staff in a survey by Twibell et al. (2008) are as follows:

- increased stress to staff
- increase in relatives' distress
- presence of relatives may influence the decision to stop resuscitation
- relatives may disrupt the resuscitation attempt
- distressed relatives may influence clinical performance of the team
- litigation
- patient confidentiality

There is little evidence to support any of these concerns and research has not shown that the resuscitation team performs less adequately when families are present (Halm 2005). Equally, the literature suggests a small decline in litigation where relatives have been present during resuscitation (Booth et al. 2004; Halm 2005; Nibert & Ondrejka 2005). This may be because of open communication with relatives who can observe that every intervention has been attempted. It cannot be assumed that patients would consent to relatives witnessing their treatment; however, few patients who have survived resuscitation have been involved in this debate (Hadfield-Law 1999). Certainly, confidentiality issues need consideration and patients who require resuscitative measures should be afforded the same rights to confidentiality as everyone else. By the very nature of their condition, it is not possible to ask patients whether they would wish relatives to witness their treatment and, in such situations, the legal and confidentiality issues are generally outweighed by humane considerations (McLauchlan 1997).

   All other areas of concern may be addressed by the development and introduction of witnessed resuscitation guidelines within organisations. These guidelines can be developed around the following principles (Eichhorn et al. 1996; RCN 2002):

- assessing the needs of the family
- preparing the family for the resuscitation environment
- supporting the family during and after resuscitation
- education of the support nurse or chaperone

The Resuscitation Council (UK) (1996) also addresses these issues in their guidelines (see Box 4.2) and advocate the presence of an appropriately trained and experienced nurse or member of the clergy to accompany or chaperone the relatives during the resuscitation. A study by Grice et al. (2003) strongly endorses

---

Box 4.2   Recommendations for relatives witnessing resuscitation attempts

These guidelines are generalised but can be adapted to most circumstances. It is important to remember that every situation is unique and every person different. The carer must be able to:

- Acknowledge the difficulty of the situation. Ensure that the relatives understand that they have a choice whether or not to be present during resuscitation. Avoid provoking feelings of guilt, whatever their decision.
- Explain that they will be accompanied by someone specifically to care for them, whether or not they enter the resuscitation room. Make sure introductions are made and names are known.
- Give a clear and honest explanation of what has happened in terms of the illness or injury and warn them of what they can expect to see when they enter the room, and particularly the procedures they may witness.
- Ensure that they understand that they will be able to leave and return at any time, and will always be accompanied.
- Ask the relative not to interfere, for the good of the patient and their own safety. They will be allowed the opportunity to touch the patient when it is safe to do so.
- Explain the procedures as they occur in terms that the relatives can understand. Ultimately, this may mean being able to explain that the patient has failed to respond and has died and that the resuscitation has had to be abandoned.
- Advise that once the relative has died, there will be a brief interval while equipment is removed after which they can return to be with the deceased in private. Under some circumstances, the Coroner may require certain tubes to be left in place.
- Offer the relatives time to think about what has happened and give them the opportunity to ask further questions.

Source: Resuscitation Council UK (1996)

---

this and recommends effective preparation and training of the chaperone to ensure the efficacy of this supportive role.

The literature supporting the inclusion of families within the resuscitation room far outweighs the concerns of the medical and nursing staff. With the implementation of strong guidelines and with appropriately trained staff, nurses can alleviate the loss of control experienced by relatives when isolated from their loved one at such a critical time. By excluding families from a dying patient's resuscitation as a matter of routine, death is portrayed merely as a clinical event. By so doing, we devalue the importance of death as a profoundly unique human event that touches the lives of others, we protect and perpetuate our own myth of control (Van der Wong 1997) and, as a medical team, we allow our own insecurities to compound the grief of the dying patient's relatives.

Summary

This chapter has outlined the importance of the early recognition of deterioration in patients and the practice guidelines for the management of cardiac arrest and peri-arrest situations. Nurses' roles in recognising and responding to cardiac arrests are fundamental in ensuring that these guidelines are effectively implemented, thereby offering the patient their best chance of survival. Despite the fact that many acute care areas have a presence of medical personnel, nurse-led cardiac arrest management has proven to improve the outcome of patients in cardiac arrest, especially out-of-hours. Similarly, the development of a ward or unit policy outlining the management of relatives witnessing resuscitation is highly recommended by many professional bodies.

References

Abella B, Alvarado J, Mykleburst H et al. (2005) Quality of cardiopulmonary resuscitation during in-hospital cardiac arrest. *Journal of the American Medical Association*, 293, 305–310.

Achleitner U, Wenzel V, Strohmenger H et al. (2001) The beneficial effects of basic life support on ventricular fibrillation mean frequency and coronary perfusion pressure. *Resuscitation*, 51, 151–158.

Aiken L, Clarke S, Sloane D et al. (2002) Hospital nurse staffing and patient mortality, nurse burnout, and job satisfaction. *Journal of the American Medical Association*, 288, 1987–1993.

Australian Commission on Safety and Quality in Healthcare (2009) *Windows into Safety and Quality in Health Care*. Sydney: ACSQHC.

Berg R, Sanders A, Kern K et al. (2001) Adverse haemodynamic effects of interrupting chest compressions for rescue breathing during cardiopulmonary resuscitation for ventricular fibrillation cardiac arrest. *Circulation*, 104, 2465–2470.

Booth M, Woolrich L & Kinsella J (2004) Family witnessed resuscitation in UK emergency departments: A survey of practice. *European Journal of Anaesthesiology*, 21(9), 725–728.

Buckman R (1992) *How to Break Bad News: A Guide for Health Care Professionals*. London: Papermac.

Cooper S & Wakelam A (1999) Leadership of resuscitation teams: Lighthouse Leadership. *Resuscitation*, 42, 27–45.

Deakin C & Ambler J (2006) Post shock myocardial stunning: A prospective randomised double-blinded comparison of monophasic and biphasic waveforms. *Resuscitation*, 68, 329–333.

Delacretaz E (2006) Clinical practice: Supraventricular tachycardias. *New England Journal of Medicine*, 354, 1039–1051.

DeVita MA, Bellomo R, Hillman K et al. (2006) Findings of the first consensus conference on medical emergency teams. *Critical Care Medicine*, 34, 2463–2478.

Duran CR, Oman KS, Abel JJ, Koziel VM & Szymanski D (2007) Attitudes toward and beliefs about family presence: A survey of healthcare providers, patients' families and patients. *American Journal of Critical Care*, 16, 270–279.

Eichhorn DJ, Meyers TA, Mitchell TG & Guzzetta CE (1996) Opening the doors: Family presence during resuscitation. *Journal of Cardiovascular Nursing*, 10(4), 59–70.

Eftestol T, Wik L, Sunde K et al. (2004) Effects of cardiopulmonary resuscitation on predictors of ventricular fibrillation defibrillation success during out-of-hospital cardiac arrest. *Circulation*, 110, 10–15.

Eftastol T, Sunde K, Steen P et al. (2002) Effects of interrupting precordial compressions on the calculated probability of defibrillation success during out-of-hospital cardiac arrest. *Circulation*, 105, 2270–2273.

European Resuscitation Council (2010) *Summary of the main changes in the Resuscitation Guidelines*. https://www.erc.edu/index.php/mainpage/en/ (accessed 10 April 2011).

Friedman D & Berger D (2004) Improving team structure and communication: a key to hospital efficiency. *Archives of Surgery*, 139(11), 1194–1198.

Gaba D (2000) Anaesthesiology as a model for patient safety in health care. *BMJ*, 320(7237), 785–788.

Goldhill D, McNarry A, Mandersloot G & McGinley A (2005) A physiologically-based early warning score for ward patients the association between score and outcome. *Anaesthesia*, 60, 547–553.

Grice A, Picton P & Deakin C (2003) Study examining attitudes of staff, patients and relatives to witnessed resuscitation in adult intensive care units. *British Journal of Anaesthesia*, 91(6), 820–824.

Hadfield-Law L (1999) Do relatives have a place in the resuscitation room? *Care of the Critically Ill*, 15(1), 19–22.

Halm M (2005) Family presence during resuscitation: A critical review of the literature. *American Journal of Critical Care*, 14, 494–513.

Hess E, Russell J, Liu P et al. (2008) A high peak current 150-J fixed-energy defibrillation protocol treats recurrent ventricular fibrillation (VF) as effectively as initial VF. *Resuscitation*, 79, 28–33.

International Liaison Committee on Resuscitation (1997) Special resuscitation situations. *Resuscitation* 34, 129–149.

Jacobs I, Nadkarni V, Bahr J et al. (2004) Cardiac arrest and cardiopulmonary resuscitation outcome reports: Update and simplification of the Utstein templates for resuscitation registries. A statement for healthcare professionals from a task force of the International Liaison Committee on resuscitation. *Resuscitation*, 63, 233–249.

Kause J, Smith G, Prytherch D et al. (2004) A comparison of antecedents to cardiac arrest, deaths and emergency intensive care admissions in Australia, New Zealand and the United Kingdom: the ACADEMIA study. *Resuscitation*, 62, 275–282.

Kaye P (1995) *Breaking Bad News: A Ten-Step Approach*. Northampton: EPL Publications.

Kidby J (2003) Family witnessed cardiopulmonary resuscitation. *Nursing Standard*, 17(51), 33–36.

Lighthall G, Marker S & Hsiung R (2009) Abnormal vital signs are associated with an increased risk for critical events in US veteran inpatients. *Resuscitation*, 80, 1264–1269.

Mazer M, Cox L & Capon A (2006) The public's attitude and perception concerning witnessed cardiopulmonary resuscitation care. *Critical Care Medicine*, 34(12), 2925–2928.

Mian P, Warchal S, Whitney S, Fitzmaurice J & Tancredi D (2007) Impact of a multifaceted intervention on nurses' and physicians' attitudes and behaviors towards family presence during resuscitation. *Critical Care Nurse*, 27(1), 52–62.

McLauchlan C (1997) Letter. *BMJ*, (314), 1044.

Meaney P, Nadkarni V, Kern K et al. (2010) Rhythm and outcomes of adult in-hospital cardiac arrest. *Critical Care Medicine*, 38, 101–108.

Meyers TA, Eichhorn DJ, Guzzetta CE et al. (2000) Family presence during invasive procedures and resuscitation: The experience of family members, nurses and physicians. *American Journal of Nursing*, 100(2), 32–41.

National Patient Safety Agency (2004) *Establishing a Standard Crash Call Telephone Number in Hospitals*. www.nrls.npsa.nhs.uk/resources/?EntryId45=59789 (accessed 10 April 2011).

National Patient Safety Agency (2007) *Recognising and Responding Appropriately to Early Signs of Deterioration in Hospital Patients*. www.nrls.npsa.nhs.uk/resources/?entryid45=59834 (accessed 10 April 2011).

Needleman J, Buerhaus P, Mattke S et al. (2002) Nurse staffing levels and the quality of care in hospitals. *New England Journal of Medicine*, 346, 1715–1722.

Nibert I & Andrej D (2005) Family presence during paediatric resuscitation: An integrative review of evidenced-based practice. *Journal of Pediatric Nursing*, 20(2), 145–147.

Nolan J, Greenwood J. & Mackintosh A (1999) *Cardiac Emergencies: A Pocket Guide*. Oxford: Butterworth-Heinemann.

Paterson R, McLeod D, Thetford D et al. (2006) Prediction of in-hospital mortality and length of stay using an early warning scoring system: Clinical audit. *Clinical Medicine*, 6, 281–284.

Peberdy M, Kaye W, Ornato J et al. (2003) Cardiopulmonary resuscitation of adults in the hospital: A report of 14720 cardiac arrests from the National Registry of Cardiopulmonary Resuscitation. *Resuscitation*, 58, 297–308.

Peberdy M, Cretikos M, Abella B et al. (2007) Recommended guidelines for monitoring, reporting and conducting research on Medical Emergency Teams. *Circulation*, 116, 2481–2500.

Resuscitation Council (UK) (1996) *Should relatives witness resuscitation? A report from a project team of the Resuscitation Council (UK)*. London: RCUK.

Resuscitation Council (UK) (2001) *Decisions relating to cardiopulmonary resuscitation – a joint statement from the British Medical Association, the Resuscitation Council (UK) and the Royal College of Nursing*. London: RCUK.

Resuscitation Council (UK) (2005) *Resuscitation Guidelines 2005*. London: RCUK.

Resuscitation Council (UK) (2008) *Cardiopulmonary Resuscitation: Standards for Clinical Practice and Training. A Joint Statement from the Royal College of Anaesthetists, the Royal College of Nursing, the Royal College of Physicians of London, the Intensive Care Society and the Resuscitation Council (UK)*. London: RCUK.

Resuscitation Council (UK) (2010a) Adult advanced life support. In *Resuscitation Guidelines 2010*. London: RCUK.

Resuscitation Council (UK) (2010b) *Resuscitation Guidelines 2010*. London: RCUK.

Resuscitation Council (UK) (2010c) Peri-arrest arrhythmias. In *Resuscitation Guidelines 2010*. London: RCUK.

Royal College of Nursing (2002) *Witnessed Resuscitation: Guidance for Nursing Staff*. London: RCN.

Salas E, Sims D, France D et al. (2005) Is there a 'Big Five' in teamwork? *Small Group Research*, 36(5), 555–599.

Sandronic C, Sanna T, Cavallaro F et al. (2008) Myocardial stunning after successful defibrillation. *European Journal of Cardiovascular Nursing*, 76, 3–4.

Shepherd G & Pharm D (2006) Treatment of poisoning caused by B-adrenergic and calcium channel blockers. *American Journal of Health-System Pharmacy*, 63(19), 1828–1835.

Smith G, Prytherch D, Scgmidt P et al. (2008) Should age be included as a component of track and trigger systems used to identify sick adult patients? *Resuscitation*, 78, 109–115.

Soar J & McKay U (1998) A revised role for the hospital cardiac arrest team? *Resuscitation*, 38, 145–149.

Spearpoint K, McLean C & Zidemann D (2000) Early defibrillation and the chain of survival in 'in hospital' adult cardiac arrest: Minutes count. *Resuscitation*, 44, 165–169.

Spearpoint K, Gruber P & Brett S (2009) Impact of the Immediate Life Support Course on the incidences and outcomes of in hospital cardiac arrest calls: An observational study over 6 years. *Resuscitation*, 80, 638–643.

Sutton R, Niles D, Nysaether J et al. (2009) Quantitative analysis of CPR quality during in-hospital resuscitation of older children and adolescents. *Paediatrics*, 124, 494–499.

Tourangeau A, Cranley L & Jeffs L (2006) Impact of nursing on hospital patient mortality: A focused review and related policy implications. *Quality Safe Health Care*, 15, 4–8.

Tsai E (2002) Should family members be present during cardiopulmonary resuscitation? *New England Journal of Medicine*, 346, 1019–1021.

Twibell RS, Siela D, Riwitis C et al. (2008) Nurses' perceptions of their self-confidence and the benefits and risks of family presence during resuscitation. *American Journal of Critical Care*, 17, 101–111.

Van der Wong M (1997) Should relatives be invited to witness a resuscitation attempt? A review of the literature. *Emergency Nursing*, 5(4), 215–218.

Walker W (1999) Do relatives have a right to witness resuscitation? *Journal of Clinical Nursing*, 8, 625–630.

Weaver W, Martin J, Wirkus M et al. (1993) Influence of external defibrillator electrode polarity on cardiac resuscitation. *Pace*, (16), 285–290.

Useful links

European Resuscitation Council. https://www.erc.edu/index.php/mainpage/en/.

Intensive Care National Audit and Research Centre. https://www.icnarc.org/Default.aspx? AspxAutoDetectCookieSupport=1

Resuscitation Council (UK).www.resus.org.uk/SiteIndx.htm

University Hospital of South Manchester NHS Foundation Trust (2010) *MEWS Escalation Policy for the Management of Acutely Ill Adult Patients*. www.uhsm.nhs.uk/.../MEWS%20 Escalation%20Policy%20V1.00.pdf (accessed 10 May 2010).

5 Shock
Judith Morgan and Ian Wood

Aims

This chapter will:

- describe the causes and pathophysiology of shock
- describe the clinical features of patients who present with shock
- outline a systematic approach to the assessment and immediate management of the shocked patient

---

Introduction

The diagnosis and treatment of shock can be one of the most challenging situations for the clinical team. Shock can be defined as a life-threatening condition where tissue metabolism is inadequate and it develops when oxygen supply is inadequate to meet oxygen demand at cellular level. Shock can be classified in many ways, however, medical nurses will mainly deal with 3 types. These are:

- hypovolaemic shock
- cardiogenic shock
- distributive shock (includes septic shock and anaphylaxis)

Common clinical features

The clinical features associated with the shocked patient vary according to the type of shock present. However, several clinical features are common to all types of shock (see Box 5.1).

Initial Management of Acute Medical Patients: A Guide for Nurses and Healthcare Practitioners,
Second Edition. Edited by Ian Wood and Michelle Garner.
© 2012 John Wiley & Sons, Ltd. Published 2012 by John Wiley & Sons, Ltd.

> **Box 5.1   Clinical features common to all types of shock**
>
> Raised respiratory rate
> Tachycardia (in initial stages)
> Altered blood pressure
> Reduced urine output
> Altered consciousness

Initial assessment

An initial assessment must identify life-threatening problems. Assessment of the patient's airway, breathing, circulation and neurological disability are of paramount importance (see Chapter 1 – Initial assessment). Gather a history of the patient's present problem and their previous medical history.

Airway

Ensure that the patient's airway is clear. If necessary, use positioning and suctioning techniques, airway adjuncts or advanced airway management techniques to maintain a patent airway.

Breathing

Respiratory rate is the first physiological parameter to be affected when shock is developing. Count the patient's respiratory rate and note their depth of respiration. Assess the adequacy of their ventilation and note any altered breathing sounds. Check that the patient has bilateral air entry and lung expansion. Record their oxygen saturation levels and commence high percentage oxygen therapy to ensure satisfactory saturations. Endotracheal intubation should be considered in the patient with altered mental status, respiratory distress and/or severe hypotension as mechanical ventilation decreases the demands on respiratory muscles and subsequently on the circulation by as much as 40% during respiratory distress (Kanaparthi et al. 2011).

Circulation

The adequacy of the patient's circulation can be assessed through several physiological parameters: pulse, blood pressure, capillary refill, skin colour (as well as appearance, turgor and texture), urine output and level of consciousness. Calculating the mean arterial pressure (MAP) is a very effective way of measuring if perfusion is adequate. The aim in fluid resuscitation should be to restore the MAP to between 70 and 80 mmHg (Moore & Woodrow 2008). Most automated

---

Box 5.2   Immediate management of the shocked patient

Administer 100% oxygen
Lie the patient flat to maintain cerebral perfusion (if appropriate)
Insert two large bore (14 G) intravenous cannulae in large veins (antecubital fossae)
Consider commencing intravenous fluids depending on the cause of shock (see later)

---

blood pressure monitors can calculate the MAP, it can also be calculated using the following formula:

$$MAP = (\tfrac{1}{3} \times \text{systolic pressure}) + (\tfrac{2}{3} \times \text{diastolic pressure}).$$

Disability (neurological)

Evidence of an altered consciousness level (e.g. irritability, confusion, drowsiness) is a late developing feature of shock caused by reduced cerebral tissue perfusion. If appropriate, emergency care should be initiated immediately and expert assistance sought from the multi-professional team (i.e. nurses, physicians, anaesthetists, medical emergency team and surgeons).

Exposure

It is important to undress the patient in order to inspect their skin for rashes that may indicate meningococcal septicaemia.

Immediate management

In suspected cases of shock, the management interventions outlined in Box 5.2 can be administered whilst the assessment is being carried out.

A: HYPOVOLAEMIC SHOCK

Causes

There are three main causes of hypovolaemia (Box 5.3).

Hypovolaemia results from a mismatch between fluid intake and fluid loss/output where fluid loss is greater than the fluid intake.

Extensive haemorrhage is an important cause of hypovolaemic shock. It is common following a gastrointestinal bleed (e.g. duodenal ulcer, gastric ulcer, oesophageal varices), ruptured or leaking aortic aneurysm, and blunt or penetrating trauma.

> **Box 5.3   Main causes of hypovolaemia**
>
> Haemorrhage
> Inadequate fluid intake
> Excessive fluid output

Inadequate fluid intake can occur in states of unconsciousness, confusion, dysphagia, mental ill health, depression, reduced mobility, loss of thirst in older people, fever, and lack of care from carers (Iggulden 1999).

Excessive fluid output can have many causes:

- increased gut motility (e.g. diarrhoea and vomiting)
- diaphoresis (i.e. sweating)
- skin loss with subsequent fluid seepage (e.g. burns, scalds)
- effusions (e.g. capillary leakage or ascites)
- acute haemorrhagic pancreatitis
- endocrine conditions (e.g. diabetes insipidus, diabetes mellitus)
- diuretic therapy or overdose (e.g. frusemide)
- excessive fluid removal during renal dialysis

Pathophysiology

In an average 70 kg male adult, there are approximately 42 litres of fluid (approx. 60% of body weight) distributed between two compartments (Brandis 2011):

- 23 litres of intracellular fluid (within the cells) that consists mainly of glucose with little or no sodium
- 19 litres of extracellular fluid which is distributed in an intravascular compartment and an interstitial fluid compartment

The intravascular compartment comprises 5 litres of blood. Of this, 3.2 litres is plasma with the remainder being made up of blood cells and proteins. Interstitial fluid (ISF) accounts for approximately 8.4 litres of fluid, mainly of water and electrolytes (e.g. potassium, magnesium, nitrates) with other dissolved substances and urea; bone water 3.2 litres; dense connective tissue water 3.2 litres; transcellular fluid 1 litre (Brandis 2011).

When fluid is lost through dehydration or blood loss, it is important to replace the fluid from each compartment with the appropriate type in order to maintain equilibrium (see Table 5.1). In haemorrhage, initial fluid loss can be replaced by using a crystalloid (a substance that is evaporated to crystals when heated) such as 0.9% sodium chloride (normal saline) or Hartmann's solution. If haemorrhage is significant, blood is the preferred replacement fluid as only blood has an oxygen-carrying capacity. In this case, the ideal treatment is to replace like with like (e.g. replace blood loss with blood). In the event of extensive blood loss, the blood pressure can be increased by using a plasma expander such as Dextran 70 (ensure blood samples and

Table 5.1   Fluid replacement suitable for compartments

Extracellular fluid Intravascular/Interstitial compartment	Intracellular fluid
Crystalloid	

0.9% sodium chloride intravenous infusion
  Isotonic solution
  Replaces fluid and sodium chloride outside
    the cell
Hartmann's solution intravenous infusion
  Contains sodium chloride, potassium chloride
    and calcium chloride
  Replaces fluid & electrolytes outside the cell
    0.9% sodium chloride and 5% glucose
    intravenous infusion
  Comprised of both dextrose, sodium and chloride
  Water from the solution will pass into the cell
  Glucose will cross into the cell
  Isotonic sodium chloride will remain extracellular
	5% glucose
	intravenous
	infusion

Colloid	

Plasma substitutes
Gelofusine® or Haemaccel®
  Animal product – gelatine-based
  Large protein molecules which stay in circulation
  Short-term volume expansion up to 2000 mL
  Haematocrit should not fall below 25%
    (BMA/RPS 2011)
Hetastarch or pentastarch
  Etherified starch-based
  Large molecules which stay in circulation
  Short-term volume expansion
  Maximum dose 20 mL/kg/24 hours
    (BMA/RPS 2011)
Dextran 70
  Starch-based solution
  Large molecules which stay in circulation
  Maximum dosage 20 mL/kg in first 24 hours
    (BMA/RPS 2011)
Blood: packed cells, rarely whole blood	

cross match is taken prior to administration as it could interfere with results), gelatine-based solutions (e.g. Geloplasma®, Gelofusine®, Isoplex® and Volplex®) or etherified starches (e.g. hetastarch, pentastarch and tetrastarch). These types of colloid are not intended to replace more than a third of the circulating volume. Care should be taken to avoid haematocrit concentration falling below 25–30% as large volumes of plasma expanders can increase risk of bleeding through lack of clotting factors. In addition, they stay for long periods in the circulation as they metabolise slowly (British Medical Association and Royal Pharmaceutical Society 2010). Plasma expanders are rarely required in water or sodium depletion as normally the shock responds to fluid and electrolyte replacement (BMA & RPS 2010).

Hypovolaemia due to blood loss

Local reaction

Vessel damage causes local vasoconstriction of the damaged area and its surrounding tissue. A platelet plug forms in an attempt to occlude the damage and to arrest bleeding. Blood flow in this area is slowed to prevent the clot from dislodging. If the damage to the vessel is greater than 5 mm, the platelet plug may not be able to form and bleeding will continue.

Systemic reaction

When blood loss reaches a critical level, baroreceptors in the carotid sinus and arch of the aorta detect a drop in blood pressure and a number of compensatory mechanisms are activated via the sympathetic and parasympathetic branches of the autonomic nervous system. This leads to vasoconstriction (increased peripheral vascular resistance) and an increase in heart rate and force of ventricular contraction which increases stroke volume, cardiac output and blood pressure; when vasoconstriction is present, care must be taken when interpreting the blood pressure as the patient my still have a significant occult hypoperfusion at tissue level (Fouche et al. 2010). Breathing becomes deeper and more rapid to ensure maximum oxygenation of remaining haemoglobin molecules. If bleeding continues and fluid loss is not replaced, there will be a steady increase in the respiratory rate, heart rate, force of ventricular contraction and peripheral vascular resistance. Only when approximately 30% of the normal blood volume is lost will the systolic blood pressure start to drop (American College of Surgeons 1997; Kolecki & Menckhoff 2010). Hypotension has physiological effects on other systems.

Renal effects

Low blood pressure affects the afferent arterioles of the kidney and causes renin production, which splits angiotensinogen (a plasma protein) to form angiotensin I. This is then converted to angiotensin II which is a very powerful vasoconstrictor. In response to the production of angiotensin I and II, aldosterone is released. This causes the renal tubules to retain sodium and water, leading to a reduced urine output, increased circulating blood volume and a rise in blood pressure.

Neurological effects

Hypotension leads to reduced cerebral oxygenation (cerebral hypotension and reduced cerebral blood flow) causing the patient to become progressively confused and, on occasions, aggressive as their consciousness level starts to deteriorate.

When the blood loss exceeds 50% of normal circulating volume, the compensatory mechanisms described above are no longer effective and haemodynamic collapse ensues (ACS 1998). Some young, fit adults are able to maintain their blood pressure until significantly more blood is lost; however, after this there is a marked drop in systolic blood pressure that can lead rapidly to cardiac arrest. In young patients especially, blood loss up to 40% of the normal circulating volume can occur before the limits of compensation are reached and then catastrophic vascular collapse occurs (Fouche et al. 2010).

Hypovolaemia due to dehydration

Dehydration can occur insidiously or acutely. Insidious onset of dehydration more commonly occurs in the older person as they may have a reduced sensation of thirst and may lose the ability to adequately concentrate urine (Benelam & Wyness 2010). Older people are more susceptible due a reduced overall fluid content (about 10% less than younger people) and some may also deliberately limit their fluid intake throughout the day so as not to get up at night to urinate. Insidious onset of dehydration can cause hypernatraemia as water is lost without some of the salts. This should be suspected when the specific gravity of the urine is at the lower limits of normal (normal range: 1.000 to 1.025). The presenting features of this type of dehydration can be confusion and/or hallucinations (Iggulden 1999) as well as the classic signs of shock (increased heart and respiratory rate with a late drop in blood pressure). Acute dehydration occurs because conditions such as vomiting (with or without diarrhoea) causes hyponatraemia in which both salts and water are depleted. The thirst reflex is absent in this type of dehydration (Watson 1996).

Presenting features

Clinical features of hypovolaemic shock will depend upon the degree of shock present. In addition to the physiological responses outlined in Table 5.2, the patient may be pale, diaphoretic (sweaty), peripherally cold and clammy. As shock progresses, the patient will show signs of cerebral hypoxia as detailed above.

Table 5.2 Physiological responses to estimated fluid loss (adapted from American College of Surgeons 1997)

	Class 1	Class 2	Class 3	Class 4
Fluid/blood loss	Up to 15%	15–30%	30–40%	>40%
Respiration rate	14–20/min	20–30/min	30–40/min	>35/min
Heart rate	<100/min	>100/min	>120/min	>140/min
Pulse pressure	Normal or increased	Decreased	Decreased	Decreased
Capillary refill	<2 seconds	>2 seconds (slow)	>2 seconds (slow)	Undetectable
Blood pressure	Normal	Systolic: normal Diastolic: raised	Systolic: decreased Diastolic: raised	Both decreased
Urine output	>30 mL/h	20–30 mL/h	5–15 mL/h	Negligible
Fluid replacement	Crystalloid/colloid	Crystalloid/colloid	Crystalloid/colloid and blood	Crystalloid/colloid and blood

Immediate management

The immediate management for all types of hypovolaemic shock is to find the cause and treat it as quickly as possible. The immediate management for the shocked or critically ill adult is outlined in Table 5.3. Aim to titrate warmed intravenous fluids to ensure that the patient's MAP remains above 70 mmHg (Moore & Woodrow 2008). This ensures that a rising blood pressure does not dislodge clots that may have formed at bleeding points and is known as 'hypotensive fluid resuscitation'.

Obtain blood samples for group and cross match (haemorrhagic shock), urea and electrolytes, clotting screen, full blood count and arterial blood gases. If the patient is bleeding and showing signs of class 3 shock (see Table 5.2), order type-specific blood. If class 4 shock is evident, consider administering type 'O' blood (universal donor). Remember that haemoglobin (Hb) results may be unreliable, as when extensive bleeding occurs, the blood is not diluted immediately. The patient's Hb may remain at a pre-haemorrhage level until fluid from the interstitial space or from the intravenous infusion dilutes the circulating volume. When this happens the Hb falls, as does the packed cell volume (PCV).

If the patient is suffering from diarrhoea and vomiting, they may need to be isolated and barrier nursed until it is known that they are not infectious.

Diagnostic investigations

If the patient is bleeding from the gastrointestinal tract, gastroscopy or sigmoidoscopy may be considered (see Chapter 9 – Abdominal pain and upper gastrointestinal bleeding). Likewise, a patient suffering from diarrhoea and vomiting will need stool samples sending for microscopy, culture and sensitivity.

Table 5.3   Immediate management for the shocked or critically ill patient

Airway	Maintain a patent airway Use suction, adjuncts and advanced techniques as appropriate
Breathing	Administer high-flow oxygen (100%) via an oxygen mask with non-rebreathe bag Record respiratory rate, depth and oxygen saturation levels Monitor respiratory effort and equality of ventilation
Circulation	Insert two 14 G intravenous cannulae in antecubital fossae Commence warmed intravenous fluid as appropriate (crystalloid 20 mL/kg or colloid 10 mL/kg); rate should be (<0.2 L/min unless blood loss >2 L) as returning the blood pressure to normal or above could dislodge clots and cause further bleeding and so blood pressure should be kept hypovolaemic (Fouche et al. 2010). Record pulse rate, volume and regularity manually Note the patient's skin colour Feel the skin for heat and moisture Consider possible causes for hypovolaemia Record a 12-lead ECG Commence continuous cardiac monitoring and observe for arrhythmias Insert a central venous catheter and record central venous pressure Insert a urinary catheter and record hourly urine output

Ongoing assessment and nursing management

Ongoing assessment is important in determining the cardiovascular state of a patient who may be developing hypovolaemic shock. If untreated, hypovolaemia can progress through four stages (classes) as the patient's condition deteriorates (Table 5.2). Early, accurate assessment and prompt intervention will prevent this happening. When using this classification system of shock, the individual's underlying state of health must be considered. For example: a fit, healthy patient with a normal resting pulse rate of 50 bpm could be considered to be tachycardic even before their pulse rate increases to 100 bpm. A core care plan for the ongoing assessment and nursing management of the shocked or critically ill adult is outlined in Table 5.4.

Table 5.4   Core nursing care plan for shocked or critically ill patient

Problem or potential problem	Plan of care
Airway Compromise or potential for	Maintain a patent airway; if appropriate use airway adjuncts Use suction as required, exercise care when suctioning endotracheal tubes as oxygen depletion can occur if suctioning extends beyond 15 seconds
Breathing Complications or potential for	Record respiratory rate and depth; initially recordings every 5–10 minutes may be necessary Record oxygen saturations continuously. Set alarms to alert when levels are < 90–95% Observe for reduced air entry on either side of chest Titrate oxygen to maintain saturation levels ≥95% Monitor arterial blood gases
Circulatory Insufficiency or potential for	Continuous cardiac monitoring of heart rate and rhythm: if a new arrhythmia presents, record serial ECGs Record heart rate; initially recordings every 5–10 minutes may be necessary Note regularity and strength of pulse Feel the skin for heat and moisture and monitor peripheral perfusion Record blood pressure; initially recordings every 5–10 minutes may be necessary Seek medical help if the systolic pressure falls below 90 mmHg or the mean arterial pressure falls below 60 mmHg Inspect intravenous cannulae for inflammation and swelling Administer warmed intravenous fluid and medications as prescribed Measure (manual or transduced) CVP every 15 minutes while patient is shocked or has the potential to become shocked Insert a urinary catheter and measure urine output every 15 minutes Record hourly fluid intake and output
Reduced consciousness level or potential for	Observe for reduced consciousness level or early signs of confusion, agitation or aggression Record neurological observations as indicated by the patient's condition
Dry sore mouth and lips due to oxygen therapy	Offer sips of water or mouth washes frequently Lubricate lips

Table 5.4   (cont'd)

Problem or potential problem	Plan of care
Potential for pressure sore development	Undertake a pressure sore risk assessment and plan care accordingly Keep skin and bedding as dry as possible
Anxiety	Keep patient informed of what is going to happen, be honest and reassure the patient even when they are confused or have a reduced consciousness level. With the patient's permission, inform relatives of condition and progress; ensure that consent is real as individuals who are shocked can argue that they were not of sound mind when they agreed to an action Reassure and support relatives
Nutrition	Consider how best to meet the patient's nutritional needs

B: CARDIOGENIC SHOCK

Causes

The definition of cardiogenic shock is a clinical state in which there is decreased cardiac output with a systolic blood pressure less than 90 mmHg producing hypoperfusion with tissue hypoxia in the presence of adequate intravascular volume (European Society of Cardiology 2008; Lenneman & Ooi 2011). It usually occurs following an acute myocardial infarction (particularly anterior) with or without ST elevation (Lenneman & Ooi 2011). The occurrence of cardiogenic shock following myocardial infarction lies at 5% to 8% but this reduces to 2.5% if percutaneous coronary intervention is used (Reynolds & Hochman 2008) with a mortality of 56 to 67% in hospital compared to 80 to 90% in the community. It is predicted that the mortality rate from cardiogenic shock will decline as treatments (thrombolysis) and interventions (primary angioplasty) advance (Lenneman & Ooi 2011). Cardiogenic shock can also occur with cardiomyopathy, mitral valve incompetence, arrhythmias, rupture of papillary muscle or ventricular septal defect. Dysfunction of the left ventricle is responsible for 85% of patients who develop cardiogenic shock. Shock occurs when more than 40% of the left ventricle is damaged. Cardiogenic shock may also develop because of cumulative damage to the left ventricle, for example due to a new infarct with previous history of acute myocardial infarction (Lenneman & Ooi 2011). The rarer causes of cardiogenic shock are those that produce low cardiac output as the heart is prevented from ejecting blood with sufficient force (e.g. cardiac tamponade, tension pneumothorax, pulmonary embolism and aortic stenosis).

Pathophysiology

When the left side of the heart fails to pump blood with sufficient force, the cardiac output drops with the result that the systolic blood pressure falls to below 90 mmHg. This hypotension triggers an autonomic nervous system response causing increased respiratory rate, increased heart rate with increased ventricular contractility and increased peripheral vascular resistance (vasoconstriction). These responses increase the diastolic blood pressure (afterload), and so more force is needed to eject blood effectively from the left ventricle. A state of persistent hypotension causes reduced urine output even though there has been no depletion in fluid volume. In the vasculature, pre-capillary vasodilation and post-capillary vasoconstriction result in circulating fluid seeping into the interstitial spaces. Hypotension can also cause cerebral underperfusion with the resultant cerebral hypoxia causing confusion, agitation or a reduced consciousness level. Poor ejection of blood from the left ventricle causes congestion within the left atrium and pulmonary veins with resultant pulmonary oedema, as the pulmonary circulation tries to empty into an already full left side of the heart. If severe, this will eventually lead to right-sided heart failure due to the high pressure within the pulmonary circulation that the right ventricle has to contract against. Right-sided heart failure subsequently causes back-pressure into the systemic venous circulation. This is characterised by neck vein distension, pitting oedema in the lower limbs or abdominal ascites.

In cardiogenic shock due to right ventricular dysfunction (which may occur when a right ventricular myocardial infarction accompanies an extensive inferior myocardial infarction), the pathophysiology is quite different. The right ventricle dilates, leading to a drop in right ventricular pressure and a subsequent fall in cardiac output from the right ventricle. This results in back-pressure into the systemic venous circulation and less blood being pumped to the left ventricle (reduced left ventricular preload). As a result, left ventricular output is reduced and blood pressure falls. Typical features include hypotension and raised neck veins without pulmonary oedema. The treatment varies considerably from the conventional treatment of cardiogenic shock and includes percutaneous coronary intervention (PCI). Ideally, this should be initiated within 90 minutes of presentation; however, it is useful up until 12 hours after onset. Reperfusion of the ischaemic myocardium by the early administration of a thrombolytic agent is used when PCI is not available (Brandler & Sinert 2010); however, there is an increased mortality as the efficacy of antithrombolytics are lower in hypotension (Reynolds & Hochman 2008). Infusion of intravenous fluids to increase right ventricular filling pressure will improve right ventricular output and, therefore, increase left ventricular filling and cardiac output leading to an increase in blood pressure. Fluid loading must be done carefully, preferably with invasive haemodynamic monitoring (including pulmonary artery pressure and pulmonary capillary wedge pressure) in either the coronary care unit or intensive care unit.

Presenting features

The presenting featurs of cardiogenic shock are summarised in Box 5.4.

A diagnosis of myocardial infarction, based on clinical symptoms and ECG evidence, may or may not have already been made. The patient will usually present with severe chest pain. Patients in cardiogenic shock will usually be pale and/or cyanosed and will have severe dyspnoea and tachypnoea. Their poor respiratory state will progress to Cheyne-Stokes breathing in the pre-terminal stage. The

> **Box 5.4   Presenting features of cardiogenic shock**
>
> Chest pain (remember, no pain in silent myocardial infarction)
> Anxiety (feeling of impending doom)
> Tachypnoea
> Severe dyspnoea (with pink, frothy sputum if acute left ventricular failure)
> Tachycardia (more rarely, bradycardia)
> Hypotension
> Pallor or cyanosis
> Cold, clammy skin
> Reduced urine output
> Pitting oedema

patient's skin is usually cold and clammy, their extremities mottled and they may have a delayed capillary refill time (>2 s). There will be decreased urine output and confusion. Cardiac arrhythmias may be present. The patient will invariably have a tachycardia or, more rarely, a bradycardia. If bradycardia follows a tachycardia, this is usually a pre-terminal sign. Persistent hypotension results in a reduced urine output of <30 mL/h that will progress to anuria. Poor cerebral perfusion will lead to restlessness and irritability. In patients with ensuing right ventricular failure, distended neck veins and pitting oedema in the lower parts of the body (legs, hands or sacral area if sitting) will be present. In the older person, the symptoms of cardiogenic shock can progress rapidly. Diagnosis is made with the help of pulmonary artery catheterisation and Doppler cardiogram which can confirm increased filling pressures in the left ventricle (Reynolds & Hochman 2008).

Immediate management

The aim of management is to identify the cause early and treat appropriately. Optimal treatment demands early reperfusion as well as haemodynamic support to prevent end organ failure and death. The aim in managing these patients is to reduce cardiac workload by reducing afterload and oxygen consumption, to correct the filling pressures and improve the contractility of the heart while reducing fluid overload. Factors which may be contributing to the hypotension must be excluded (see Box 5.5).

As these patients require invasive monitoring to enable effective treatment, they should be moved at the earliest opportunity to a level 2 or level 3 critical care facility. Here, invasive monitoring and treatment can occur as the best prognosis is achieved when aggressive supportive therapy can be used.

An ABCDE approach should be adopted.

Airway and breathing

Assess the airway for patency and breathing for effectiveness. High flow oxygen at 15 litres/min should be administered via a reservoir mask (British Thoracic Society 2008) as this reduces the work of the heart as the tissue demands of oxygen drops.

Box 5.5   Other factors which may contribute to hypotension (Hands 1997)

Hypovolaemia
Sepsis
Acidosis
Hypoxaemia
Arrhythmias
Narcotics such as diamorphine
Nitrates
Beta-blockers
Calcium antagonists

If more comfortable, nurse the patient upright or semi-recumbent if pulmonary oedema or air hunger is present. In critically ill patients, it is recommended that the oxygen saturation level should be maintained between 94 and 98% with urgent blood gas analysis to guide further management in those with chronic obstructive pulmonary disease or other risk factors for hypercapnic (type II) respiratory failure (British Thoracic Society 2008).

If there is an excessive increase in work of breathing, endotracheal intubation and mechanical ventilation should be considered; however, this may compromise venous return (preload). In the presence of acute pulmonary oedema, non-invasive ventilation has been found to improve haemodynamics and reduce intubation rates (Brandler & Sinert 2010).

If the patient has pulmonary oedema or is in pain, administer an intravenous opioid (e.g. diamorphine 2.5–5 mg or morphine 5–10 mg). This will reduce pain, anxiety, ventricular preload (increases venous capacitance) and afterload (causes mild arterial vasodilation). Combined, these effects should help to reduce the heart's oxygen demand, but may cause a drop in blood pressure. Diuretics are beneficial in pulmonary oedema. Furosemide (frusemide) 40 mg is usually given intravenously but this can be increased to 80–120 mg for patients on long-term diuretics (Cleland et al. 2010).

Circulation

The aim is to improve myocardial perfusion and increase cardiac output (Brandler & Sinert 2010). This may be achieved as follows.

- Intravenous fluid resuscitation should only be used to maintain adequate preload (Brandler & Sinert 2010) and should be avoided if pulmonary oedema, hypotension and normal JVP are present (Bedside Clinical Guidelines Partnership 2010). Fluid resuscitation should be monitored and titrated according to central venous pressures and pulmonary wedge pressure (Brandler & Sinert 2010). Invasive monitoring is required and this normally includes central venous and arterial lines, and Swan-Ganz catheterisation.

- Correction of electrolyte and acid–base abnormalities, such as hypokalaemia, hypomagnesaemia, and acidosis, are essential (Lenneman & Ooi 2011).
- Reperfusion of the coronary arteries through emergency angiography or, preferably, primary PCI should be done at the earliest opportunity (ESC 2008; Lenneman & Ooi 2011). Once cardiogenic shock has occurred, thrombolysis has not been found to improve prognosis and is, therefore, not routinely indicated (Lenneman & Ooi 2011).

A number of medications may be used to support the patient's circulation, as follows.

- Nitrates may be given to help to alleviate pain and to reduce preload by their vasodilatory effects, however, they should be administered with caution as they can exacerbate hypotension (Brandler & Sinert 2010).
- For bradycardia, intravenous atropine should be administered in 500 μg doses every 3 to 5 minutes up to a maximum of 3 mg. If not effective, temporary transvenous pacing may be required (RCUK 2010).
- Inotropes (drugs that increase the contractility of the heart) and vasopressors are usually indicated if the MAP falls below 60 mmHg. They are necessary to maintain essential blood flow to vital organs during periods of inadequate cardiac output (Krenn & Karth 2011). The following inotropes and vasopressors may be considered:
  o Dopamine should be given via a central line due to its vasoconstriction effects (if the former is not available, a large peripheral vein should be used, preferably a large vein high up on a limb) (BCGP 2010). Given at a does <3 μg/kg/min, dopamine may be given to improve renal function. At a rate of 1–5 μg/kg/min, dopamine causes renal vasodilation, improving renal perfusion and inducing a diuresis. At higher infusion rates (2–10 μg/kg/min), dopamine will increase the heart rate and contractility (similar effects to dobutamine). At rates greater than 10 μg/kg/min, dopamine causes widespread vasoconstriction which is disadvantageous in a failing heart.
  o Dobutamine should also be given via a central line – a large peripheral vein may be used if necessary (BCGP 2010). Doses range from 5 to 20 μg/kg/min to improve or stabilise the haemodynamic state (ESC 2008). Dobutamine increases the contractility of the heart without significantly increasing the heart rate at lower doses. It causes mild peripheral vasodilation (decrease in afterload) but, unfortunately, increases myocardial oxygen consumption and could increase size of a myocardial infarction. In general, it should be avoided in moderate or severe hypotension (systolic blood pressure is <80 mmHg) due to the peripheral dilation caused (Lenneman & Ooi 2011).

In patients who are unresponsive to other vasopressors, lidocaine or norepinephrine infusions may be used with caution (Brandler & Sinert 2008; Lenneman & Ooi 2010). On giving any of these drugs careful observation must be made of heart rate as any marked increase will raise myocardial oxygen consumption and may extend the size of the myocardial infarction (Brandler & Sinert 2010).

Anticoagulants (such as heparin) and anti-platelets (such as aspirin) should be used as in other cases of acute myocardial infarction; however, clopidogrel may be postponed until after angiography (Reynolds & Hochman 2008).

Diagnostic investigations

- Record a 12-lead ECG and right-sided ECG to check for cardiac abnormalities or pulmonary embolism (Brandler & Sinert 2010).
- Take blood samples for full blood count, urea and electrolytes, blood gases, cardiac enzymes and clotting. Serial samples may be needed.
- Obtain a chest X-ray to check for heart size, pulmonary vascularity, co-existing pulmonary pathology and pulmonary oedema. A chest X-ray also provides a rough estimate of mediastinal and aortic sizes in the event that aortic aetiology is being considered (Brandler & Sinert 2010).
- Doppler echocardiograms should be used to determine ventricular function. This should be should be recorded as early as possible (ESC 2008) unless the patient has an acute anterior myocardial infarction when PCI should be a priority (Reynolds & Hochman 2008).
- Monitor central venous pressure. Measurements will be higher than normal (i.e. >10 cm water when measured at a mid-axillary point with a manometer or >8 mmHg with a transducer.
- Swan-Ganz catheter will determine the pulmonary wedge pressure.

Ongoing assessment and nursing management

- A core care plan for the shocked or critically ill adult (Table 5.4).
- Regular 12-lead ECG recordings should be taken as well as at every rhythm change.

C: DISTRIBUTIVE SHOCK

Distributive shock encapsulates different types of shock. In the context of acute medical settings, this chapter will look at septic shock and anaphylactic shock.

SEPTIC SHOCK

Causes

Septic shock is life-threatening sepsis-induced hypotension (National Institute for Health & Clinical Excellence 2011) that does not respond to intravenous fluid resuscitation. It is a medical emergency in the same way as an acute myocardial infarction or stroke.

In England and Wales, there are said to be approximately 31,000 cases of severe sepsis per year (NICE 2011) with a mortality rate of 30–50%. This mirrors a mortality rate of 20–50% in the United States, outlined by Pinsky et al. (2011). The prevention, assessment and management of sepsis (and subsequently, septic shock) has become an integral part of working in any hospital, with prevention campaigns being introduced in recent years (for example, 100,000 Lives campaign 2004, Surviving Sepsis campaign 2008).

According to the Surviving Sepsis Group (2011), everyone is at risk of developing sepsis; however, the very young, older patients, those who are immunosuppressed, alcoholics, drug addicts, patients with catheters or drains or those who have wounds from burns are more prone to developing sepsis. Hospital in-patients with serious diseases are said to be most at risk because of their disease, previous use of antibiotics, drug-resistant organisms and the invasive interventions they require.

Patients may be admitted to hospital with an infection (community-based infection) that may originate from a range of sources. Alternatively, an infection can be acquired in hospital (healthcare acquired infection; HCAI). Sepsis can be caused by an infection in any part of the body though the respiratory, gastrointestinal, urinary tract and skin are most common. Most commonly, sepsis is caused by Gram-negative organisms (e.g. *Escherichia coli, Klebsiella, Pseudomonas, Bacteroides, Proteus*) although Gram-positive organisms (e.g. *Staphylococcus, Streptococcus, Pneumococcus*) now cause similar numbers as multi-resistant organism have become increasingly common (Kanaparthi et al. 2011). Sepsis is also caused by yeasts, viruses and fungi. In approximately 20% of cases the cause of sepsis is not found (Surviving Sepsis Campaign 2010). When the causative agent is a Gram-positive bacillus (usually *Staphylococcus aureus*), a rare type of septic shock called toxic shock syndrome can occur. Toxic shock syndrome most frequently occurs in those who have had nasal piercing or in menstruating women who use tampons. It can also be found subsequent to surgical and non-surgical infections of the skin, subcutaneous or osseous tissue.

Pathophysiology

Generalised fever is a significant response to localised infection or inflammation. This fever increases the body's basal metabolic rate as the temperature is reset by the hypothalamus to balance heat production and loss in favour of a higher temperature. Chills are felt as muscle movement produces heat and increases the temperature (Kunert 2009). Increased metabolic rate increases oxygen demand and, as a result, there is an increase in respiratory rate and depth. When respiratory acidosis is present, there is also hyperventilation as an effort is made to reduce acidosis through expelling carbon dioxide. When the infection cannot be contained locally and the body is no longer able to defend itself, a generalised bacteraemia (haematogenous spread) occurs and the organism is widely distributed to many organs in the body. This causes widespread and indiscriminate vascular (arterial and venous) dilation. This dilation leads to fluid leaking from the vessels into the interstitial compartment (third space) with the subsequent hypovolaemia causing reduced tissue perfusion and hypotension. This hypotensive state (hypovolaemia) initiates an autonomic nervous system response, which causes an increase in heart rate and cardiac output. If untreated, when the hypovolaemia reaches a critical level, the patient's consciousness level will decrease (cerebral hypoxia), haemodynamic collapse (lack of perfusion to the tissues) and renal failure with oliguria will ensue (Collins 2000). In the early stages, hyperglycaemia is frequently found (increase in gluconeogenesis and insulin resistance which prevent glucose moving into the cell); however, in more advanced states this becomes hypoglycaemia as the glycogen stores become depleted. In the elderly and patients who are immunosuppressed, they may not have subclinical ranges of the symptoms as they are not able to respond to the stressors in the same way.

The localised inflammation or infection causes activation of body's defence mechanisms with an influx of neutrophils and monocytes which have a phagocytic action thus forming pus, and a microphagic action respectively. There is subsequent release of inflammatory mediators which cause local vasodilation, increased endothelial permeability and activation of coagulation pathways. In severe sepsis and septic shock, changes occur at a microvascular and cellular level with widespread activation of inflammatory and coagulation cascades, vasodilation and vascular maldistribution, capillary endothelial leak, and dysfunctional use of oxygen and nutrients at the cellular level (Pinsky et al. 2011).

Activation of the coagulation cascade can lead to widespread consumption of the clotting factors with resultant bleeding as these factors become depleted and disseminated intravascular coagulopathy (DIC) develops. During septic shock, increased microvascular permeability occurs in the lungs as well as other tissues. In the lungs, this causes interstitial and alveolar oedema. The ensuing neutrophil invasion causes injury to the alveolar capillary membrane and subsequently adult respiratory distress syndrome occurs in about 40% of patients (Pinsky et al. 2011). Eventually, all of these factors in a patient unresponsive to treatment will ultimately lead to death.

Presenting features

The clinical history will give the first indication that sepsis is the cause of the shock. If the patient is unconscious, the absence of another cause having used the ABCDE approach will lead the clinician to suspect an infection. Patients generally have the following presenting features:

- Pyrexia (see Table 5.5) often associated with shaking chills, especially in the early phase. In some cases, pyrexia may be absent and some patients may even be hypothermic (especially the young, or older people)
- Dyspnoea with possible hyperventilation
- Warm skin (sometimes with a skin rash)
- Sweating
- Tachycardia

Table 5.5 Grades of hypothermia and pyrexia
(adapted from Dougherty & Lister 2008)

<28°C	Severe hypothermia
28°C–32°C	Moderate hypothermia
32°C–35°C	Mild hypothermia
37°C–38°C	Low grade pyrexia
38°C–40°C	Moderate to high grade pyrexia
>40°C	Hyperpyrexia
>41°C	Convulsions can occur
>43°C	Death can occur

- General weakness, fatigue, malaise
- Anxiety, confusion
- Raised white cell count (however, in severe sepsis WCC may be low)

Site-specific presenting features of sepsis include:

- With lung infection, there may be dyspnoea and/or purulent sputum, pleuritic chest pain, wheeze
- With urinary tract or gynaecological infections, there may be dysuria, smelly urine, frequency of micturition, urgency, purulent discharge and lower abdominal pain
- With a central nervous system infection such as meningitis, the patient may have a severe headache, photophobia, sore throat, neck stiffness and confusion
- With abdominal infections (e.g. appendicitis), patients may have nausea, vomiting, cramping abdominal pain and guarding
- With skin infections, there may be skin heat, swelling, lymphangitis, redness, swelling and offensive discharge (Surviving Sepsis Campaign 2011)

Immediate management

Since the 100,000 Lives and Surviving Sepsis campaigns, the recognition and management of sepsis now follows a systematic process so that the different degrees of sepsis and septic shock are identified and treated early. The path in which the illness is likely to progress is clearly defined by the Surviving Sepsis Campaign and follows three stages: uncomplicated sepsis, severe sepsis and septic shock.

Uncomplicated sepsis is suffered by many patients per year and includes viral infections, flu, dental abscesses or gastroenteritis, these patients do not require hospitalisation.

In severe sepsis, patients have one or more vital organs affected (heart, lung, kidneys, liver) and consequently are very ill and have a 35% increased risk of dying in comparison to those with uncomplicated sepsis.

Septic shock is where the organ failure leads to a low blood pressure even in the presence of fluid resuscitation and vasopressors.

The treatment of patients with septic shock consists of the following three major goals: (1) resuscitate the patient from septic shock using supportive measures to correct hypoxia, hypotension, and impaired tissue oxygenation; (2) identify the source of infection and treat with antimicrobial therapy, surgery, or both; (3) maintain adequate organ system function guided by cardiovascular monitoring and interrupt the pathogenesis of multi-organ system dysfunction (Pinsky et al. 2011).

In the current Resuscitation Care Bundle (Surviving Sepsis 2011), the goal is to perform all the following tasks 100% of the time within the first 6 hours of identification of severe sepsis.

The tasks are:

1   Measure serum lactate
2   Obtain blood cultures prior to antibiotic administration
3   Administer broad-spectrum antibiotic within 1 hour
4   Treat hypotension and/or a serum lactate > 4 mmol/L with fluids
    a   Deliver an initial minimum of 20 mL/kg of crystalloid or an equivalent
    b   Administer vasopressors for hypotension not responding to initial fluid resuscitation to maintain mean arterial pressure (MAP) > 65 mmHg
5   In the event of persistent hypotension despite fluid resuscitation (septic shock) and/or lactate > 4 mmol/litre, maintain adequate central venous pressure and central venous oxygen saturation:
    a   Achieve central venous pressure of > 8 mmHg
    b   Achieve central venous oxygen saturation ($ScvO_2$) > 70% or mixed venous oxygen saturation (SvO_2) > 65%

The current Sepsis Management Bundle (Surviving Sepsis 2011) consists of four tasks to be completed within 24 hours of the onset of severe sepsis. This management will generally be delivered in a Critical Care area but it should not be viewed as following on from the Resuscitation Bundle as efforts should be made to implement it concurrently. The four tasks are:

1   Consider low-dose steroids for patients with septic shock which is refractory to fluids and vasopressors.
2   Consider activated Protein C in patients with severe sepsis and high risk of death unless are contra-indications.
3   Consider the use of insulin therapy to control blood glucose in the event of hyperglycaemia.
4   Prevent excessive inspiratory pressure in patients who are mechanically ventilated.

A quick and easy to remember approach that summarises the above immediate management approach is called the 'Sepsis 6' (Survive Sepsis 2010). This approach can be adopted by any member of the healthcare team and should be completed within the first hour following recognition of sepsis. The six elements are:

1   Give high-flow oxygen (via non-rebreathe mask)
2   Take blood cultures before
3   Give intravenous antibiotics
4   Start intravenous fluid resuscitation (with Hartmann's or equivalent)
5   Check haemoglobin and lactate
6   Monitor hourly urine output accurately (may require urinary catheter)

ANAPHYLACTIC SHOCK

Anaphylaxis can be defined as an excessive response to a foreign substance (i.e. a severe allergic reaction to an antigen). The severity of an allergic reaction can range from very mild symptoms (e.g. a mild skin reaction) to circulatory collapse and subsequent death.

Causes

Anaphylactic shock refers to the state when a severe, whole-body allergic reaction causes circulatory collapse. The speed of onset of the shock is related to the route by which the antigen enters the body. The quickest response follows injection of the substance (Henderson 1998). Antigens are substances foreign to the body, for example, proteins (such as nuts), drugs (especially antibiotics), latex and insect bites/stings.

Pathophysiology

There are four types of allergic reaction:

- Type I (anaphylaxis)
- Type II (cytotoxic)
- Type III (immunocomplex)
- Type IV (cell-mediated)

Both types I and II provoke an anaphylactic reaction.

Type I occurs when a foreign substance called an antigen enters the body. These antigens bind to antibodies (immunoglobulin – IgE) on the surface of basophils in the blood and mast cells in body tissue. On first encounter, they do not usually cause a noticeable reaction but, in some individuals, a subsequent exposure to the antigen is recognised by the antibodies and an immune response starts. The antigen (now known as an allergen because it causes an allergic reaction) causes the cell membrane of the basophils and mast cells to rupture, thus releasing allergy producing mediators (e.g. histamine, prostaglandins and leukotrienes) (Guyton & Hall 2005; Porth 2009). Subsequently, histamine, heparin and other chemical mediators are released that cause an inflammatory allergic response. Histamine

---

Box 5.6   Possible presenting features of anaphylaxis

Airway swelling (e.g. swelling of the tongue, pharyngeal/laryngeal oedema)
Drooling (difficulty in swallowing)
Hoarseness of the voice
Stridor
Shortness of breath (increased respiratory rate)
Wheezing
Cyanosis (usually a late sign)
Confusion (due to hypoxia)
Feeling faint or collapse with tachycardia, tachypnoea and/or hypotension
Tightness of the chest
Urticarial rashes with or without pruritus (itching)
Warm skin that may be erythematous
Abdominal spasm with or without diarrhoea
Extremities may be cold and clammy due to peripheral shutdown

---

causes widespread vasodilation and increased permeability of the capillaries and venules. This increased permeability results in loss of plasma from the circulation, a drop in blood pressure, increased heart rate and oedema. Leukotrienes cause spasm of the smooth muscles of the bronchioles with subsequent stridor and increased vascular permeability (Copstead & Banasik 2009). When the reaction is severe, if it is untreated, death may rapidly follow.

Type II is known as an anaphylactoid reaction (pseudoanaphylaxis). It results from non-specific degranulation of mast cells that release allergy-producing mediators. This reaction is not an IgE-based sensitivity. It is, however, impossible in an emergency situation to identify which type is presenting and, as the initial management is the same, identifying the type of reaction is not relevant in this situation.

Presenting features

Any of the following features may be present or absent depending upon the site and source of the allergen (Box 5.6).

Stridor may be especially severe due to bronchospasm that presents as wheezing. In these cases, the patient may only be able to complete short sentences, or a few words, or may even have insufficient expiratory force to produce any sound at all.

Immediate management

The aim is to reduce the allergic response while supporting the circulation. In addition to the emergency treatment outlined in Figure 5.1, consider the following:

- The drug of choice in severe anaphylactic reactions is adrenaline as it is a bronchodilator and vasoconstrictor. It is quickly absorbed, increases the force of cardiac contraction and suppresses histamine and leukotriene release. Administer

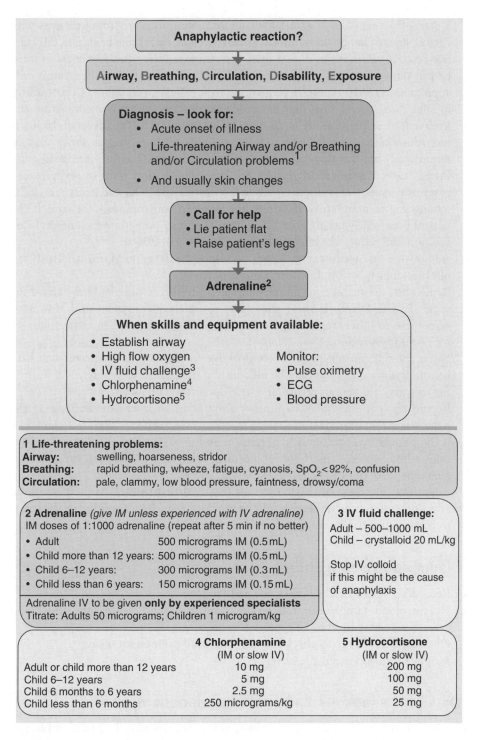

Figure 5.1 Emergency treatment of anaphylactic reactions: guidelines for health care providers (RCUK 2009). Reproduced with the kind permission of the Resuscitation Council (UK).

a dose of 0.5 mg (0.5 mL of 1:1000 solution) intramuscularly to all patients with clinical signs of anaphylactic shock, airway swelling or definite breathing difficulty (see Box 5.6). Repeat this dose if there is no improvement after 5 minutes or if the patient shows any signs of deterioration. The effective half-life of adrenaline is only approximately 5–10 minutes depending upon the patient's metabolism. Consequently, in some cases several doses may be needed, particularly if improvement is transient.

- Intravenous adrenaline in a dilution of at least 1:10,000 (never 1:1000) is hazardous and must be reserved for patients with profound shock that is immediately life-threatening and for special indications (e.g. during anaesthesia). In this case, the injection should be given slowly and only by experienced practitioners (e.g. anaesthetists) while monitoring the ECG and heart rate. ECG monitoring is mandatory if adrenaline is given intravenously. Beware if the patient is currently taking beta-blockers as they may potentiate the anaphylactic reaction and reduce the effects of adrenaline (RCUK 2009).
- Administer an antihistamine such as chlorpheniramine (Piriton) 10–20 mg intramuscularly, or by slow intravenous infusion.
- Remember, the features of anaphylaxis and life-threatening asthma can be the same (RCUK 2009). If the patient has severe bronchospasm and was non-responsive to other treatment, consider a nebuliser. Use oxygen rather than air for its administration.
- Nurse the patient in a position comfortable for them. Sitting upright will help breathing difficulties but may be unhelpful if the patient is hypotensive. Raising the legs may aid venous return and help correct hypotension.
- Record the patient's peak expiratory flow prior to treatment as long as the patient is not in extremis.
- If the patient has profound hypotension and does not respond to the medications administered, rapid fluid replacement with 500–1000 mL of crystalloid is recommended as a fluid challenge (RCUK 2009).
- Administer intravenous corticosteroids (e.g. hydrocortisone). As their optimum effect takes 4–6 hours, these should be the last on the list of routine medications to be administered for anaphylaxis.

Diagnostic investigations

- Record a 12-lead ECG to check for arrhythmias.
- Obtain blood samples for full blood count, urea and electrolytes and blood gases. These may need to be repeated frequently.
- Obtain a chest X-ray to check for heart size and pulmonary oedema.
- Monitor central venous pressure.

Ongoing assessment and nursing management

In addition to the core care plan for the shocked or critically ill adult in Table 5.4, record peak expiratory flow every 4 hours or before and after the administration of nebulisers.

Summary

The recognition of the early signs of shock and its effective management are vital if mortality and morbidity are to be reduced. This chapter has outlined the initial assessment and management of patients who develop shock. It is important to remember that the presenting features of shock can be caused by 'non-medical' conditions (e.g. ruptured abdominal aortic aneurysm) that require 'non-medical' treatment. In this context, it is important for nurses to have a high index of suspicion for both medical and non-medical causes when patients present with signs of shock. Initial assessment and management is only the first component of a successful outcome for the patient. Treatment of the underlying cause of shock is vital and can only be successfully achieved through effective teamwork from all members of the healthcare team.

References

American College of Surgeons (1997) Committee on Trauma. *Advanced Trauma Life Support for Doctors* (6th edition). Chicago: ACS.

Bedside Clinical Guidelines Partnership (BCGP) (2010) *Medical Guidelines*. Stoke on Trent: Bedside Clinical Guidelines Partnership.

Benelam B & Wyness L (2010) Hydration and health: a review *Nutrition Bulletin*, 35(1), 3–25.

Brandler E & Sinert R (2010) Cardiogenic shock in emergency medicine. *Emedicine*. http://emedicine.medscape.com/article/759992-overview (accessed 21 April 2011).

Brandis K (2011) *Fluid compartments*. www.anaesthesiamcq.com/FluidBook/fl2_1.php (accessed 5 April 2011).

British Medical Association & Royal Pharmaceutical Society (2011) *British National Formulary* 61 (March). http://bnf.org/bnf/bnf/60/5001.htm?q=hetastarch&t=search&ss=text&p=2#_hit (accessed 20 April 2011).

British Thoracic Society (2008) *British Thoracic Society Guideline for emergency oxygen use in adult patients*. www.brit-thoracic.org.uk/clinical-information/emergency-oxygen/emergency-oxygen-use-in-adult-patients.aspx (accessed 20 April 2011).

Cleland J, Yassin A & Khadjooi K (2010) Acute heart failure: Focusing on acute cardiogenic pulmonary oedema. *Clinical Medicine*, 10(1), 59–64.

Collins T (2000) Understanding shock. *Nursing Standard*, 14(49), 35–41.

Copstead L-E & Banasik J (2009) *Pathophysiology* (4th edition). Philadelphia: W.B. Saunders.

Dougherty L & Lister S (2008) *The Royal Marsden Hospital Manual of Clinical Nursing Procedures* (7th edition). Oxford: Wiley-Blackwell.

European Society of Cardiology (ESC) (2008) Management of acute myocardial infarction in patients presenting with persistent ST-segment elevation. *European Society of Cardiology Guidelines. European Heart Journal* 29, 2909–2945. www.escardio.org/guidelines-surveys/esc-guidelines/GuidelinesDocuments/guidelines-AMI-FT.pdf (accessed 22 March 2011).

Fouche Y, Sikorski R & Dutton R. (2010) Changing paradigms in surgical resuscitation. *Critical Care Medicine*. 38(9) (Suppl.), s411–s420.

Guyton A & Hall J (2005) *Textbook of Medical Physiology* (11th edition). Philadelphia: Elsevier Saunders.

Henderson N (1998) Anaphylaxis. *Nursing Standard*, 12(47), 49–55.

Iggulden H (1999) Dehydration and electronic disturbance. *Nursing Standard*, 13(19), 48–56.

Kanaparthi L, Lessnau K-D, Peralta R, Langenfeld S & Neeley S (2011) Distributive shock: Treatment and medication. *Emedicine*. http://emedicine.medscape.com/article/168689-overview (accessed 23 February 2011).

Kolecki P & Menckhoff C (2010) Hypovolemic shock. *Emedicine*. http://emedicine.medscape.com/article/760145-overview (accessed 23 February 2011).

Krenn L & Karth G (2011) Essential lessons in cardiogenic shock: Epinephrine versus norepinephrine/dobutamine. *Critical Care Medicine*, 39(3), 583–584.

Kunert M (2009) Alterations in temperature regulation In: Porth C & Matfin G (eds), *Pathophysiology: Concepts of Altered Health State* (8th edition). Philadelphia: Lippincott, Williams & Wilkins.

Lenneman A & Ooi H (2011) Cardiogenic shock: Treatment and management *Emedicine*. http://emedicine.medscape.com/article/152191-overview (accessed 13 March 2011).

Moore T & Woodrow P (2008) *High Dependency Nursing Care: Observation, intervention and support for Level 2 patients* (2nd edition). Oxford: Routledge.

National Institute for Health & Clinical Excellence (2011) Septic shock. www.cks.nhs.uk/patient_information_leaflet/septic_shock#-464753 (accessed 10 April 2011).

Pinsky M, Al Faresi F, Brenner B, Filbin M et al. (2011) Septic shock. *Emedicine*. http://emedicine.medscape.com/article/168402-overview#a0101 (accessed 7 April 2011).

Porth C (2009) Disorders of the immune response In: Porth C & Matfin G (eds), *Pathophysiology: Concepts of Altered Health State* (8th edition). Philadelphia: Lippincott, Williams & Wilkins.

Resuscitation Council (UK) (2009) *Emergency treatment of anaphylactic reactions: Guidelines for health care providers*. www.resus.org.uk/pages/mediMain.htm (accessed 20 April 2011).

Resuscitation Council (UK) (2010) Adult bradycardia algorithm. www.resus.org.uk/pages/glalgos.htm (accessed 26 April 2011).

Reynolds H & Hochman J (2008) Cardiogenic shock: Current concepts and improving outcomes. *Circulation*, 117, 586–697.

Survive Sepsis (2010) The Sepsis 6. www.survivesepsis.org/#/sepsis-six/3525187 (accessed 10 April 2011).

Surviving Sepsis Campaign (2011) About sepsis. www.survivingsepsis.org/Introduction/Pages/default.aspx#howdoessepsisshow (accessed 10 April 2011).

Watson R (1996) Thirst and dehydration in elderly people. *Elderly Care*, 8(3), 23–26.

Further reading

Institute for Healthcare Improvement (2004) *The 100,000 Lives Campaign*. www.ihi.org/IHI/Programs/Campaign/100kCampaignOverviewArchive.htm (accessed 10 April 2011).

Migliozzi J (2009) Shock. In Nair M & Peate I (eds) (2009) *Fundamentals of Applied Pathophysiology*. Oxford: Wiley-Blackwell.

Porth C & Matfin G (eds) (2009) *Pathophysiology: Concepts of Altered Health State* (8th edition). Philadelphia: Lippincott, Williams & Wilkins.

6 Altered Consciousness
Ian Wood and Carole Donaldson

Aims

This chapter will:

- describe a systematic approach to the initial assessment and management of patients presenting with altered consciousness
- outline the clinical features of acute stroke, acute subarachnoid haemorrhage, tonic-clonic status epilepticus and bacterial meningitis
- describe the clinical features of hypoglycaemia, hyperglycaemia and diabetic ketoacidosis (DKA) and hyperosmolar hyperglycaemic state (HHS)
- describe the clinical features associated with common overdoses causing altered consciousness and their assessment and management

---

Introduction

Alteration of conscious level is a common feature of patients with acute illness and often presents as a medical or neurological emergency. Patient management is determined by the underlying cause but an initial ABCDE assessment should always be performed to identify and treat immediately or potentially life-threatening problems. There are several medical and neurological disorders that may need to be considered and can be partially suspected on the basis of associated clinical features (Table 6.1). The presence or absence of focal weakness, meningeal irritation or previously known pre-morbid illnesses (e.g. a prior diagnosis of epilepsy) may point towards the underlying aetiology.

The cause of altered consciousness may be better understood and identified if the initial assessment considers the following common presentations:

- Short-lived/transient (seconds to minutes) or episodic impairment of consciousness. This often suggests an episode of syncope, an epileptic seizure or, rarely, other causes (e.g. TIA if focal symptoms, cataplexy, or hydrocephalic attacks).

Initial Management of Acute Medical Patients: A Guide for Nurses and Healthcare Practitioners, Second Edition. Edited by Ian Wood and Michelle Garner.
© 2012 John Wiley & Sons, Ltd. Published 2012 by John Wiley & Sons, Ltd.

Table 6.1 Common causes of altered consciousness and associated clinical features

Causes of altered consciousness	Typical clinical features
Neurological emergencies	
Stroke/cerebrovascular disease	**Anterior (carotid) circulation**
	Hemiparesis
	Hemisensory disturbance
	Visual field loss
	Dysphasia
	Sensory inattention and neglect
	Eye deviation away from the hemiparesis
	Posterior (vertebrobasilar) circulation
	Quadriparesis
	Limb or gait ataxia
	Dysphagia
	Bilateral visual loss
	Diplopia
	Facial sensory loss
	Eye deviation towards the hemiparesis
Subarachnoid haemorrhage	Sudden, severe headache
	Neck stiffness, photophobia – may take hours to develop
	Nausea and vomiting
	Epileptic seizure
	Transient loss of consciousness
	Coma
Epileptic seizure	Abrupt onset, usually preceded by a warning symptom
	Tonic-clonic movements affecting all four limbs*
	Impaired consciousness
	Incontinence
	Tongue biting
Meningitis	Acute fever
	Malaise
	Worsening headache
	Neck stiffness, photophobia, nausea
	Non-blanching skin rash
	Loss of consciousness
Diabetic emergencies	
Hypoglycaemia	Shaking
	Sweating
	Pins and needles in lips, tongue
	Hunger
	Palpitations
	Double vision
	Difficulty concentrating
	Slurred speech
	Confusion
	Loss of consciousness
Hyperglycaemia and diabetic ketoacidosis (DKA)	Polydipsia
	Polyuria
	Smell of 'pear drops' (ketones) on breath
	Hunger (polyphagia)
	Fatigue

Table 6.1 (cont'd)

Causes of altered consciousness	Typical clinical features	
	Nausea and vomiting Abdominal pain Kussmaul's breathing Confusion	
Hyperosmolar hyperglycaemic state (HSS)	Severe dehydration Altered consciousness Seizures	
Overdose of drugs or alcohol		
Aspirin	Restlessness Tinnitus Sweating Epigastric pain Hyperventilation Dehydration Hypotension Convulsions**	Tachycardia Deafness Blurred vision Nausea and vomiting Hyperpyrexia Confusion Unconsciousness**
Paracetamol	Few if any presenting features Nausea and vomiting (if >24 hours after ingestion)	
Tricyclic antidepressants	Dry mouth Drowsiness Muscle twitching Hypertonia/hyperreflexia Hypothermia or hyperpyrexia Excitement/visual hallucinations	Urinary retention Depressed respiration** Tachycardia/arrhythmias** Hypotension** Convulsions** Unconsciousness**
Alcohol	Slurred speech Loss of inhibitions Aggression Red conjunctivae Smell of alcohol on breath Altered consciousness level Postural hypotension	Ataxia Loss of judgement Irritability Hypoglycaemia Gastric irritation Nausea and vomiting Respiratory depression
Narcotics	Altered consciousness level Respiratory depression Hypothermia Non-cardiogenic pulmonary oedema Bradycardia Hypotension Pinpoint pupils (miosis)	

* Multiple tonic-clonic seizures lasting >20 minutes with no recovery of consciousness, indicates tonic-clonic status epilepticus.
** Indicates severe toxicity.

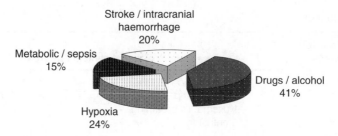

Figure 6.1 Relative frequency of presenting causes of altered consciousness (fits, syncope and hypoglycaemia excluded).

- Persistent and/or worsening impairment of consciousness level. This may suggest an **intracranial** (e.g. meningitis, encephalitis, raised intracranial pressure, cerebral venous sinus thrombosis), **systemic** (e.g. hypoxic brain injury, substance or alcohol intoxication, hypothermia, septicaemia) or **metabolic** cause of altered consciousness. Metabolic causes include diabetic coma (e.g. hypoglycaemia, hyperglycaemia with ketoacidosis or hyperosmolar non-ketotic coma) or hyponatraemia.

The relative frequency of common causes is shown in Figure 6.1.

Initial assessment of the patient with altered consciousness

Airway

Assessment and management of airway problems is of paramount importance in patients who present with altered consciousness.

- Listen for stridor/wheeze.
- Observe for and remove foreign bodies in the airway.

Breathing

- Assess respiratory rate and depth.
- Observe for chest movement.
- Observe for peripheral and central cyanosis.
- Measure oxygen saturations/arterial blood gases.
- Smell the breath for unusual odours.

Circulation

- Measure the heart rate.
- Assess pulse volume and regularity.

- Measure the blood pressure.
- Observe for signs of haemorrhage.
- Feel the patient's skin for warmth and texture.

Disability

- Confirm the level of consciousness using AVPU (**A**lert, responds to **V**erbal stimulus, responds to **P**ainful stimulus or **U**nresponsive) and/or Glasgow Coma Score (GCS).
- Check pupil size and reaction to light.
- Measure the patient's capillary blood sugar (e.g. BM stix, glucostix).
- Observe for obvious signs of facial/postural weakness.

Exposure

- Undress the patient.
- Observe for rashes/puncture wounds/injuries.
- Record the temperature.
- Perform urinalysis.

Initial management of the patient with altered consciousness

- Use appropriate airway management techniques (Chapter 1 – Initial assessment).
- Give high-flow oxygen via non-rebreathe mask or bag-valve-mask (if ventilatory support is required to assist breathing).
- Monitor cardiac rate and rhythm.
- Secure intravenous access.
- Consider possible causes of altered consciousness.
- Measure the patient's capillary blood sugar and correct if necessary.

A: NEUROLOGICAL EMERGENCIES
(Ian Wood, based on the original chapter by Brendan Davies)

Stroke/cerebrovascular disease (excluding subarachnoid haemorrhage)

A stroke is a clinical syndrome characterised by symptoms and signs of acute focal, neurological disturbance with loss of function lasting more than 24 hours. It has an underlying vascular cause and is the third commonest cause of death and disability in adults after cancer and ischaemic heart disease. Stroke is distinguished from a transient ischaemic attack (TIA) by the duration of symptoms. A TIA lasts less than 24 hours and usually less than 60 minutes. The clinical distinction between a TIA and mild stroke is important from an epidemiological viewpoint but not particularly useful when considering future prognosis and investigation as both necessitate emergency assessment to minimise the risk of future disabling stroke.

The concept of therapeutic nihilism in stroke care is changing and stroke should now be considered an acute medical emergency. The term 'brain attack' and the concept of 'Time is brain' are analogous to the commonly accepted notion of 'heart attack' where 'Time is muscle'. These principles become ever more important as therapies emerge that make the time to initiation of treatment for stroke a fundamental consideration (National Institute of Neurological Disorders and Stroke study group 1995, 1997; Hacke et al. 1998; Department of Health 2007).

Pathophysiology

The pathological subtype of stroke is important because treatment, prognosis and secondary prevention may differ. In general, most strokes are ischaemic (approximately 85%) with the remainder being due to primary intracerebral haemorrhage. The majority of ischaemic strokes occur as a complication of atherosclerosis. There may be artery-to-artery thrombo-embolism (e.g. from the carotid or vertebrobasilar arteries to the cerebral circulation), embolism from the heart (e.g. cardiac thrombus or endocarditis) or in-situ intracranial small vessel disease and arteriosclerosis. Haemorrhagic stroke usually results from uncontrolled hypertension, rupture of a saccular aneurysm or arteriovenous malformation. Rarely, stroke may occur as a result of venous occlusion due to thrombosis of the cerebral venous sinuses and may reflect an inherited thrombophilic tendency. Cerebral venous occlusion should always be considered as a cause of stroke occurring in pregnancy.

The pathophysiology of stroke may also vary with age, with atherosclerosis the commonest cause of stroke in patients over the age of 45–50 years. There are several common reversible risk factors for stroke that include hypertension, smoking and hypercholesterolaemia, and several irreversible factors including increasing age, male sex and Afro-Caribbean origin. In younger patients, stroke may otherwise occur as a result of arterial tearing (dissection), especially following minor trauma or as a result of cardiac defects (e.g. atrial septal defects) and rarely due to genetic inheritance (MELAS and CADASIL) or thrombophilia.

The pathological consequence of stroke is reduced oxygen delivery to the brain and thus cerebral infarction and irreversible tissue damage. The area of infarction and irreversible tissue damage usually results in clinical disability. In the early stages of cerebral infarction the area of irreversible tissue infarction is surrounded by an area of reversible tissue ischaemia called the 'ischaemic penumbra'. This area of brain may potentially be salvaged with appropriate early and continuing stroke care and thus there is the potential to limit physical disability with appropriate care.

> **Box 6.1   Typical presenting features of anterior and posterior cerebral circulatory dysfunction**
>
> **Anterior (carotid) circulation**
> Hemiparesis
> Hemisensory disturbance
> Visual field loss
> Dysphasia
> Sensory inattention and neglect
> Eye deviation away from the hemiparesis
>
> **Posterior (vertebrobasilar) circulation**
> Quadraparesis
> Limb or gait ataxia
> Dysphagia
> Bilateral visual loss
> Diplopia
> Facial sensory loss
> Eye deviation towards the hemiparesis

Presenting features

It is difficult to differentiate without brain imaging whether patients have suffered an ischaemic or haemorrhagic stroke (Muir 2001). Patients typically present with acute onset, focal negative symptoms i.e. loss of function (compared with the slowly spreading, positive symptoms of migraine or sensory epileptic seizure). The pattern of symptoms and signs help differentiate whether the stroke has affected the anterior (carotid) or posterior (vertebrobasilar) circulation. In addition, headache is more common with haemorrhagic and posterior circulation ischaemic stroke. Typical presenting features are outlined in Box 6.1.

Alteration of consciousness with stroke is extremely unusual unless there is raised intracranial pressure, involvement of the brainstem, bilateral cerebral hemisphere disease or co-morbid disease. Possible scenarios include:

- large haemorrhagic stroke with secondary raised intracranial pressure
- massive anterior circulation stroke with dense hemiparesis and secondary raised intracranial pressure (usually 2–3 days after onset)
- posterior circulation, brainstem stroke with involvement of the reticular formation
- subarachnoid haemorrhage (see below)

Thus, impaired consciousness in the context of stroke suggests the need for more extensive medical assessment to exclude other metabolic factors and early brain scan to exclude cerebral haemorrhage or alternative intracerebral pathology.

Box 6.2   ROSIER Scale for assessing likelihood of stroke versus stroke mimic

Has there been loss of consciousness or syncope?		Yes (−1)	No (0)
Has there been seizure activity?		Yes (−1)	No (0)
Is there a NEW ACUTE onset (or on awakening from sleep)?			
i	Asymmetric facial weakness	Yes (+1)	No (0)
ii	Asymmetric arm weakness	Yes (+1)	No (0)
iii	Asymmetric leg weakness	Yes (+1)	No (0)
iv	Speech disturbance	Yes (+1)	No (0)
v	Visual field defect	Yes (+1)	No (0)
Total score (range −2 to +5) =			

If total score > 0 (i.e. 1 to 5), a diagnosis of acute stroke is likely. If total scores equal 0, −1 or −2, stroke is unlikely but is not excluded.

Initial assessment

Patients suspected of having suffered acute stroke require rapid initial assessment if the benefits of early treatment interventions are to be optimised. The use of assessment tools such as ROSIER (Nor et al. 2005) (see Box 6.2) may be appropriate in differentiating a stroke from those conditions that can mimic a stroke (e.g. seizure and syncope). The initial medical assessment involves detailed history taking of the acute event from the patient (or witness if the patient has dysphasia). A relevant past medical history of hypertension, diabetes mellitus, ischaemic heart disease or atrial fibrillation should be sought in addition to any family history of stroke. A smoking, alcohol and drug history may be relevant. In younger patients, a history of recent drug ingestion may identify illicit drugs that can cause stroke (e.g. cocaine, amphetamine). In addition, a recent history of neck trauma or rotational injury may suggest arterial dissection as a potential cause of stroke in young patients.

General examination should specifically include an assessment of ABCDE, temperature, pulse rate, rhythm and arterial blood pressure (in both arms if pulse asymmetry) and heart auscultation in addition to a more general assessment of the patient's condition. The initial neurological assessment should include Glasgow Coma Scale, speech (for dysarthria or dysphasia) and orientation.

Neurological examination should characterise visual fields, oculomotor abnormalities, pupil size and reactivity, swallowing ability, and the pattern and severity of focal weakness and/or sensory loss both in the cranial nerves and in limbs. Walking ability or disturbances of co-ordination and balance should preferably be included in the assessment. A capillary blood sugar measurement and urine dipstick test should be included in the examination of patients presenting with stroke.

Immediate management and investigations

Acute stroke is a medical emergency. Brain scan should be performed as soon as possible to exclude haemorrhagic stroke and differentiate stroke from non-vascular brain disorders (Muir 2001). This scan should be performed within 15 minutes for the following patients:

- potential thrombolysis candidates (clinical diagnosis of stroke, previously independent and well, onset time known and 4.5 hours or less)
- those who are anticoagulated or have known bleeding disorder (platelets <100×10⁹/L, INR >1.2)
- those with depressed level of consciousness (GCS< 13)
- those with unexplained progressive or fluctuating symptoms
- those with papilloedema, neck stiffness, or fever
- those with severe headache at onset of stroke

Bedside Clinical Guidelines Partnership (2010)

Basic screening tests for the cause of stroke should be performed on admission and should include a full blood count, clotting studies, ESR, glucose, urea and electrolytes, ECG and cholesterol (if within 12 hours of symptom onset). Patients who are taking warfarin should have an immediate INR.

After the exclusion of intracranial haemorrhage by the prompt use of imaging techniques, where appropriate, thrombolysis should start within 3 hours of the onset of the stroke symptoms. Once primary intracerebral haemorrhage has been excluded, aspirin (75–300 mg) should be given. Combined data from three trials (Chen et al. 2000) indicate that early initiation of aspirin:

- prevents early recurrence of stroke
- reduces death and disability at 3–6 months
- increases the proportion making a full recovery at the expense of a small increase in intracranial and extracranial haemorrhage risk

All stroke patients should have access to an acute stroke unit that provides rapid treatment and high-dependency care including physiological and neurological monitoring of their condition and its associated complications. Early rehabilitation such as early mobilisation, early feeding and measures to prevent aspiration, and palliative care services should also be available (Department of Health 2007).

Patients with a TIA and non-disabling stroke may be suitable for urgent outpatient assessment only if appropriate investigations and rehabilitation services can be accessed promptly.

Ongoing assessment and treatment

The long-term clinical outcome and increased mortality of stroke can be adversely affected by several physiological variables that need monitoring within an acute setting and, subsequently, on transfer to a stroke unit or ward. High body temperature, low diastolic blood pressure, hyperglycaemia and hypoxia have detrimental effects on stroke outcome and should be monitored and treated accordingly.

Continued assessment of neurological status is imperative with treatment of secondary stroke complications such as seizures (2% of strokes at onset) and infection (e.g. aspiration or hypostatic pneumonia) and early involvement of appropriate paramedical services (i.e. occupational therapy and physiotherapy).

Subarachnoid haemorrhage

Subarachnoid haemorrhage (SAH) accounts for 3% of all strokes and 5% of all stroke deaths. It is a common neurological emergency and has an approximate incidence of 11 per 100,000 person years; appropriate recognition is important to avoid a potentially fatal outcome (van Gijn & Rinkel 2001).

Pathophysiology

Subarachnoid haemorrhage most commonly occurs due to rupture of an intracranial saccular aneurysm and less commonly an arteriovenous malformation. Such aneurysms are not congenital but develop during life, usually at the bifurcation of cerebral arteries. It is largely unknown why different individuals develop an aneurysm but smoking, hypertension and excess alcohol consumption are all risk factors. In some cases an abnormality of connective tissue in the blood vessel wall may play a role (e.g. Ehlers-Danlos type IV). In addition, there may be a genetic element in some families either independent of other diseases or as part of an inherited disease affecting other organs (e.g. autosomal dominant polycystic kidney disease, neurofibromatosis type I).

Presenting features

The classic history of SAH consists of sudden-onset (within seconds), severe (worst ever) headache. This may be the only initial presenting feature as meningism (neck stiffness and photophobia) may take several hours to develop and vomiting, although often present, can also be associated with other conditions that may mimic SAH. Less commonly, an epileptic seizure may occur at onset in up to 16% of cases and the presence of an unusually severe headache following a first seizure should raise the suspicion of SAH. Presentation with an acute confusional state is less frequent (1–2%) but transient loss of consciousness of more than 1 hour's duration is reported in more than 50% of patients in case series. There is often no complaint of focal weakness and in its mildest form (grade I SAH) there is only headache with otherwise intact neurological status. Massive SAH may cause coma and extensive focal neurological deficits and 25% of patients die within the first 24 hours of onset.

Initial assessment

Initial assessment should ensure adequate assessment and stabilisation of patient ABCDE's and subsequent confirmation of an appropriate history for SAH. The presence of co-morbid illness that may be associated with aneursymal SAH should be sought and any recent history of trauma or drug ingestion recorded to exclude a provoked cause for SAH.

Examination should record baseline GCS (airway management if consciousness is impaired), neurological observations, vital signs (e.g. pulse, BP, respiratory rate and temperature) and ECG. The presence or absence of neck stiffness, photophobia, focal neurological deficit and conjunctival haemorrhage should be noted.

Immediate management and investigations

Appropriate supportive care is needed to avoid secondary brain insults following SAH and to minimise the risk of subsequent vasospasm. Patients should be nursed in dimmed light, in a quiet environment and complete bed rest to avoid the risk of early rebleeding. General measures should include intravenous hydration (at least 2.5–3.5 litres of 0.9% saline per 24 hours), avoidance of hypotension and adequate analgesia (e.g. paracetamol or codeine phosphate). Specific treatment should be aimed at limiting vasospasm and secondary ischaemia, and reducing the re-bleed risk (e.g. nimodipine orally, via nasogastric tube, or intravenously).

CT brain imaging should occur at the earliest opportunity after the onset of symptoms to confirm radiological evidence of SAH. In addition, this enables prompt management decisions about future angiography in confirmed SAH.

CT scanning may be negative in 2% of patients with subsequent confirmed SAH even when it is performed within the optimum time of 12 hours from headache onset. In patients whose CT scan is negative, lumbar puncture is mandatory to detect or exclude the presence/absence of xanthochromia in suspected SAH before a diagnosis can be confirmed or refuted (van der Wee et al. 1995). Lumbar puncture, if needed, should not be performed less than 12 hours after the onset of headache as xanthochromia takes time to develop and earlier lumbar puncture may produce a false negative result (Vermeulen & van Gijn 1990). Xanthochromia represents the breakdown products of red blood cell haemoglobin (i.e. bilirubin and oxyhaemoglobin) in the cerebrospinal fluid (CSF). It can only be detected reliably in-vivo 12 hours after SAH. The introduction of blood into the subarachnoid space can occur by a difficult-to-perform, and thus traumatic, tap procedure. Similarly, xanthochromia can develop in-vitro if CSF samples from a lumbar puncture are allowed to stand for several hours without appropriate analysis. Thus, it is imperative to differentiate SAH-related xanthochromia from traumatic or in-vitro xanthochromia using the following steps. The CSF sample should be processed by the laboratory at the earliest opportunity and centrifuged immediately after lumbar puncture in order to test for xanthochromia properly and to avoid a false positive diagnosis of SAH as the three-tube test for a traumatic tap is unreliable. Immediate centrifugation avoids the in-vitro development of xanthochromia as a result of a traumatic tap (van Gijn & Rinkel 2001).

Ongoing assessment and treatment

Patients with confirmed SAH should be transferred to specialist neurological or neurosurgical care promptly following diagnosis. Cerebral angiography should be instituted at an early stage to plan neurosurgical management and limit the risks of morbidity and mortality that can result from rebleeding. Continued monitoring of the GCS and pupillary responses allows detection of clinical change and directs the need for reassessment and investigation. The continuing assessment of neurological status permits the early detection of secondary complications of SAH (e.g. early rebleeding, intracerebral haematoma, hydrocephalus, secondary ischaemia due to vasospasm). Consider anti-embolism stockings.

Epileptic seizures

Patients presenting to an emergency care setting with an apparent epileptic seizure are a common clinical occurrence. They may present with an isolated first seizure which may be symptomatic, provoked (e.g. due to alcohol intoxication or withdrawal, or head injury) or may have no apparent cause. The episode may be a seizure in the context of established epilepsy. Alternatively, patients may present with an increasing frequency of seizures or even status epilepticus. Each of these circumstances necessitates structured assessment and management. The main purpose of treatment is to prevent cerebral damage and patient morbidity caused by uncontrolled seizure activity. The following relates predominantly to tonic-clonic status epilepticus.

Pathophysiology

The physiological status of the brain is markedly disturbed in status epilepticus. In the initial stages, there are compensatory mechanisms for increased seizure activity with matching of the brain energy requirements by increased cerebral blood flow and cerebral auto-regulation and increased autonomic activity. This initially protects the brain from the damaging effects of hypoxia, acidosis and hypoglycaemia and, if seizure activity is terminated at this stage, there is unlikely to be long-term cerebral damage. With continued seizure activity, particularly for more than 60 min, these compensatory mechanisms start to fail, with consequent brain-tissue hypoxia and inability to maintain brain metabolism homeostasis. This leads to secondary effects on the systemic control of other body organ systems. Ultimately this results in impaired brain metabolism and function from continuing seizure activity and the increasing risk of permanent, irreversible brain damage and even death. The loss of autonomic control due to continued seizure-induced brain dysfunction may cause worsening systemic metabolic changes (e.g. hypogly-caemia, acidosis, tissue hypoxia, hypothermia and disseminated intravascular coagulation or DIC). This may cause progressive multi-organ failure with respira-tory failure, hypotension and hepato-renal failure in addition to cerebral oedema and death (Shorvon 2001).

The recognition of early status epilepticus and initiation of appropriate therapy, therefore, provides a window of opportunity to avoid the potentially fatal consequences.

Presenting features

The commonest presentation in an acute care setting is following one or more tonic-clonic seizures. The first and most important issue is whether the patient's episode was a definite epileptic seizure rather than an alternative paroxysmal episode such as syncope (vasovagal or drug-induced), cataplexy (as part of narcolepsy), migraine or, rarely, a TIA (if there are other focal, usually brainstem, symptoms).

Typically with a tonic-clonic seizure there is an abrupt onset, sometimes with a preceding warning that may be brief (e.g. an uncomfortable epigastric sensation or sensation of *deja vu* in focal epilepsy originating from the temporal lobe). In generalised seizures, tonic-clonic movements affect all four limbs and occur with associated impaired consciousness. Incontinence and severe (especially lateral) tongue biting may be seen. Tonic-clonic seizures usually have duration of 1–3 minutes before self-termination. Following a tonic-clonic seizure there is usually post-ictal confusion that may be prolonged, and recovery to the patient's normal state may be slow in contrast to the rapid recovery following syncope. Less commonly transient, focal weakness following a generalised tonic-clonic seizure may occur (e.g. Todd's paresis). Prolonged impairment of consciousness following seizures is uncommon unless there have been multiple seizures.

If multiple tonic-clonic seizures occur with no recovery of consciousness (arbitrarily defined as lasting more than 20 minutes), this is termed 'tonic-clonic status epilepticus' and constitutes a neurological emergency.

Acute symptomatic seizures account for up to one-third of all new-onset seizures and are not classified as epilepsy. In such patients, several causes may be apparent. Equally precipitants may induce seizures in patients with known epilepsy and include:

- alcohol (intoxication and/or withdrawal)
- drugs (illicit and pro-convulsant prescribed drugs)
- CNS or systemic infection
- trauma
- stroke
- acute metabolic disorder (e.g. hypoxia, hyponatraemia, hypocalcaemia, hypomagnesaemia)

The annual incidence of tonic-clonic status epilepticus is 18–28 cases per 100,000 persons and occurs most commonly in children, individuals with learning disability and patients with intracranial structural pathology. Most cases of 'status' develop without a prior history of epilepsy and can also be caused by all the conditions described above (Shorvon 2001). In patients with established epilepsy, drug withdrawal, intercurrent illness or metabolic disturbance are the commonest provoking factors. The possibility of non-epileptic seizure disorder should always be considered in patients with a past history of psychiatric disorder, particularly if there are atypical features or the patient presents with status epilepticus.

Important conditions to differentiate from isolated seizures include syncope (both vasovagal and cardiac), hypoglycaemic attacks, postural hypotension and, rarely, cataplexy or intracranial disorders that cause intermittent obstructive hydro-cephalus. Patients in ventricular fibrillation may also exhibit twitching or signs of convulsion.

Syncope is the commonest missed diagnosis and is characterized by pre-syncopal symptoms (e.g. feeling lightheaded, hot, sweaty, blurring or dimming of vision and tinnitus before loss of consciousness) and subsequent short-lived loss of conscious-ness with rapid recovery without confusion. Some patients who experience syncope may exhibit short-lived tonic-clonic or myoclonic involuntary limb movements that may be mistaken for epileptic seizures. This is termed 'convulsive syncope' (Lempert et al. 1994). Incontinence can also occur with syncope and thus does not discriminate between a seizure and syncope.

Initial assessment

Initial ABCDE assessment aims to identify immediate and potentially life-threatening problems with subsequent history-taking confirming the likelihood of a seizure. As the patient usually has no recollection of events, an account of the circumstances should be sought from witnesses. This is imperative for the adequate recognition of a seizure.

Recording of vital signs and GCS (especially pupillary responses and motor function) are important. Similarly, it is important to evaluate whether there is evidence of head trauma, skin rash (especially if non-blanching – indicative of meningococcal septicaemia), meningism, venous puncture wounds or abnormal breath odour (e.g. alcohol, ketones). Identify any mouth trauma (e.g. bitten tongue or inner cheeks) and the presence or absence of urinary or faecal incontinence. Gain intravenous access, check the blood sugar level and perform a cardiovascular assessment including an ECG to exclude possible alternative causes of transient loss of consciousness.

Immediate management and investigations

With patients presenting in status epilepticus, once the ABCDEs have been managed, give appropriate intravenous or rectal medication to stop the fit. Nasopharyngeal airways are particularly well suited for use during a convulsion as they are easily inserted and are well tolerated. Administration of high-flow oxygen is beneficial. If the patient suffers a convulsion, ensure they are safe by removing or padding equipment that may cause injury. The treatment of status can be divided into three

Stage 1
Early status epilepticus
Immediate measures:
Secure airway, assess &
manage breathing &
circulation, give oxygen,
secure IV access, take
bloods (glucose, FBC, U&E,
LFT, calcium, clotting, anti-
epileptic drug levels, ABGs)

Lorazepam 4 mg IV bolus into a large vein
or
Diazemuls 10 mg IV (given over 2–5 min) or rectally
Repeated once only after 10 min if no cessation of seizures
Caution due to prolonged sedative effects of diazemuls

If continued seizures

Stage 2
Established 'status'
Within 10–30 minutes since
seizure onset

Call ICU to inform them of
the patient

IV infusion of phenytoin (18 mg/kg at a rate of 50 mg/min) with ECG monitoring
or (and)
IV infusion of phenobarbital (15 mg/kg at a rate of 100 mg/min)
or
IV fosphenytoin (18 mg/kg at a rate of up to 150 mg/min) with ECG monitoring

If continued seizures

Stage 3
Refractory 'status'
60 min or more following
seizure onset without
recovery

With EEG monitoring to
identify burst-suppression
pattern

Intensive care/anaesthetic support Treat with general anaesthesia
Either: Propofol 2 mg/kg IV bolus followed by infusion according to local/national protocols to control seizures
or
Thiopental 100–250 mg IV bolus and subsequent induction regime until seizures are controlled
and
then maintenance regime with IV infusion until a burst suppression pattern is seen on the EEG
Both anaesthetic drugs should be slowly withdrawn 12 hours after the last seizure

Figure 6.2 Emergency drug treatment for a patient presenting with continuing seizure activity in status epilepticus.

stages (Scottish Intercollegiate Guidelines Network 2005) and is outlined in Figure 6.2. Continuing generalised tonic-clonic status epilepticus increases the risk of irreversible brain damage and systemic decompensation; thus aggressive intervention and the need to step up therapy should occur within the first 2 hours of presentation with status epilepticus.

In conjunction with the emergency management outlined above, consider performing the following investigations:

- blood glucose, sodium, calcium and magnesium
- renal and hepatic function
- full blood count and clotting studies
- blood anticonvulsant drug levels (if appropriate medications are being taken)
- toxicology screening (blood and urine)
- arterial blood gases (for hypoxia and acidosis)
- ECG
- saved sera (for subsequent virology if needed)

Ensure full resuscitation facilities are available in case of respiratory compromise secondary to benzodiazepines or phenytoin. Correct metabolic abnormalities if present. Administer intravenous glucose and thiamine if there is a possibility of hypoglycaemia or alcoholism.

Ongoing assessment and treatment

If tonic-clonic seizures continue despite initial drug treatment, early anaesthetic review and subsequent transfer to an intensive care unit is needed. An EEG needs to be performed for three reasons: first, to confirm the clinical impression of generalised electrical status, particularly if there is any suspicion of non-epileptic pseudo-status in patients with tonic-clonic motor activity; second, in comatose and ventilated patients where motor activity has ceased but electrical status may be continuing; and third, to identify burst suppression on the EEG and assess the response to anticonvulsant treatment.

When the patient has been stabilised, and in cases of refractory status, CT brain imaging as well as lumbar puncture needs to be performed to identify the aetiology of status epilepticus when the cause is not readily apparent.

If patients fail to respond to therapy, reassessment is needed to ensure:

- sufficient anticonvulsant drug dosages have been used
- maintenance anticonvulsant drug therapy has been initiated
- co-morbid medical conditions have been treated, especially the underlying cause
- there is no persisting metabolic problem provoking seizures
- the diagnosis is correct and the patient is not having 'pseudoseizures'

Meningitis

Few clinical conditions merit more prompt assessment and immediate treatment than bacterial meningitis. There are several recognised causes of meningitis but an infective cause (i.e. bacterial meningitis) is the most common aetiology with approximately 1000 adult cases per year in the UK (Moller & Skinhoj 2000). It is a neurological emergency that should always be considered in anyone presenting with headache and fever. Any delay in the recognition and treatment of this condition is always associated with a poor prognosis. One in four adults with bacterial meningitis will die or sustain significant neurological deficit even with early treatment.

Table 6.2 Age at presentation and bacterial pathogens commonly responsible for bacterial meningitis

Clinical setting and age	Likely organism	Drug sensitivity
Children and adults	*Neisseria meningitides* *Streptococcus pneumoniae*	IV benzyl penicillin or third-generation cephalosporin (± rifampacin)
Head trauma (e.g. penetrating skull injury/fracture)	Staphylococci Gram-negative bacteria *S. pneumoniae*	Vancomycin ± rifampacin
Immunocompromised and pregnancy	As above for adults plus *Listeria monocytogenes* Opportunistic organisms e.g. *Nocardia asteroides*	Ampicillin and third-generation cephalosporin As per local protocol
Neonates (less than 3 months old)	Group B streptococcus *Escherichia coli* (*E. coli*) *Listeria monocytogenes*	Ampicillin and third-generation cephalosporin (e.g. ceftriaxone/cefotaxime)

Infective meningitis represents an inflammatory response to an infection of the leptomeninges and sometimes the brain parenchyma (known as meningo-encephalitis). It can be caused by both bacterial and viral agents. The former can prove rapidly fatal whereas the latter may have a more benign prognosis. The remainder of this section will concentrate on acute bacterial meningitis and will not consider viral, tuberculous, fungal or auto-immune meningitis.

Pathophysiology

The commonest bacterial pathogens responsible for acute bacterial meningitis vary according to different age groups in society. The *Haemophilus influenzae* (type B) and *Neisseria meningitidis* (type C) vaccination programmes in the UK may change the relative incidence of infection in the future. Currently meningococcal infection in UK adults is caused in equal measure by serotypes B and C organisms with no vaccination available against the B strain. Pneumococcal infection is an equally common bacterial pathogen in adults. *Staphylococcus aureus*, *Listeria monocytogenes*, *Streptococcus pyogenes*, *Escherichia coli* and other organisms are less common but may affect certain patient groups, for example, after neurosurgical procedures or penetrating head injuries (*Staphylococcus aureus*), pregnant women and the elderly (*Listeria monocytogenes*) and children (*E coli*, *Haemophilus*, *Streptococcus pyogenes*).

The organisms responsible for meningitis often colonise the host's (i.e. the patient's) mucosal surfaces (e.g. nasal mucosa, sinuses, mastoids) before spreading either locally from adjacent structures or as a complication of bacteraemia from a more distant source of infection. Meningitis may also result from a localised collection within the skull (e.g. a subdural empyema or cerebral abscess).

Table 6.2 sets out the commonest bacterial pathogens according to age and immunocompetence (e.g. pregnancy, immunocompromised secondary to hereditary or acquired causes).

Presenting features

Patients with acute bacterial meningitis usually present with an acute (hours to a few days) fever, malaise and worsening headache (often occipital or generalised) associated with meningism (neck stiffness, photophobia and nausea). Abnormal mental states with confusion and disorientation are often seen (80% of patients) and patients may sometimes present hyperacutely with acute onset, severe headache resembling acute SAH but with a high fever. Coma with high fever is also a recognised presentation. A characteristic non-blanching rash on the skin may be a 'tell-tale' sign of meningococcal infection and should provoke high diagnostic suspicion in conjunction with the appropriate history. Approximately 15% of patients (especially the elderly) may complain of focal neurological symptoms and up to 50% may have seizures during the course of their illness, particularly in pneumococcal meningitis.

Important conditions that may sometimes mimic bacterial meningitis include viral encephalitis and intracerebral focal infection (e.g. a cerebral abscess or subdural collection). The former often follows a prodromal viral illness and often has confusion, impaired consciousness, dysphasia and focal seizures as prominent parts of the history in conjunction with fever, headache and meningism. Focal infection in the brain often produces rapidly progressive focal neurological deficits often associated with seizures and high fever.

Initial assessment

A rapid assessment of ABCDE precedes appropriate history taking. For those patients with headache and fever, carry out a rapid assessment looking for meningism, rash and depressed conscious level using the GCS. Evaluate the patient's orientation, alertness and speech. Note cardiovascular signs of sepsis or instability (e.g. sinus tachycardia, arterial hypotension) and act promptly. An initial low baseline GCS and the presence of double vision, ocular motility dysfunction and focal signs in the limbs may suggest a more severe pathological disease process and raise the possibility of alternative diagnoses. Establish intravenous access at an early stage. The occurrence of seizures warrants early appropriate intervention to control them.

In suspected bacterial meningitis, the initial assessment should be brief so that antibiotic therapy can be initiated at the earliest opportunity. Further clinical information should be gained later to avoid delaying antibiotic therapy. Ideally, pre-hospital antibiotics will have been given by the patient's GP prior to their arrival.

Immediate management and investigations

If bacterial meningitis is suspected, empirical antibiotics should always be given pending later confirmation of the diagnosis using nationally or locally agreed antibiotic protocols for meningitis. These should take into account local microbiology

Patient with suspected bacterial meningitis

↓

Pre hospital antibiotics   IV or IM benzyl penicillin 1200 mg (2 mega units) by
GP/paramedic with subsequent transfer urgently to
hospital
(cefotaxime or ceftriaxone 1 g if penicillin allergic)

↓

On arrival in hospital   Brief clinical assessment and supportive care
as above
Immediate blood sampling for:
- cultures
- basic haematology and clotting studies
- serological blood testing for bacterial
  organisms with PCR
- rapid initiation of appropriate antibacterial
  treatment

IV 2.4 g benzyl penicillin 4-hourly
or
IV 2 g ceftriaxone 12-hourly
or
IV 2 g cefotaxime 6-hourly

±IV 2 g ampicillin 4-hourly

↓

Early brain imaging (CT scan) once patient stabilized
Exclude other causes
Lumbar puncture
If no contraindications to establish/confirm
diagnosis
Identify organism responsible (Gram stain and PCR)
Nasal and posterior pharyngeal wall swabs

Early involvement of ICU/HDU if problems with:
- cardiovascular or respiratory instability
- seizures and impaired conscious level
- septicaemia (especially meningococcal)

Consider steroids: dexamethasone 4–6 mg 6-hourly
(Coyle 1999) in adults with:
- impaired consciousness, focal signs or
- evidence of raised intracranial pressure

Figure 6.3   Management of bacterial meningitis (adapted from Begg et al. 1999).

advice and knowledge of local drug resistance. A suggested general management plan for the treatment of adult bacterial meningitis is shown in Figure 6.3.

The early involvement of specialist infectious disease, neurology and anaesthetic specialty care should be encouraged to advise on management, particularly if complications are apparent. Seizures, hydrocephalus, raised intracranial pressure, acidosis, coagulopathy and any other co-morbidity should be treated conventionally.

Ongoing assessment and treatment

Following stabilisation, patients should be transferred to specialised care (infectious diseases or neurology department) for continued bacterial chemotherapy and monitoring. The relevant consultant in communicable disease control (CCDC) should be informed of the diagnosis without delay. This enables contact tracing and chemoprophylaxis to be arranged for recent close contacts, if appropriate, to prevent cases of secondary meningitis. General principles of fluid balance monitoring and intervention should be continued. Changes in alertness, worsening GCS and the development of new neurological deficit or focal seizures should prompt further review including brain imaging to look for secondary complications of meningitis (e.g. hydrocephalus, localised subdural empyema, stroke and cerebral venous sinus thrombosis).

B: DIABETIC EMERGENCIES
(Carole Donaldson)

Introduction

Diabetes mellitus is a metabolic condition with an increasing incidence world-wide (Kisiel & Marsons 2009). It is characterised by hyperglycaemia due to a deficit, or complete lack, of insulin production by the pancreas. Nurses must be aware that patients admitted to hospital may have previously diagnosed or undiagnosed diabetes type 1 (insulin-dependent diabetes mellitus, IDDM) or type 2 (non insulin-dependent diabetes mellitus, NIDDM). IDDM occurs due to the inability of the pancreatic beta cells to produce insulin, whereas NIDDM is caused by peripheral insulin resistance due to defective insulin secretion (Yehia et al. 2008).

The management of the patient with diabetes mellitus requires careful control of blood glucose levels that can often be affected by illness, anxiety and a change in diet and routine (Soal et al. 2006). These precipitating factors occur regularly in patients admitted to hospital and may lead to hypoglycaemia, hyperglycaemia, diabetic ketoacidosis (DKA) or hyperosmolar hyperglycaemic syndrome (HHS), formerly classified as hyperosmolar non-ketotic hyperglycaemia (HONK) (Kearney & Dang 2007).

Hypoglycaemia

Hypoglycaemia is a biochemical diagnosis defined as a blood glucose level <2.5 mmol/L (Kearney & Dang 2007); however, it should be noted that patients with chronic hyperglycaemia may have autonomic symptoms of hypoglycaemia at much higher blood glucose levels (Lingenfelter et al. 1995). In a hospital environment, the usual cause of a hypoglycaemic event in a normally well-controlled diabetic is due to alterations in insulin dosage or oral hypoglycaemic drug regimes (Kearney & Dang, 2007). Hypoglycaemia is an inevitable consequence of tight

Table 6.3   Counter-regulatory hormones

Glucagon	Released by the Alpha cells of the pancreas in response to low blood glucose levels. Glucagon converts glycogen to glucose.
Adrenaline and noradrenaline	Catecholamines promote glycogenolysis by stimulating the conversion of glycogen in the liver and muscle to glucose. Adrenaline stimulates glucagon secretion, inhibits insulin release from the beta cells and increases the utilization of fatty acids to preserve glucose.
Cortisol	Stimulates gluconeogenesis, increasing hepatic glucose production.
Growth hormone	Normally inhibited by insulin, decreases the uptake of glucose by cells, therefore increasing blood glucose levels.

glycaemic control in critically ill patients, with the NICE SUGAR (Normoglycaemic in Intensive Care Evaluation and Survival Using Glucose Algorithm Regulation) Trial (Finfer et al. 2009) showing a 6.8% increase in episodes of hypoglycaemia in the intensively treated type 1 diabetic patient. Although IDDM patients are more prone to hypoglycaemic events than those with NIDDM, sulphonylurea medications can also lead to hypoglycaemic episodes (Shorr et al. 1997).

Pathophysiology

The body's normal response to low levels of blood glucose is to release stored glucose in the form of glycogen from the liver and muscles. Alpha cells in the pancreas secrete glucagon, one of the counter-regulator hormones released in response to low blood glucose levels (see Table 6.3) which converts glycogen to glucose by a process known as glycogenolysis (Porth 2007). Gluconeogenesis also takes place whereby amino acids and fats are converted to glucose to be used by the body for energy. Incorrect doses of insulin administered to in-patients may lead to a hypoglycaemic event whereby the demand for glucose outweighs the body's ability to convert stored glucose to the cells (Yale et al. 2001).

Presenting features

The onset of hypoglycaemia is often rapid, occurring within 15–30 minutes after the administration of subcutaneous insulin, but can be rapidly reversed if the nurse is aware of the initial signs and symptoms of hypoglycaemia and is able to initiate treatment quickly (Yale et al. 2001) (Box 6.3). Signs and symptoms of hypoglycaemia vary widely between each individual and can be grouped as either autonomic: sweating, anxiety, palpitations, warm sensation and nausea; or neuroglycopenic: yawning, tiredness, unco-ordinated movements, slurred speech, double vision, confusion, altered behaviour, coma and seizures (Kearney & Dang 2007). Neuroglycopenic symptoms usually occur first at blood glucose levels of 3.3–3.6 mml/L (Kearney & Dang 2007) but hypoglycaemia should be suspected in any patient who exhibits acute agitation, abnormal behaviour or impaired consciousness.

Box 6.3   Presenting features of hypoglycaemia

Shaking	Slurred speech
Cold, clammy skin	Difficulty in concentrating
Pins and needles in lips and tongue	Confusion or restlessness
Hunger and palpitations	Coma
Double vision	

Initial assessment and management

When assessing any patient with suspected hypoglycaemia, the ABCDE approach should be adopted (see Chapter 1 – Initial assessment). Adopt airway interventions that are appropriate for the patient's level of consciousness. Assess breathing and administer oxygen at 15 l/minute via a reservoir mask to unconscious patients. When administering oxygen in an emergency situation, it is important that local hospital guidelines are followed and that oxygen saturation is continuously monitored. The aim is to maintain SpO_2 between 94–98%. Secure intravenous access with a minimum 18 G cannula in a large peripheral vein and measure capillary blood glucose. This should be followed up with a laboratory blood glucose measurement. Measure and record the blood pressure and heart rate.

For patients who are conscious, 2–6 dextrose tablets or 15 g of a fast-acting carbohydrate should be given with a drink of milk to increase the blood glucose levels quickly. Those who are semi-conscious should be given glucose gel (e.g. GlucoGel) applied to their buccal mucosa (Baker et al. 2006). This should be repeated after 10–15 minutes as necessary.

If the patient is unconscious, give intravenous glucose solution via a large cannula according to local medical guidelines. Highly viscous glucose solutions (e.g. 50%) should be avoided due to their irritant effects on peripheral veins (Yale et al. 2001). Response to this treatment is usually rapid but if not, a repeat dose can be given. Once conscious, oral glucose or carbohydrate should be given and repeat blood glucose measurements recorded. If the hypoglycaemic episode is thought to have been caused by excess of oral medication or insulin, consider an intravenous infusion of 5–10% glucose as a maintenance regime.

After the initial management of any hypoglycaemic event, it is important to identify the cause in order to prevent further episodes. All patients with a severe hypoglycaemic event should be admitted for observation.

Hyperglycaemia and diabetic ketoacidosis

In any patient known to have diabetes, any acute illness may lead to hyperglycaemia and diabetic ketoacidosis (DKA) (Kitabchi et al. 2009). Classic signs of hyperglycaemia include increased thirst (polydipsia), urinary frequency (polyuria), increased hunger (polyphagia) and general fatigue. Once the cause of the raised blood sugar has been established and treatment commenced, patients

---

Box 6.4   Causes of DKA and HHS

Acute illness: myocardial infarction, pancreatitis, cerebrovascular accident
Severe trauma
Newly diagnosed type 1 diabetes mellitus
Surgery
Poor compliance with insulin regimes
Malfunction of insulin infusion devices
Psychological problems: eating disorders, purposeful insulin omission, acute stress
Infection: diarrhoea and vomiting, sepsis
Excessive alcohol intake
Cocaine use and other substance abuse
Medications that affect carbohydrate metabolism: glucocorticoids, thiazide diuretics, dobutamine, terbutaline, second-generation antipsychotics

---

usually recover quickly. If left untreated, however, hyperglycaemia can lead to the patient developing DKA.

Worldwide the most common precipitating cause of DKA and hyperosmolar hyperglycaemic syndrome (HHS) (see later) is infection, being responsible for nearly a quarter of all cases (Yehia et al. 2008). Other causes are outlined in Box 6.4. Patients with type 1 diabetes are at a significantly higher risk of developing DKA than those with type 2; however, patients with type 2 diabetes can develop DKA due to catabolic stress during an episode of critical illness. The incidence of this is low (Kisiel & Marsons 2009).

Pathophysiology

DKA is a medical emergency and a life-threatening condition usually developing over 24 hours or less (Trachtenbarg 2005). It is characterised by blood glucose above 12 mmol/L, the presence of ketonuria and an arterial blood pH of < 7.35. As such, it is a metabolic disorder consisting of co-existing hyperglycaemia, hyperketonaemia and metabolic acidosis. Glucose is an essential source of energy for body tissues, especially the brain and nervous system. In the absence of insulin, the body is unable to utilise glucose for cellular energy as insulin is needed to increase the permeability of cell membranes to glucose and other major electrolytes (Porth 2007). Under these circumstances, the body attempts to produce more glucose by the release of counter-regulatory hormones (Table 6.3) that initiate the processes of glycogenolysis (conversion of glycogen to glucose), gluconeogenesis (conversion of non-carbohydrates such as amino acids to glucose) and lipolysis (conversion of fats to fatty acids and glucose). These processes further increase blood glucose levels, leading to hyperglycaemia, which increases plasma osmolarity, thus shifting fluid from the intracellular and extracellular compartments into the intravascular space. This leads to extreme cellular dehydration. There is a resultant loss of cellular potassium, sodium and, to a lesser extent, phosphate due to osmotic fluid shift (Kisiel & Marsons 2009). This leads

---

Box 6.5   Degrees of acidosis associated with DKA

Mild: pH 7.25–7.30; HCO_3^- 15–18 mEq/L; mental state alert; blood glucose > 12 mmol/L
Moderate: pH 7.00–7.25; HCO_3^- 10–15 mEq/L; mental state drowsy; blood glucose > 12 mmol/L
Severe: pH <7.0; HCO_3^- <10 mEq/L; mental state – stupor, coma; blood glucose > 12 mmol/L

---

to cellular hypokalaemia and hyponatraemia but initial plasma hyperkalaemia and hypernatraemia.

Ketogenesis occurs due to the metabolism of fats leading to the formation of acetoacetic acid, acetone and beta-hydroxybutyric acid that precipitates a metabolic acidosis. Nitrogen is produced as a by-product of protein metabolism and leads to raised urea and blood nitrogen urea (BUN), thus compounding the metabolic acidosis as blood pH falls below normal ranges (7.35–7.45). The movement of potassium from the cells to the intravascular compartment leads to an increase in cellular hydrogen ions, thus compounding the acidosis. Ketone bodies are excreted in the urine and, collectively, with glucosuria, an osmotic diuresis ensues with resultant loss of serum sodium, potassium, phosphate and magnesium. The body's buffering system attempts to restore blood pH to normal limits by utilising bicarbonate and by excreting ketone bodies through the respiratory system (giving the characteristic 'pear drops' smell). Tidal volumes also increase leading to deep, laboured breathing (Kussmaul's respirations) (Porth 2007). If left untreated the neurological effects of osmotic fluid loss and acidosis leads to coma and death (see Box 6.5).

Presenting features

The classic features of DKA are polydipsia, polyuria initially, and polyphagia. Other presenting features include hyperglycaemia, nausea, vomiting, abdominal pain, lethargy, weight loss, increased respirations, palpitations, tachycardia, hypotension, dehydration and/or confusion, as explained in Box 6.6. symptoms of underlying infection may also be present.

Initial assessment and management

As with hypoglycaemia, assessment should be based upon the ABCDE approach and interventions made according to assessment findings. Monitoring and recording of airway patency and respiratory rate, depth and effort, along with administration of high-flow oxygen in accordance with hospital protocols, should be priorities of care. An arterial blood sample should be obtained to ascertain the level of metabolic acidosis and to identify any respiratory alkalosis, which may occur due to hyperventilation and lowered CO_2 levels. Cardiovascular status should be assessed promptly and intravenous access obtained quickly, ideally with two large-bore cannulae in large veins to enable fluid resuscitation if hypovolaemia is evident (De Beer et al. 2008). The patient should be monitored for cardiac arrhythmias and a 12-lead ECG obtained.

Blood samples should be obtained for serum glucose, urea and electrolytes, BUN, full blood count, amylase, blood cultures (should infection be considered as a

---

Box 6.6   Presenting features of hyperglycaemia and DKA

Polydipsia: due to osmotic diuresis and dehydration
Polyuria: due to osmotic diuresis secondary to hyperglycaemia
Hyperglycaemia: due to absolute deficiency in insulin and release of counter-regulatory hormones
Nausea, vomiting and abdominal pain: due to the production of ketone bodies
Lethargy and weight loss: due to lack of glucose available for the tissues to use as energy secondary to absolute insulin deficiency
Kussmaul's respirations: respiratory compensation for metabolic acidosis
Tachycardia: release of counter-regulatory hormones and stimulation of the sympathetic nervous system
Hypotension: secondary to dehydration, osmotic diuresis
Palpitations: due to alterations in potassium and other cellular electrolytes
Confusion/obtundation: due to cellular dehydration, altered sodium levels and acidosis of brain cells

---

potential cause) and liver function tests. Use the GCS to assess the patient's conscious level every 15 minutes and check the patient's urine by dipstick for the presence of ketones. Abdominal pain is a common presenting symptom of DKA and often resolves when the patient is managed with insulin and fluid resuscitation. Persistent abdominal pain despite correction of acidosis should be investigated to exclude pancreatitis and acute abdominal conditions (Nattrass 2002).

Treatment protocols may vary from hospital to hospital. This has led to the formulation of clinical guidelines outlining the management of DKA and HHS by the American Diabetes Association (De Beer et al. 2008; Yehia et al. 2008) in order to provide a standardised approach (Figure 6.4). The management of DKA incorporates the administration of insulin and fluids intravenously and the correction of electrolyte imbalances (in particular, potassium). To this end, intravenous insulin should be given by syringe pump at a rate of 0.1 iu/kg/h aimed at reducing blood glucose levels by no more than 4 mmol/h. It is important that blood glucose levels are not lowered too rapidly, to avoid potential complications of cerebral oedema (Brenner 2006). Patients with moderate to severe DKA may have an estimated total fluid loss of 5–8 litres with resultant hypovolaemic shock (Yehia et al. 2008). Consequently, fluid resuscitation is also a prime treatment objective with the overall goal being to replace half of the fluid deficit over the first 8 hours and the remaining fluid over the next 16 hours (Brenner 2006). There is a general consensus that one litre of 0.9% saline should be administered over the first hour to replace intracellular and extracellular volume and restore renal perfusion (Kitabchi et al. 2009). The degree of electrolyte imbalance must be assessed prior to the administration of potassium and insulin. Electrolytes should be re-checked hourly. Insulin should be withheld if serum potassium is below 3.3 mmol/L as serum potassium levels will fall with the administration of insulin. Likewise, if serum potassium is greater than 5.5 mmol/L, intravenous potassium should not be administered. Phosphate and magnesium levels are often altered in DKA (and HHS), however, replacement therapy is not routinely administered unless patients

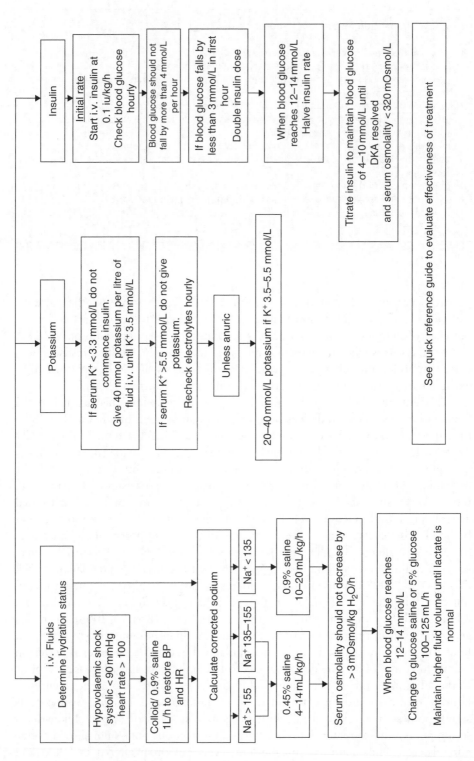

Figure 6.4 Diagnosis and management of diabetic ketoacidosis.

show signs of cardiac compromise or associated respiratory compromise (Kitabchi et al. 2006). Sudden falls in serum sodium levels can lead to cerebral oedema, therefore, the choice of resuscitation fluid must be carefully considered (Keays 2003). It is important to point out that local, evidence-based management regimes should be used according to the patient's situation.

Hyperosmolar hyperglycaemic state

Hyperosmolar hyperglycaemic state (HHS) is a diabetic emergency that is predominantly associated with type 2 diabetes managed by diet and/or oral medication. It is primarily observed in older patients and develops more insidiously than DKA, usually evolving over days or weeks (Kisiel & Marsons 2009). As with DKA, precipitating factors include concurrent or co-existing illness (e.g. infection) (see Box 6.4 above) and medications that affect carbohydrate metabolism, e.g. corticosteroids (Moore 2004). The slow evolution of HHS and co-existing underlying disease often makes this condition difficult to recognise and diagnose (Kisiel & Marsons 2009).

Pathophysiology

Both DKA and HHS manifest due to the elevation of counter-regulatory hormones, secondary to insulin deficiency leading to hyperglycaemia. The marked difference with HHS is minimal ketosis because of the small amounts of insulin present which suppresses lipolysis; hence, ketones are not produced. Ketonuria and metabolic acidosis, if present, are usually mild with a blood pH not less than 7.30 (Kitabchi et al. 2009). Compared to DKA, blood glucose is usually grossly elevated as residual insulin limits ketone production but is insufficient to control hyperglycaemia (Chiasson et al. 2003). The hyperosmolar state results in dehydration over days and weeks which can lead to poor renal function that exacerbates the hyperglycaemia due to poor glucose excretion.

Presenting features

Presenting features are common with those for DKA and include those associated with severe dehydration, neurological symptoms (e.g. seizures and/or coma), hyperglycaemia, hyperosmolality in the context of absent or minimal metabolic acidosis (Charalambous et al. 1999).

Initial assessment and management

Assessment is again based on ABCDE principles. Blood sugar levels are usually very high, often up to 80–100 mmol/L. It is rare for the patient with HHS to progress to unconsciousness; however, the same assessment and management strategies should be employed for the patients with HHS as for those with DKA, with the main difference being a reduced insulin dosage. Patients with HHS are very sensitive to insulin and there is a considerable risk of serum glucose levels falling too rapidly. Glucose levels may not decline initially and obese patients with type 2 diabetes may require larger doses of insulin to reduce serum glucose levels (Matz 1999; De Beer et al. 2008).

Nurses can play a pivotal role in recognising and responding to diabetic emergencies. With the integration of evidence-based protocols for the management of diabetic emergencies, the diabetic patient can be managed optimally, leading to better long-term outcomes and decreased length of stay in hospital.

C: DRUGS AND/OR ALCOHOL AS A CAUSE OF ALTERED CONSCIOUSNESS
(Ian Wood)

As previously indicated (Figure 6.1), 47% of the presenting causes of altered consciousness (excluding fits, syncope and hypoglycaemia) relate to the effects of drugs or alcohol; therefore, overdose of drugs and/or alcohol should be considered as a potential cause in any patient who is unconscious. The taking of a deliberate overdose may relate to the patient's pre-existing psychological problems in an attempt to cause self-harm or may be a spontaneous attempt to gain help. Accidental overdoses can occur when a patient unwittingly takes more than their usual dose of medication but it is important to remember that non-accidental overdoses occur when patients are deliberately given excessive amounts of medication (e.g. Munchausen's syndrome by proxy). The number of drugs that can cause an alteration in consciousness level is immense. For this reason, this chapter focuses on those agents which are most commonly associated with overdose, which are:

- aspirin (salicylate)
- paracetamol
- tricyclic anti-depressants
- alcohol
- opioids

Detailed information regarding poisons is available from National Poisons Centres (www.npis.org, www.toxbase.org).

Initial assessment

Assess all patients who have taken an overdose according to ABCDE principles, though initial assessment, treatment and investigations will usually have been carried out in the emergency department. It is important, however, to understand the importance of accurate history taking in cases of overdose. History should include details about the substance, how much was taken, when it was taken, whether it was taken with any other substances (e.g. alcohol) and why it was taken. Some patients will freely volunteer such information while others will deliberately withhold information or may try to mislead the history taker. All patients who have taken an overdose should receive a psychiatric referral to allow expert assessment of their mental health status.

Overdose of aspirin (salicylates)

Four categories may be used when assessing the potential severity of an acute, single event of non-enteric-coated, salicylate ingestion:

- Less than 150 mg/kg – no toxicity to mild toxicity
- From 150–300 mg/kg – mild to moderate toxicity
- From 301–500 mg/kg – serious toxicity
- Greater than 500 mg/kg – potentially lethal toxicity

Kreplick (2009)

Pathophysiology

After ingestion, aspirin is rapidly metabolised to form salicylic acid. Large overdoses can result in the development of a large mass of tablets in the stomach, with a resultant rise in serum salicylate levels for up to 20 hours after ingestion. Salicylate causes disruption of cellular function leading to catabolism secondary to the inhibition of ATP-dependent reactions with the following physiological results:

- increased oxygen consumption
- increased carbon dioxide production
- depletion of hepatic glycogen
- hyperpyrexia

Acid–base disturbances vary depending on the form of ingested aspirin (e.g. enteric-coated products are more slowly absorbed), the patient's age and their previous renal function, and the severity of the intoxication. Initially, a respiratory alkalosis develops secondary to direct stimulation of the respiratory centre. This may be the only consequence of a mild overdose. The kidneys excrete potassium, sodium and bicarbonate resulting in alkaline urine. A severe metabolic acidosis with compensatory respiratory alkalosis may develop in cases of severe overdose. Resulting excretion of hydrogen ions produces acidic urine (Kreplick 2009).

Presenting features

Clinical features that may be evident when a patient has ingested an overdose of aspirin are shown in Box 6.7.

Immediate management and investigations

Management priorities follow the ABCDE principles and specifically include prevention of absorption, correction of fluid deficits and acid–base abnormalities, and enhancement of excretion and elimination. To this end, consider gastric lavage

---

Box 6.7   Presenting features of aspirin (salicylate) overdose

Restlessness	Hyperventilation
Tachycardia	Hyperpyrexia
Tinnitus	Dehydration
Deafness	Confusion
Sweating	Hypotension
Blurred vision	Unconsciousness*
Epigastric pain	Seizures*
Nausea/vomiting	*Indicates severe toxicity.

---

if > 10 g has been ingested and the patient attends within 1 hour of ingestion. Give 50 g activated charcoal orally or via gastric tube after lavage. If the patient has features of salicylate toxicity, give further doses of 12.5 g activated charcoal every hour to a total dose of 200 g (Bedside Clinical Guidelines Partnership 2009). If the patient has taken < 10 g of aspirin, simply give 50 g of activated charcoal. Activated charcoal acts by absorbing drugs but only absorbs 10% of its own weight (i.e. 50 g of charcoal will absorb 5 g of drug).

Results of investigations will determine further treatment. Take blood samples for urea and electrolytes, creatinine, glucose and salicylate levels. Measure arterial blood gases and urine pH. If plasma salicylate levels are ≤ 3.6 mmol/L, rehydrate with oral fluids or intravenously if vomiting. If levels are > 3.6 mmol/L, consider alkaline diuresis provided renal function is within normal limits (creatinine < 150 μmol/L) and heart failure or shock are not present. Forced diuresis is not recommended as alkalinisation of the urine is more difficult when urine flow is greater. If the patient has taken a potentially fatal dose of modified-release or enteric-coated aspirin, consider whole bowel irrigation (e.g. using polyethylene glycol) to decrease the transit time of the tablets through the gut. Patients who fail to respond or show continuing deterioration may require haemodialysis.

Overdose of paracetamol

In England and Wales, on average approximately 130 deaths per year can be directly attributed to paracetamol alone (Office for National Statistics 2009). It is a relatively common presenting complaint to emergency departments.

Pathophysiology

The maximum recommended dose of paracetamol is 4 g per day in adults. In these therapeutic doses, the drug is mostly metabolised by the liver although 5% is excreted by the kidney. In cases of overdose (> 12 g or 150 mg/kg body weight), the normal metabolic processes within the liver become saturated, causing depletion of hepatic glutathione and the production of toxic metabolites. These metabolites cause hepatocellular death and subsequent centrilobular liver necrosis (Farrell 2010).

Presenting features

Many people have a misguided belief that an overdose of paracetamol will cause unconsciousness. It does not; indeed, it causes few, if any, presenting features. Nausea and vomiting may be present if a hepatotoxic dose has been ingested but these features usually occur more than 24 hours after ingestion. Serious liver complications of an overdose usually occur 3–4 days after an overdose; right subcostal pain along with nausea, vomiting and/or jaundice may indicate liver necrosis. Occasionally, patients may present even later with complications such as hypoglycaemia, bleeding and confusion (Moulton & Yates 2006).

Immediate management and investigations

Gastric lavage is no longer indicated for paracetamol overdose, as activated charcoal is more effective at reducing absorption. If the patient has taken > 12 g or 150 mg/kg and presents within 2 hours of ingestion, give 50 g activated charcoal either orally or via a nasogastric tube (BCGP 2009).

Collect blood samples for paracetamol levels 4 hours after ingestion. This time can be extended up to 16 hours after ingestion if the patient has delayed their presentation to hospital. Compare levels with the treatment graph in Figure 6.5. Treat patients whose levels are above, on or even slightly below the treatment line with intravenous N-acetylcysteine in 5% glucose. The treatment regime is as follows:

- 150 mg/kg in 150 mL 5% glucose over 15 minutes followed by
- 50 mg/kg in 500 mL 5% glucose over 4 hours followed by
- 100 mg/kg in 1000 mL 5% glucose over 16 hours

BCGP (2009)

In patients who present 24–36 hours after an overdose (where time of ingestion is confirmed), detection of paracetamol in the plasma indicates a very substantial overdose or one that has been taken over a period of time. Ongoing management of all patients who have taken significant paracetamol overdoses includes measurement of their FBC, INR (international normalised ratio), liver function tests, urea and electrolytes (in particular, creatinine and phosphate) and blood glucose.

Overdose of tricyclic antidepressants

Overdose of tricyclic antidepressants (TCAs) can be dangerous, with over 20% of fatal ingestions involving this category of drug (e.g. dothiepin and amitriptyline). In 2009, 107 deaths in England and Wales resulted from overdose of TCAs (Office of National Statistics 2009).

Pathophysiology

TCAs are rapidly absorbed in the alkaline conditions of the gastrointestinal tract and, consequently, toxicity may become apparent as early as the first hour after an

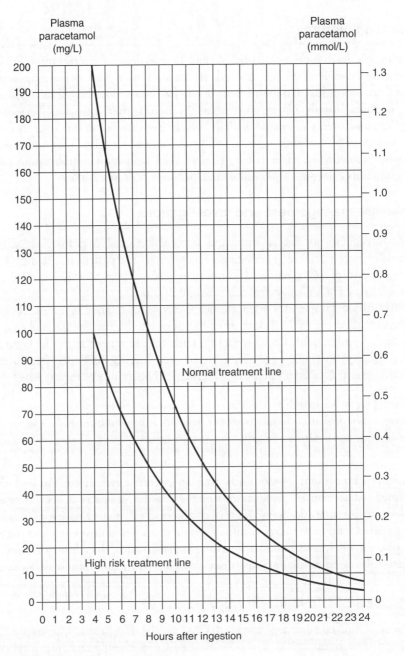

Plasma
paracetamol
(mg/L)

Plasma
paracetamol
(mmol/L)

Normal treatment line

High risk treatment line

Hours after ingestion

Figure 6.5   Treatment graph for paracetamol overdose.

overdose. In cases of mixed overdose, symptoms may take several hours to appear
if the combination of ingested drugs has caused delayed gastric emptying. Toxic
levels of TCAs have peripheral and central anticholinergic effects and cause cardiac
depression due to sodium channel blockade. The latter leads to delayed myocardial

Box 6.8   Presenting features of tricyclic antidepressant overdose

Dry mouth	Urinary retention
Blurred vision	Depressed respiration*
Drowsiness	Tachycardia/arrhythmias*
Dilated pupils	Hypotension*
Muscle twitching	Seizures*
Hypertonia/hyperreflexia	Unconsciousness*
Hypothermia or hyperpyrexia	
Excitement/visual hallucinations	*Indicates severe toxicity.

conduction with prolonged PR, QRS and QT intervals on the ECG. Progressive toxicity leads to tachycardia, ventricular bigeminy and ventricular fibrillation.

Presenting features

The effects of a TCA overdose usually occur within 12 hours of ingestion and presenting features are varied (see Box 6.8).

Immediate management and investigations

As always, assessment and management of ABCDE priorities is fundamental. Consider gastric lavage if patient presents within 1 hour of ingestion and if the overdose is potentially serious (>750 mg). Give 50 g of activated charcoal orally or via a nasogastric tube. Monitor the patient and record a 12-lead ECG. Measure arterial blood gases and correct metabolic acidosis if accompanied by hypotension. Further treatment and management is dependent on presenting features.

Overdose of alcohol (ethanol)

Ingestion of alcohol is a common cause of altered consciousness. Alcohol may be taken in isolation but may also accompany ingestion of other substances. It may also be associated with a head injury.

Pathophysiology

Ethanol has sedative-hypnotic effects on the CNS which cause many of the features above. It is rapidly absorbed by the gastrointestinal tract and is metabolised by the liver to form water and carbon dioxide. Alcohol also suppresses gluconeogenesis in the liver, which leads to hypoglycaemia.

Presenting features

The features of alcohol ingestion (see Box 6.9) depend upon the amount taken and how well the patient tolerates its physiological effects.

Box 6.9   Presenting features of alcohol overdose

Slurred speech	Smell of alcohol on breath
Ataxia	Altered consciousness level
Loss of inhibitions	Hypoglycaemia
Loss of judgement	Gastric irritation
Aggression	Nausea/vomiting
Irritability	Postural hypotension
Red conjunctivae	Respiratory depression

It is important to remember that the smell of alcohol on a patient's breath does not necessarily mean that they are intoxicated. Other causes of altered consciousness must be considered especially if a head injury exists.

Immediate management and investigations

Management is based on ABCDE principles. In the patient with altered conscious level, ensure that their airway is maintained and supplemental oxygen given if tolerated. Ensure that breathing and circulatory status are satisfactory. Measure capillary blood glucose and send blood samples for laboratory investigation. Record the patient's GCS regularly, especially if a head injury is suspected. If wounds are present, check the patient's antitetanus status.

Overdose of opioids

Opioids can be divided into natural (e.g. morphine and codeine), semi-synthetic (e.g. heroin) and synthetic substances (e.g. methadone). Opioids which can be taken by oral or intravenous routes may result in overdose following therapeutic administration or recreational use.

Pathophysiology

Opioids have effects on neurotransmission in the CNS and peripheral nervous system (PNS). Physiological effects include analgesia, euphoria, respiratory depression, pinpoint pupils and sedation (Stephens 2010).

Presenting features

Features of narcotic overdose usually appear within minutes of intravenous administration or within 20–30 minutes if taken orally. The features outlined in Box 6.10 may be present.

> **Box 6.10   Presenting features of opioid overdose**
>
> Altered consciousness level
> Respiratory depression
> Hypothermia
> Non-cardiogenic pulmonary oedema
>
> Bradycardia
> Hypotension
> Pinpoint pupils (miosis)
> Reduced gut motility

Immediate management and investigations

Management of the patient's airway, breathing and circulation is particularly important as the support of breathing with a bag-valve-mask and oxygen will be required if respiratory depression is evident. Administration of intravenous naloxone 0.4–2.0 mg restores CNS and cardiopulmonary functions rapidly. If no response, repeat doses every 2–3 minutes may be given to a maximum of 10 mg. If respiratory function deteriorates, further doses may be required and, in cases of severe opioid intoxication, a naloxone infusion may be commenced.

Summary

This chapter has focused on a range of conditions that may cause an alteration in the patient's conscious level. In some cases, identification of the underlying condition may be relatively simple while in others there may be no obvious cause. It is important to reiterate that, whatever the cause of the altered consciousness, assessment and management of the patient's airway, breathing, circulation and neurological disability is of paramount importance. Similarly, once a diagnosis has been made and treatment given, management of the patient's ABCDEs must continue until definitive care is given.

References

Baker H, Horton A, Low P et al. (2006) 'HYPOBOX' a practical aid in the Management of hypoglycaemia in hospital. *Diabetic Medicine*, 23, 186.

Bedside Clinical Guidelines Partnership (2010) *Medical Guidelines: General Adult Medicine*. West Mercia: Bedside Clinical Guidelines Partnership.

Begg N, Cartwright K, Cohen J et al. (1999) Consensus Statement on Diagnosis, Investigation, Treatment and Prevention of Acute Bacterial Meningitis in Immunocompetent Adults. *Journal of Infection*, (39), 1–15.

Brenner Z (2006) Management of hyperglycaemic emergencies. *AACN Clinical issue* 17(1), 56–65.

Charalambous C, Schofield I & Malik R (1999) Acute diabetic emergencies and their management. *Care of the Critically Ill* 15(4), 132–135.

Chen Z, Sandercock P & Pan H (2000) Indications for early aspirin use in acute ischaemic stroke: A combined analysis of 40,000 randomised patients from the Chinese acute stroke trial and the international stroke trial. On behalf of the CAST and IST collaborative groups. *Stroke* (31): 1240–1249.

Chiasson J, Aris-Jilwan N, Belanger R et al. (2003). Diagnosis and management of diabetic ketoacidosis and the hyperglycaemic hyperosmolar state *Canadian Medical Association Journal*, 168(7), 859–866.

Coyle P (1999) Glucocorticoids in central nervous system bacterial infection. *Archives of Neurology*, (56), 796–801.

De Beer K, Michael S, Thacker M et al. (2008) Diabetic ketoacidosis and hyperglycaemic hyperosmolar syndrome – clinical guidelines. *Nursing in Critical Care*, 13(1), 5–11.

Department of Health (2007) *National Stroke Strategy*. London: Department of Health. www.dh.gov.uk/en/Publicationsandstatistics/Publications/PublicationsPolicyAnd Guidance/DH_081062 (accessed 25 October 2010).

Farrell S (2010) Acetaminophen toxicity. *Emedicine*. www.emedicine.com/emerg/topic819. htm (accessed 11 June 2011).

Finfer S, Chittock DR, Su Sy et al. (2009) The NICE-SUGAR Study: Intensive versus conventional glucose control in critically ill patients. *New England Journal of Medicine*, 360, 1283–1297.

Hacke W, Kaste M, Fieschi C and the Second European-Australasian Acute Stroke Study Investigators (1998) Randomised double-blind placebo controlled trial of thrombolytic therapy with intravenous alteplase in acute ischemic stroke (ECASS II). *Lancet*, 352, 1245–1251.

Kearney T & Dang C (2007) Diabetic and endocrine emergencies. *Postgraduate Medical Journal*, 83, 79–86.

Keays R (2003) Diabetic emergencies. In: Bersten A, Oh TE & Soni N (eds), *Oh's Intensive Care Manual* (5th edition). Oxford: Butterworth-Heinemann.

Kisiel M & Marsons L (2009) Recognizing and responding to hyperglycaemic emergencies. *British Journal of Nursing*, 18(18), 1094–1098.

Kitabchi A, Murphy M, Umpierrez G & Kreisberg R (2006) Hyperglycaemic crisis in adult patients with diabetes: A consensus statement from the American Diabetes Association. *Diabetes Care*, 29(12), 2739–2748.

Kitabchi A, Miles J, Umpierrez G & Fisher J (2009). Hyperglycaemic crisis in adult patients with diabetes. *Diabetes Care*, 32(7), 1335–1343.

Kreplick L (2009) Salicylate toxicity. *Emedicine*. www.emedicine.com/emerg/topic514.htm (accessed 11 June 2011).

Lempert T, Bauer M & Schmidt D (1994) Syncope: A videometric analysis of 56 episodes of transient cerebral hypoxia. *Annals of Neurology*, (36), 233–237.

Lingenfelter T, Buettner U, Martin J et al. (1995) Improvement of impaired counter regulatory hormone response and symptom perception by short-term avoidance of hypoglycaemia in IDDM. *Diabetes Care*, 18, 321–325.

Matz R (1999) Management of hyperosmolar hyperglycaemic syndrome. *American Family Physician*, 60, 1468–1476.

Moller K & Skinhoj P (2000) Guidelines for managing acute bacterial meningitis. *BMJ* (320), 1290.

Moore T (2004) Diabetic emergencies in adults. *Nursing Standard*, 18(46), 45–52.

Moulton C & Yates D (2006) *Lecture Notes on Emergency Medicine* (3rd edition). Oxford: Blackwell Science.

Muir K (2001) Medical management of Stroke. *Journal of Neurology, Neurosurgery and Psychiatry* (70):i12–16.

National Institute of Neurological Disorders and Stroke rt-PA Stroke Study Group (1995) Tissue plasminogen activator for acute ischemic stroke. *New England Journal of Medicine*, (333), 1581–1587.

National Institute of Neurological Disorders and Stroke tPA Stroke Study Group (1997) Generalized efficacy of tPA for acute stroke: Subgroup analysis of the NINDS tPA stroke trial. *Stroke*, 28, 2119–2125.

Nattrass M (2002) Diabetic ketoacidosis. *Medicine Publishing*, 34(3), 51–53.

Nor A, Davis J, Sen B, et al. (2005) The Recognition of Stroke in the Emergency Room (ROSIER) scale: Development and validation of a stroke recognition instrument. *Lancet Neurology*, 4(11), 727–734.

Office for National Statistics (2009) *Numbers of deaths from drug-related poisoning by sex and underlying cause of death, England and Wales 1993–2009*. www.statistics.gov.uk/ (accessed 11 November 2010).

Porth C (2007) *Essential of Pathophysiology: Concepts of Altered Health Status*. Philadelphia: Lippincott Williams & Wilkins.

Scottish Intercollegiate Guidelines Network (2005) *Diagnosis and Management of Epilepsy in Adults: A national clinical guideline*. Edinburgh: SIGN.

Shorr R, Ray W, Daugherty J et al. (1997) Incidence and risk factors for serious hypoglycaemia in older persons using insulin or sulfonylureas. *Archives of International Medicine*, 157, 1681–1686.

Shorvon S (2001) The management of status epilepticus. *Journal of Neurology, Neurosurgery and Psychiatry (Suppl. II)* (70), ii22–27.

Soal E, Garzons S, Garcia-Torres S et al. (2006) Management of diabetic ketoacidosis in a tertiary hospital. *Acta Diabetologia*, 43, 127–130.

Stephens E (2010) Opioids toxicity. www.emedicine.com/emerg/topic330.htm (accessed 11 June 2011).

Trachtenbarg D (2005) Diabetic ketoacidosis. *American Family Physician*, 71(9), 1705–1714.

Van Gijn J & Rinkel G (2001) Subarachnoid haemorrhage: Diagnosis, causes and management. *Brain*, (124), 249–278.

Van der Wee N, Rinkel G, Hasan D & van Gijn J (1995) Detection of subarachnoid haemorhage on early CT: Is lumbar puncture still needed after a negative scan? *Journal of Neurology, Neurosurgery and Psychiatry*, 58; 357–359.

Vermeulen M & van Gijn J (1990) The diagnosis of subarachnoid haemorrhage [Review]. *Journal of Neurology, Neurosurgery and Psychiatry*, 53, 365–372.

Yale J, Begg L, Gerstein H, et al. (2001) Canadian Diabetes Association Clinical practice guidelines for the prevention and management of hypoglycaemia in diabetes. *Canadian Journal of Diabetes*, 26(1), 22–23.

Yehia B, Epps K & Golden S (2008) Diagnosis and management of diabetic ketoacidosis in adults. *Hospital Physician*, 35, 21–26.

7 Shortness of Breath

Michelle Garner, Susan Hope and Ian Wood

Aims

This chapter will:

- describe the initial assessment and management of patients who present with shortness of breath
- describe the causes, pathophysiology, investigations and immediate management of the most common causes of shortness of breath

---

Causes

The most common causes of acute shortness of breath are outlined in Box 7.1.

Box 7.1 Most common causes of acute shortness of breath

Acute respiratory failure
Chronic obstructive pulmonary disease
Asthma
Community acquired pneumonia
Pneumothorax
Acute heart failure
Cardiac arrhythmia (see Chapter 4 – Cardiac arrest)
Pulmonary embolism (see Chapter 8 – Chest pain)
Myocardial infarction (see Chapter 8 – Chest pain)

Clinical features

Table 7.1 outlines the clinical features that commonly accompany shortness of breath due to a specific cause.

Initial Management of Acute Medical Patients: A Guide for Nurses and Healthcare Practitioners,
Second Edition. Edited by Ian Wood and Michelle Garner.
© 2012 John Wiley & Sons, Ltd. Published 2012 by John Wiley & Sons, Ltd.

Table 7.1 Clinical features that commonly accompany shortness of breath due to a specific cause

Condition causing shortness of breath	Associated features
Acute respiratory failure	Cyanosis Drowsiness Confusion Tiredness Reduced respiratory rate and effort Loss of consciousness and respiratory arrest
Exacerbation of COPD (GOLD 2010)	Increased shortness of breath Increased cough Increased sputum purulence Increased sputum volume Chest tightness Increased wheeze Pyrexia *Signs associated with very severe COPD*: Pyrexia Purulent sputum Severe airways obstruction with audible wheeze Use of accessory muscles Paradoxical chest wall movements Peripheral oedema Haemodynamic instability Signs of right-sided heart failure Worsening or new-onset cyanosis Reduced alertness or change in mental status
Asthma (British Thoracic Society/ Scottish Intercollegiate Guidelines Network 2011)	*Acute severe*: Peak expiratory flow (PEF) <50% of predicted or best Can't complete sentences in one breath $SpO_2 \geq 92\%$ Respirations ≥25 breaths per minute Heart rate ≥110 bpm *Life-threatening*: PEF <33% of predicted or best $SpO_2 < 92\%$ Silent chest, cyanosis, or feeble respiratory effort Bradycardia, arrhythmia or hypotension Exhaustion, confusion or coma
Spontaneous pneumothorax	Dyspnoea Pain on inspiration Reduced breath sounds on affected side
Tension pneumothorax	Increased respiratory rate and effort Tachycardia Sweating Inability to speak Inequality of chest movement Distended neck veins Cyanosis Tracheal deviation

(continued)

Table 7.1   (cont'd)

Condition causing shortness of breath	Associated features
Acute heart failure	Dyspnoea
	Tachypnoea
	Pallor or cyanosis
	Diaphoresis
	Anxiety
	Tachycardia
	Cool peripheries
	Possible hypotension
	Cough
	Pink, frothy sputum
	Oliguria

Initial assessment

Assessment of patients presenting with shortness of breath (defined as a respiratory rate greater than 20 breaths per minute) (Adam et al. 2010) is based on the ABCDE principles outlined in Chapter 1 – Initial assessment. The following items relate specifically to the assessment of patients who are short of breath. It is important to remember that an elevated respiratory rate is often one of the first signs of deterioration in a patient's condition.

Airway

- Ensure that the cause of shortness of breath is not related to an airway obstruction
- Treat any airway obstruction

Breathing

- Record respiratory rate, depth and pattern of breathing
- Record and monitor SpO_2 by pulse oximetry
- Assess equality of chest expansion
- Auscultate for equality of air entry
- Assess use of accessory muscles – is the patient making a lot of effort to breathe? Is breathing paradoxical?
- Observe for signs of fatigue or respiratory distress including mouth opening, pursed-lip breathing and flaring of the nostrils
- Observe for skin retraction around ribs and clavicles
- Is the patient short of breath at rest?
- Is this a new or sudden onset of shortness of breath?
- Assess the patient's ability to complete sentences or to voice single words only

- Listen for wheeze (inspiratory and/or expiratory) or other breath sounds. (Rattling and crackles occur with secretions, while a high-pitched stridor suggests partial obstruction of the upper airway)
- Observe the patient's position. (Are they sitting upright to maximise lung capacity? Is the shortness of breath worse when lying flat?)
- Feel the position of the patient's trachea (deviation may indicate tension pneumothorax)
- Is there any pain associated with breathing?
- Record peak expiratory flow rate (PEFR)
- Assess any cough and the nature and volume of sputum
- Observe skin colour for central and peripheral cyanosis

Circulation

- Measure capillary refill (normal < 2 seconds)
- Record heart rate, rhythm and strength of pulse
- Record blood pressure

Disability

- Assess consciousness level and changes in consciousness
- Check pupil reactions
- Assess anxiety level
- Assess pain (i.e. on inspiration, expiration, associated with activity) using the PQRST mnemonic

Exposure

- Undress the patient
- Record temperature
- Assess skin temperature and appearance
- Record capillary blood glucose (e.g. BM stix, glucostix)

Concurrent to the initial ABCDE assessment, gather a history of the patient's presenting complaint and previous medical history (see Chapter 1 – Initial assessment). Information from family and friends can give a valuable insight into the following issues relating to respiratory problems:

- known risk factors for respiratory disease
- previous admissions
- social history
- smoking habits
- recent changes in respiratory status
- prescribed medications (e.g. nebulisers, theophyllines, long-term oxygen therapy)

Table 7.2 Emergency oxygen use in adult patients (British Thoracic Society 2008)

Recommendation	Critical illness	Critically ill patients with COPD
In critical illness, initially give oxygen via a reservoir mask at 15 L/min Once stable, reduce oxygen and maintain SpO_2 at 94–98%	Cardiac arrest/resuscitation Shock, sepsis or anaphylaxis Major pulmonary haemorrhage Major head injury Carbon monoxide poisoning Near drowning Major trauma	In patients with COPD, aim for same target SpO_2 initially, but take urgent ABGs. Give controlled oxygen or non-invasive ventilation if severe hypoxaemia with respiratory acidosis
	In seriously ill patients with $SpO_2 <85\%$, give initial oxygen via reservoir mask at 15 L/min	
	Specific guidance for patients with COPD	
First step for all patients with risk factors for hypercapnia but no past history of respiratory acidosis: Prior to ABGs give 28% oxygen via venturi mask at 4 L/min. Maintain SpO_2 88–92%	If history of respiratory acidosis, give oxygen at 24% via venturi mask at 2–4 L/min. Maintain SpO_2 88–92% pending urgent ABGs	Or, give oxygen to the pre-determined SpO_2 levels specified by the patient's oxygen alert card using their own venturi mask (if they have one)
Second step once ABGs available: If $PaCO_2$ normal and no past history of respiratory acidosis, give oxygen to maintain SpO_2 94–98%. Re-check ABGs after 30–60 min or if deterioration	If $PaCO_2$ raised but pH 7.35 or more, maintain SpO_2 88–92%, re-check ABGs 30–60 min	If $PaCO_2$ raised and pH <7.35 (acidosis) consider non-invasive ventilation

- recent changes in medication
- recent exposure to allergens or chemicals
- occupational hazards
- recent illness or injury

Immediate management

Position the patient so that they are in the best possible position to breathe (usually upright, well-supported by pillows) in a well-ventilated area. Give oxygen therapy according to British Thoracic Society (2008) guidelines (see Table 7.2). Initial oxygen therapy should be given via nasal cannulae at 2–6 L/min or via simple face mask at 5–10 L/min to maintain SpO_2 at 94–98% (92–98% in patients over 70 years of age). Change to a reservoir mask at 15 L/min if target range is not achieved or if the patient is critically ill. For patients with COPD or other risk factors for hypercapnia (including previous treatment with non-invasive ventilation, tracheal intubation or past history of acidosis), the initial target SpO_2 is 88–92%. If ABGs reveal normal pCO_2 in patients with COPD then target SpO2 is 94–98%. It is important to note that if a diagnosis or past history is unavailable, all patients experiencing a life-threatening emergency should be given high concentrations of oxygen. In patients with a known past history of COPD, a useful assessment, while waiting for the ABG result, is to look for signs of carbon dioxide retention which include flushing, dilated peripheral veins (warm peripheries), bounding pulse, headache, altered consciousness, drowsiness and flapping tremor (Esmond & Mikelsons 2009).

Observe for signs of central and peripheral cyanosis. Give nebulised salbutamol 2.5–5 mg or terbutaline 5–10 mg to patients with suspected asthma or COPD. Record a 12-lead ECG if acute heart failure, pulmonary embolism or a cardiac arrhythmia are suspected and commence continuous cardiac monitoring of heart rate and rhythm. Ensure that intravenous access is secured. Monitor SpO_2, respiratory rate and effort continuously and observe for signs of deterioration (see Box 7.2). Gain senior medical advice if any symptoms of deterioration occur.

Box 7.2   Signs of respiratory deterioration

Increased respiratory rate (especially over 30 breaths per min)
Reduced SpO_2
Increasing oxygen required to keep SpO_2 in target range
Raised early warning/trigger score
CO_2 retention
Drowsiness
Headache
Flushed face
Tremor

Source: British Thoracic Society (2008)

A: RESPIRATORY FAILURE
(Michelle Garner, based on the original chapter
by Jacqueline Mitchell)

Introduction

Respiratory failure can be broadly defined as the impairment of pulmonary gas exchange leading to hypoxaemia (low arterial oxygen $PaO_2 < 8$ kPa) and/or hypercapnia (high arterial carbon dioxide $PaCO_2 > 6.5$ kPa) (Francis 2006).

Causes

The main causes of respiratory failure are listed in Box 7.3.

Box 7.3   Possible causes of respiratory failure

Respiratory system
Asthma
ARDS
Pneumonia
COPD/emphysema
Infection
Trauma/contusions
Pneumothorax
Haemothorax
Fibrosis
Aspiration
Near drowning
Thoracic surgery
Sleep apnoea

Central/peripheral nervous system
Cerebrovascular accident
Raised intracranial pressure
Drugs (sedatives/opiates)
Neurological injury
Guillain Barré syndrome
Tetanus
Failure to reverse anaesthesia

Circulatory system
Pulmonary oedema
Heart failure
Pulmonary embolus
Myocardial infarction

Neuromuscular system
Motor neurone disease
Multiple sclerosis
Myasthenia gravis

Chest wall deformity
Muscular dystrophy
Kyphoscoliosis
Chest wall deformity

Other causes
Cardiorespiratory arrest
Airway obstruction
Poisons (carbon monoxide, organophosphates)
Muscle relaxant drugs
Anaphylaxis
Fat embolism
Morbid obesity
Smoke inhalation
Status epilepticus

Pathophysiology

In broad terms, respiratory failure is caused by a failure in oxygenation and/or ventilation. Failure in oxygenation is usually due to a ventilation/perfusion (V/Q) mismatch. There may be adequate perfusion with inadequate ventilation (for example, in pneumonia) or adequate ventilation with inadequate perfusion (for example, in pulmonary embolism) (Hurst 2009). Failure in ventilation, for example due to hypoventilation, may occur due to depression of the respiratory centre caused by drugs, or may be caused by trauma, neuromuscular skeletal disorders or morbid obesity (Francis 2006). In practical terms, respiratory failure is said to exist when arterial oxygen (pO_2) is < 8.0 kPa and arterial carbon dioxide (pCO_2) is > 6.5–7.0 kPa. The pathophysiological mechanism of respiratory failure depends on the underlying condition(s) (Box 7.3). The most common primary lung disorders causing respiratory failure are COPD, asthma, chest infection (pneumonia) and adult respiratory distress syndrome (ARDS) (Copstead & Banasik 2000). It is important to remember that a satisfactory cardiac output is required to maintain optimal respiratory function. In addition, an adequate haemoglobin level is needed to deliver cellular oxygen (Field 2000).

Respiratory failure, or failure to breathe adequately, can be categorised into two types.

Type I respiratory failure

Type I failure is essentially acute hypoxaemia (low arterial oxygen) with a normal carbon dioxide level. This type of respiratory failure is usually due to a sudden acute cause (e.g. hypoventilation [RR < 10/min], acute pulmonary oedema, pneumonia, asthma, pulmonary embolism, pneumothorax) in a patient with previously 'normal' lungs and is, therefore, usually reversible (Esmond & Mikelsons 2009).

Table 7.3   Classification of respiratory failure

Normal values	Type I respiratory failure	Type II respiratory failure
pO_2 10–13.3 kPa	$pO_2 < 8$ kPa	$pO_2 < 8$ kPa
pCO_2 4.8–6.1 kPa	Normal or low PCO_2	$pCO_2 > 6.5$ kPa
pH 7.35–7.45	Normal pH	Low pH < 7.35
SpO_2	$<92\%$	$<92\%$

NB: A stable high pCO_2 can occur in patients with severe stable COPD.
ABG values represent the patient's condition at the time of assessment only and will change according to the treatment and/or underlying condition.

Box 7.4   Presenting features of respiratory failure

Alteration of breathing pattern
Tachypnoea
Bradypnoea
Cough
Noisy breathing
Pursed lip breathing
Cyanosis
Upright positioning/orthopnoea (i.e. inability to lie flat)
Inability to complete sentences
Use of accessory muscles
Apnoea/periods of apnoea
Drowsiness/confusion/agitation
Headache
Hypertension
Hypotension
Cardiac arrhythmias/tachycardia/bradycardia
Cool, clammy skin
Warm, pink skin
Pyrexia
Pain on breathing

Type II respiratory failure

Type II failure is characterised by hypoxaemia in addition to elevated pCO_2 level (usually > 6.5 kPa). This occurs when alveolar ventilation is insufficient to excrete the volume of CO_2 being produced by tissue metabolism (Field 2000) and is usually a consequence of a long-term disease such as COPD (Table 7.3).

Presenting features

The presenting features of respiratory failure depend on the underlying cause. Box 7.4 outlines the most important features of respiratory failure.

Noisy breathing may be heard on auscultation or often without a stethoscope. Stridor is a high-pitched noise often associated with the presence of a foreign body or obstruction or by presence of laryngeal oedema, often associated with the upper airway. A wheeze is another high-pitched sound that can occur during inspiration and/or expiration, associated with air moving through narrowed airways (Adam et al. 2010). Persistent cough may be apparent in the presence of infection and may be very distressing (Francis 2006).

Shortness of breath may be characterised by tachypnoea or bradypnoea. Tachypnoea (RR > 20/min) indicates increased work of breathing and is usually one of the first indications of respiratory distress (Adam et al. 2010). Bradypnoea (RR < 10/min) can indicate hypoventilation or deterioration in condition often due to sedatives, opiates or hypothermia. The patient may be so breathless that they are unable to complete full sentences. Similarly, there may be alteration to the breathing pattern. Respirations may be deep or shallow. Cheyne-Stokes breathing involves a mixture of deep breaths, shallow breaths and periods of apnoea, caused by changes in blood flow to the respiratory centre (Bucher & Melander 1999). In Kussmaul's breathing, deep regular breaths are caused by the respiratory system's response to a metabolic imbalance (e.g. diabetic ketoacidosis) in an attempt to excrete CO_2 via the respiratory system (Bucher & Melander 1999).

Upright positioning may be observed as the patient attempts to relieve dyspnoea and increase the capacity of the lungs. The use of accessory muscles (in the neck, shoulders and abdomen) indicates increased work of breathing due to an increase in oxygen demand. The patient may experience difficulty breathing in (when upper airway obstruction is present, for example) and on breathing out (in asthma, for example) (Adam et al. 2010). Pursed-lip breathing and open-mouth breathing may be seen together. Open-mouth breathing is an attempt to decrease dead space (within the upper respiratory system) and pursed-lip breathing occurs on expiration in an attempt to increase lung compliance and increase gas exchange (Field 2000).

Cyanosis may be peripheral (e.g. nail beds) or central (e.g. lips, oral cavity, tongue). The bluish skin colour is caused by the circulation of unoxygenated blood (appearing blue rather than red). Central cyanosis of the lips and tongue indicates a very serious problem and requires immediate treatment with high concentration oxygen.

Cough may be productive or non-productive and may involve haemoptysis. Pink frothy secretions are associated with pulmonary oedema (Lewis 1999) (see section E – Acute Heart Failure, below).

Hypertension is an early sign of increased work of breathing; however, hypotension develops as respiratory distress increases and oxygen demands are not met. As a result, myocardial contractility will be impaired which can lead to decreased tissue perfusion and signs of shock (Field 2000).

Cardiac arrhythmias, including tachycardia or bradycardia, can occur if hypoxaemia progresses to critical levels (SpO_2 < 90%) and the myocardium becomes hypoxic (Woodruff 1999). Increased heart rate, anxiety or pain will increase oxygen demand further. Acid–base imbalances may also exacerbate arrhythmias.

Cool and clammy skin is caused by decreased tissue perfusion. The skin may appear pale as hypoxia (oxygen deficiency in the tissues) causes vasoconstriction (Adam et al. 2010). Vasoconstriction lowers the skin temperature, reducing its ability to evaporate sweat. Conversely, the skin may feel warm and look well-perfused as elevated CO_2 levels cause vasodilation of blood vessels resulting in warm peripheries and a bounding pulse.

Drowsiness, confusion and/or agitation may be caused by decreased cerebral oxygenation. Headache may be due to CO_2 retention.

Pyrexia may indicate infection. A raised temperature will increase oxygen demand that may further exacerbate respiratory failure.

Pain may be due to surgery, trauma, chest infection, pulmonary embolism or cardiac disease and may be exacerbated by exhaustion, anxiety and deep breathing or increased respiratory rate. Pain increases oxygen demand and may worsen respiratory failure.

Periods of apnoea, usually lasting for 15–20 seconds, may be a result of damage to the respiratory centre in the brain (e.g. neurological insult or head injury), airway obstruction or post cardiorespiratory arrest.

Initial assessment

As previously described, initial assessment focuses on the identification and correction of life-threatening and potentially life-threatening conditions using the ABCDE approach.

Immediate management and investigations

Initial strategies must be prioritised to include management of the patient's airway according to their level of consciousness. Use of oral/nasal airways or tracheal intubation may be needed if the patient is obtunded. Treatment of respiratory failure takes two approaches; including treatment of the underlying cause (for example, with antibiotics for pneumonia or bronchodilators for asthma) and support of respiratory function, for example, with oxygen therapy and non-invasive ventilation (NIV) or continuous positive airway pressure (CPAP) or invasive ventilation (Hurst 2009). The goal of treatment is to restore sufficient oxygen supply to the tissues (Cooper et al. 2006). Give high concentration oxygen via a non-rebreathe mask or bag-valve-mask according to the British Thoracic Society (2008) guidance (see Table 7.2). Exercise care if the patient is likely to have COPD. Oxygen is the primary treatment for acute or chronic respiratory failure as it helps correct hypoxia, reduces the work of breathing and decreases myocardial workload (Field 2000). Ensure that the length of oxygen tubing is not too long as this can increase dead space and increase the patient's work of breathing. Consider applying humidified oxygen as this reduces the drying of the mucous membranes and will aid expectoration of sputum and secretions.

Nurse the patient in the most appropriate position that will aid their respiration. Fully conscious patients are likely to be sitting upright with backrest support. Those with altered conscious levels will require a position that aids breathing at the same time as ensuring a clear airway. For patients who are unconscious, regular turning not only reduces the incidence of pressure sores but aids the mobilisation of secretions and may improve gas exchange by improving ventilation and perfusion. The supine position reduces the patient's functional residual capacity (Moore 2000) and, therefore, the lateral position may be useful to mobilise secretions. Position

---

Box 7.5   Limitations of pulse oximetry (SpO$_2$)

Pulse oximetry determines the saturation of oxygen (SaO$_2$) by reflecting light off haemoglobin. The normal SpO$_2$ is approximately >95%. Pulse oximetry is an extremely useful assessment tool, but it does have limitations. The following limitations should therefore be considered when using pulse oximetry:

- Pulse oximetry does not provide an indication of ventilation or lung performance
- An SpO$_2$ within normal limits does not exclude hypoxaemia or hypoventilation (Lowton 1999)
- Altered reading can occur due to poor peripheral perfusion, hypothermia, hypotension, arrhythmias (e.g. atrial fibrillation), vascular disease, peripheral oedema, nail varnish and blood pressure cuff inflation (Moore 2000)
- Pulse oximetry does not indicate the presence of carbon monoxide or increasing levels of carbon dioxide (Bourke & Brewis 1998)
- Anaemic patients may display a normal SpO$_2$ even though the oxygen-carrying capacity of red blood cells is reduced. A patient with low haemoglobin may still be 97% saturated with oxygen; however, their arterial blood gas may reveal a low pO$_2$
- Probes can cause skin damage due to pressure and need to be repositioned every few hours (Barker & Shah 1996)
- The effects of motion (e.g. shivering) and excessive light can cause altered readings
- False readings can lead to inappropriate management. Readings can be severely altered as hypoxaemia progresses (Place 2000)

---

patients with unilateral lung disease with their unaffected lung down-most (Thelan et al. 1998). It must be remembered that any alteration of position increases oxygen demand. Document positional changes and any effect they may have upon SpO$_2$ and respiratory rate. Liaise with physiotherapists to enhance respiratory function.

Measure arterial blood gases (ABGs) to monitor the effectiveness of oxygen delivery, CO$_2$ removal and effects on acid–base balance. ABGs should be taken 30–60 minutes after any change in oxygen concentration and if signs of deterioration are apparent.

Measure and record the patient's respiratory rate and depth, and monitor SpO$_2$ (see Box 7.5). Record heart rate, blood pressure and feel the quality of peripheral pulse volume regularly. Record the patient's temperature and reduce any pyrexia with use of fan therapy or antipyretics. Tepid sponging can cause shivering and increase oxygen demands.

Obtain a portable chest X-ray to assess heart position and size, lung fields and any focus of infection or pathology (e.g. pneumothorax). Take blood samples for full blood count (FBC), white cell count (WCC), urea and electrolytes and glucose.

Observe for presence or development of peripheral oedema. Patients with poor peripheral perfusion due to respiratory failure are already at high risk of developing pressure sores.

Drug treatment in respiratory failure

Depending upon the severity of the respiratory failure, measured by ABGs, several approaches can be taken to drug therapy. A nebulised beta$_2$-agonist bronchodilator (e.g. salbutamol) may relieve bronchospasm and aid ventilation. An antimuscarinic bronchodilator (e.g. ipratropium) may also be given concurrently with a beta$_2$-agonist. Oral or intravenous theophylline may be used if response to nebulised bronchodilators is poor (also relax bronchial smooth muscle) (British Medical Association and the Royal Pharmaceutical Society of Great Britain 2011).

Respiratory stimulants (such as doxapram hydrochloride) have a limited role in chronic respiratory failure, having been replaced by respiratory support therapies. However, where non-invasive ventilation is contra-indicated and the patient is becoming drowsy or comatose, a short-term intravenous infusion of doxapram in combination with oxygen therapy and active physiotherapy may be useful in rousing the patient, encouraging coughing and expectoration (BMA & RPSGB 2011).

In addition to the medications outlined above, consider the use of intravenous steroids (e.g. hydrocortisone) and appropriate antibiotics if infection is identified.

Give appropriate analgesia for pain but exercise care with opiates due to their respiratory depressant effect. Monitor and document the effect of analgesia on respiratory rate and neurological status.

Liaise with respiratory physicians and/or intensivists depending upon the patient's condition. Physiotherapists may have a role to play if appropriate.

Respiratory support therapies

In addition to oxygen therapy and treatment of the underlying cause of respiratory failure, respiratory support using non-invasive ventilation or invasive ventilation is indicated if:

- respiratory status (acidosis) fails to improve despite full medical treatment
- the patient develops signs of respiratory deterioration (see Box 7.2 above) (Cooper et al. 2006)

Indications for different modes of respiratory support are outlined in Table 7.4.

Alternatively, non-invasive respiratory support may be used to support the patient's existing respiratory effort and avoid tracheal intubation. There are two types of non-invasive support: non-invasive ventilation, also called bi-level positive airway pressure (BiPAP) or non-invasive positive pressure ventilation (NiPPV); and continuous positive airway pressure (CPAP). Both types are used to promote greater alveolar ventilation without the need for endotracheal intubation and are achieved by using a close-fitting, well-sealed nasal or face mask. They allow the patient to be nursed on a ward or high dependency area, thus avoiding admission to the intensive care unit. In addition, the patient is able to eat, drink and communicate. NiPPV is used in mild to moderate respiratory acidosis, usually because of an exacerbation of COPD (Cooper et al. 2006).

Various modes of NIV are in use and include volume-cycled ventilation or pressure support ventilation. The choice of mode will be dependent on the availability of equipment and the care location (Esmond & Mikelsons 2009). In BiPAP, the ventilator cycles between two different pressures which are triggered by inspiration and expiration. NiPPV reduces the work of breathing and enhances gas

Table 7.4   Indications for different modes of respiratory support (Cooper et al. 2006)

Tracheal intubation	Non-invasive ventilation (NiPPV or BiPAP)	Non-invasive CPAP
Asthma	COPD with respiratory acidosis (pH 7.25–7.35)	Acute cardiogenic pulmonary oedema
ARDS (acute respiratory distress syndrome)	Decompensated sleep apnoea	Hypoxaemia in chest trauma/atelectasis
Severe respiratory acidosis (pH < 7.25)	Acute on chronic hypercapnic respiratory failure due to chest wall deformity or neuromuscular disease	
Any impaired consciousness level		
Pneumonia		

Box 7.6   Contraindications to non-invasive respiratory support

Recent facial or upper airway surgery, facial burns or trauma
Vomiting
Recent upper gastrointestinal surgery or bowel obstruction
Inability to protect own airway
Fixed obstruction of the upper airway
Acute asthma
Copious respiratory secretions or epistaxis
Other organ failure (such as haemodynamic instability)
Severe confusion/agitation
Life-threatening hypoxaemia
Severe co-morbidity
Unresolved pneumothorax

Source: Esmond & Mikelsons (2009)

---

exchange, thereby increasing oxygenation and correcting respiratory acidosis (Esmond & Mikelsons 2009).

CPAP is used to correct hypoxaemia, typically in acute respiratory failure caused by conditions such as pneumonia and cardiogenic pulmonary oedema. CPAP delivers a high flow of oxygen which generates positive pressure throughout the respiratory cycle. This splints open the alveoli, allowing more time for gas exchange, thus increasing oxygenation but not necessarily reducing carbon dioxide levels (Esmond & Mikelsons 2009).

There are a number of contra-indications to non-invasive respiratory support, as outlined in Box 7.6.

Invasive ventilation

Tracheal intubation may be considered if respiratory function continues to deteriorate despite non-invasive therapies or where these are contra-indicated. Invasive ventilation is able to offer a variety of ventilator modes and is more responsive to the clinical situation. It can, however, cause haemodynamic compromise and can lead to ventilator induced lung injury (Cooper et al. 2006).

B: CHRONIC OBSTRUCTIVE PULMONARY DISEASE
(Susan Hope, based on the original chapter by Helen Whitehouse)

Introduction

Chronic obstructive pulmonary disease (COPD) is a leading cause of morbidity and mortality worldwide and results in substantial economic and social burden (GOLD 2010). It is one of the common chronic diseases where the prevalence has not declined; it continues to increase in women, but appears to have reached a plateau in men (Office for National Statistics 2000; NICE 2010). COPD accounts for approximately 30,000 deaths per year in the UK (BTS 2006) and is an important co-morbidity in those dying from other smoking-related diseases such as lung cancer and ischaemic heart disease (Hansell et al. 2003; NICE 2010).

COPD exacerbations are associated with worse quality of life (Seemungal et al. 1998), faster disease progression (Donaldson et al. 2002), increased mortality (Soler-Cataluna et al. 2005) and considerable healthcare costs (Garcia-Aymerich et al. 2003). While most COPD exacerbations are treated in primary care with only a small proportion of people admitted to hospital, it accounts for one in eight emergency admissions, the second largest cause of emergency admission in the UK. About 30% of patients admitted with COPD for the first time will be readmitted within three months (BTS 2006; NICE 2010).

COPD is a heterogeneous disease that affects different patients in different ways and it is believed that about two million people in England have undiagnosed COPD (Healthcare Commission 2006). Patients may present for the first time with an exacerbation of COPD. In previously untreated patients features from the history such as age, smoking history, chronic cough and variability of symptoms should be taken into account to differentiate between COPD and asthma. COPD should be confirmed by post-bronchodilator spirometry with an $FEV_1/FVC < 0.7$ (NICE 2010). If patients report a marked improvement in symptoms in response to continued inhaled therapy, the diagnosis of COPD should be reconsidered (NICE 2010).

Definition of COPD

The Global Initiative for Chronic Obstructive Lung Disease (GOLD) describes COPD as a preventable and treatable disease with some significant extrapulmonary effects that may contribute to the severity in individual patients. Its pulmonary component is characterised by airflow obstruction that is not fully reversible. The airflow limitation is usually progressive and associated with an abnormal

Box 7.7   Definition of diseases associated with COPD

Chronic obstructive pulmonary disease
Chronic airflow limitation that is not fully reversible. This is caused by a mixture of small airway disease and emphysema. COPD is associated with significant co-morbidities

Chronic bronchitis
Cough and sputum for at least 3 months for two consecutive years

Emphysema
Destruction of the alveoli. One of several pathological changes present in patients with COPD

Asthma
COPD and asthma can co-exist. Patients with asthma who smoke and patients with long-standing asthma may develop fixed airflow limitation

Source: GOLD (2010)

inflammatory response of the lung to noxious particles or gases (GOLD 2010). Box 7.7 provides definitions of diseases associated with COPD.

Causes of COPD

Cigarette smoking is the most common risk factor for COPD and smoking cessation programmes are a key element of COPD prevention. It is believed the risk results from a gene–environment interaction as not all smokers go on to develop COPD (GOLD 2010).

Risk factors for COPD:

- Genes
- Exposure to particles
- Tobacco smoke
- Occupational dusts, organic and inorganic
- Indoor air pollution from heating and cooking with biomass in poorly ventilated dwellings
- Outdoor air pollution
- Lung growth and development
- Oxidative stress
- Gender
- Age
- Respiratory Infections
- Previous tuberculosis
- Socioeconomic status
- Nutrition
- Co-morbidities

GOLD (2010)

Pathophysiology of COPD

The clinical manifestations of COPD, which first become evident on strenuous activity and later occur at rest, include symptoms associated with airway irritation and altered lung mechanics, and vary considerably between patients. For example, patients may have chronic sputum production with no breathlessness, while other patients may have severe airway obstruction and shortness of breath without any sputum production. The diversity in symptoms serves to highlight the different underlying disease pathologies associated with COPD, which affect the conducting airways (trachea, bronchi and bronchioles), the alveoli, lung parenchyma (tissue) and the pulmonary vasculature. The physiological impact of these changes is described below (Celli et al. 1999).

Physiological changes affecting the large or central airways (>2 mm radius), trachea, bronchi and bronchioles

Exposure to irritants (e.g. cigarette smoking) leads to:

- enlargement of mucus-secreting glands and an increase in the number of goblet cells. This is associated with mucus hypersecretion which leads to sputum production and chronic cough. These changes have minimal effect on airflow limitation
- infiltration of the surface epithelium by inflammatory cells, macrophages, T lymphocytes and neutophils
- impaired clearance of mucus due to damaged cilia

Physiological changes associated with a change in lung mechanics

1. Changes in small or peripheral airways (<2 mm in diameter), bronchioles and terminal bronchioles

- As in the large airways, inflammatory cells, macrophages, T lymphocytes and neutrophils infiltrate the surface epithelium.
- Activated inflammatory cells release a variety of mediators which may damage lung structures and sustain inflammation.
- Chronic inflammation can lead to injury and repair of the airway wall. This may result in structural remodelling of the airway wall with increasing collagen content and scar tissue formation which narrows the lumen.
- Semi-solid mucus plugs may occlude some small bronchi.
- Bronchoconstriction and smooth muscle contraction occur due to inflammation. This accounts for a limited amount of airflow limitation in COPD.
- Loss of alveolar attachments due to destructive changes in emphysema lead to airflow limitation. As they contain no cartilage, there is a tendency for bronchioles to collapse when they are compressed.

2.   Changes within the alveoli

Emphysema involves the pathological destruction of the alveoli due to irreversible enzymatic destruction of the protein elastin. Loss of elastin results in disruption of alveolar attachments to the bronchioles which reduces their ability to maintain patency. This leads to their collapse or narrowing which in turn limits airflow out of the lungs. Destruction of elastin also causes loss of elastic recoil and damage to alveoli. Damaged alveoli can merge into bullae that are relatively inefficient at gas exchange due to a loss of surface area.

3.   Changes to airway resistance

Resistance from the conducting airways depends predominantly on their radius. A small change in radius results in a significant increase in the resistance. Halving the radius will increase resistance by a factor of 16. Consequently, in COPD, narrowing of the airway lumen due to inflammation, remodelling and to a lesser degree bronchoconstriction and the tendency of small airways to narrow or collapse, has a huge impact on the airway's resistance to the flow of air. Pushing air through narrowed obstructed airways becomes progressively more difficult and exhausts the respiratory muscles. This increased work of breathing results in dyspnoea. The elevated airway resistance seen in COPD causes particular difficulty on exhalation.

When expiratory flow is severely limited, alveolar hyperinflation occurs due to slow and incomplete emptying and closure of the small airways. This increase in lung volume supplements elastic recoil and is associated with an increase in end-expiratory alveolar pressure. As a consequence, the inadequate supply of fresh air results in alveolar hypoventilation. Hyperinflation also forces the respiratory muscles to work at a length that reduces their contractile strength. This has the effect of flattening the diaphragm and results in a large barrel-shaped chest.

4.   Changes to compliance

Lung compliance is a measure of the ease with which the lungs can be inflated and is affected by the elasticity of lung tissue. Both normal and emphysematous lungs distend more easily at lower volumes. This is because, at high lung volumes, the distensible components of the alveolar walls have already been stretched out and large increases in pressure only create a small increase in volume. The compliance of the emphysematous lung is increased because, as previously described, the alveolar septae that normally oppose lung expansion have been destroyed. The increased compliance seen in emphysema causes the most over-distended areas (i.e. with a higher lung volume) to receive the least ventilation. Elastic recoil usually helps the lung to return to its normal unstretched volume but, in COPD, the decreased elastic recoil of the alveoli leads to a decreased pressure gradient for expiration. Hypoventilation of the alveoli leads to impaired gas exchange because areas are being perfused but not ventilated (i.e. a ventilation-perfusion mismatch).

5.   Changes to ventilation and perfusion

Ventilation.   In the early stages of COPD, as the lung function declines, the level of oxygen in the circulation falls and the respiratory centre triggers an increase in respiratory effort. This causes the sensation of breathlessness. Accessory muscles, not usually involved in quiet inspiration, help to increase the dimensions of the chest in order to create an adequate pressure gradient. Abdominal muscles, usually passive in quiet breathing, contract and compress the abdominal contents against the relaxed diaphragm, forcing it up in expiration. Respiratory frequency increases as does the tidal volume. These measures ensure that PO_2 and PCO_2 remain at normal levels. As lung damage progresses and resistance to airflow increases, these mechanisms prove inadequate with the respiratory rate continuing to increase, tidal volume decreasing and arterial gases becoming abnormal. Too little O_2 (hypoxia) and too much CO_2 (hypercapnia) affect brain function leading to headache, insomnia, irritability and confusion. In some patients, the PO_2 falls but CO_2 is still exhaled (type 1 respiratory failure). In others, the response to low PO_2 is impaired and a dysfunctional respiratory drive develops, whereby PO_2 falls and PCO_2 rises (type 2 respiratory failure).

Perfusion.   Optimal gas exchange occurs when the ratio of lung ventilation (V) to blood flow (Q) is equal (i.e. V/Q ratio = 1). In patients with COPD, the alveoli can become hypoventilated. Initially, the local PO_2 will drop which results in vasoconstriction and a consequent fall in perfusion to that area. This has the effect of matching blood flow to ventilation; however, worsening airflow limitation results in uneven V/Q with an ensuing reduction in PO_2 (hypoxic hypoxia).

Chronic hypoxia-induced vasoconstriction of the pulmonary capillaries and damage to or destruction of many of the small blood vessels in the lungs leads to increased pulmonary vascular resistance. As a result, the heart (particularly the right ventricle) must work harder in order to pump blood through the pulmonary vessels. Over time, this leads to right ventricular hypertrophy and right ventricular failure (i.e. cor pulmonale). Eventually, blood that is unable to empty completely from the right ventricle becomes congested in the venous system. Presence of peripheral oedema associated with this process is indicative of a poor prognosis.

6.   Other physiological changes associated with COPD

Polycythaemia.   Another physiological response to inadequate oxygenation is secondary polycythaemia. Here, an increased production of red blood cells raises the oxygen-carrying capacity of the blood but the associated rise in blood viscosity increases the risk of pulmonary embolus.

Pneumothorax.   Presence of air in the pleural cavity can occur spontaneously due to emphysema. Bullae formed from damaged alveoli may rupture, causing deflation of the affected lung as air enters the pleural space.

Systemic features

It has been increasingly recognised that COPD has significant extrapulmonary effects, particularly in patients with severe disease. Loss of fat-free mass and muscle weakness are commonly seen. Patients with COPD also have increased risk of osteoporosis, depression, chronic normocytic anaemia and cardiovascular disease. It is thought that these systemic effects may be due to increased concentrations of inflammatory mediators including TNF-a, IL-6 and oxygen-derived free radicals (GOLD 2010).

Definition of an exacerbation

An exacerbation is described as a sustained worsening of the patient's symptoms from his or her usual stable state that is beyond normal day-to-day variations and is acute in onset. Commonly reported symptoms are worsening breathlessness, cough, increased sputum production and change in sputum colour. The change in these symptoms often necessitates a change in medication (NICE 2010).

Causes of an exacerbation

The cause may be unidentifiable in up to 30% of cases of exacerbations. Although bacteria can be cultured in patients with stable COPD, bacteria may also be responsible for exacerbation. Viruses are also important particularly in the winter months. Non-infectious agents, common pollutants such as nitrogen dioxide, particulates, sulphur dioxide and ozone can also cause exacerbations (GOLD 2010; NICE 2010).

Initial assessment of the patient with an exacerbation of COPD

The aim of the initial assessment is to determine and record the patient's usual stable respiratory state and the severity of their current respiratory problem. This is achieved by observation, limited verbal questioning (history) and physical examination. Assessment comprises the usual ABCDE framework with the addition of the following specific components. The assessment of breathing should include observations, history and physical examination.

Observations

- Respiratory rate
- Depth and pattern of breathing (shallow, rapid breathing indicates severe ventilatory failure and respiratory fatigue)
- Use of accessory (sternomastoid and scalene) muscles on inspiration. These accessory muscles elevate the sternum and help increase the dimensions of the chest
- Use of accessory muscles of expiration (prominent abdominal movements)

- Pursed-lip breathing
- Ability to speak in sentences
- Skin colour for pallor, cyanosis and/or sweating. Cyanosis is an insensitive physical finding. Although it is useful for alerting and detecting hypoxaemia, absence of peripheral or central cyanosis does not rule out hypoxaemia
- Wheeze caused by the sound generated by turbulent airflow through conducting airways. Wheezing may be audible and is particularly common in patients affected by emphysema and over-inflated lungs. The wheeze is usually prominent on expiration
- Use a breathlessness questionnaire (e.g. BORG score (Borg 1982) or a more detailed questionnaire such as the Baseline and Transition Dyspnoea Index (Mahler et al. 1984)
- Signs of hypercapnia such as:
  - o vasodilatation causing warm, flushed skin
  - o tachycardia with a strong, bounding pulse
  - o deteriorating level of consciousness (confusion, agitation and drowsiness may all signify hypercapnia)
  - o flapping tremor

History

- Ask about previous mobility distances and whether there has been a reduction.
- Has the patient's sleep been disturbed (i.e. orthopnoea)? How many pillows are required to sleep?
- Use of long-term oxygen therapy (LTOT) which would indicate that PO_2 is continually below 7.3 kPa and their forced expiratory volume in 1 second (FEV_1) is less than 1.5 litres (both criteria for LTOT)
- Headache may indicate hypercapnia
- Has there been increased use of inhaled/nebulised therapy prior to admission?
- Was the onset of breathlessness sudden or insidious?
- What was previous lung function or blood gas analysis in a stable state? Access reports for comparison.

Physical examination

- Lung auscultation
- Presence of rhonchi especially on expiration

The assessment of cough and sputum should include:

- Is the cough new or has their usual cough increased?
- How frequent is coughing? Is it constant or intermittent?
- What triggers coughing?
- What type of cough is it? Is it dry, hacking or productive?
- Is sputum production new or has volume or colour changed?
- What is the colour? (e.g. mucoid, mucopurulent or purulent)

> **Box 7.8   Presenting features of an exacerbation of COPD**
>
> Increasing breathlessness
> Increased sputum purulence, volume and tenacity
> Increased cough
> Upper airway symptoms (e.g. colds, sore throats)
> Pyrexia
> Chest tightness
> Increased wheeze
> Fluid retention
> Pursed lip breathing
> Prominent abdominal movement
> Predominant use of accessory muscles
> Tachycardia
> Reduced exercise tolerance
> Anorexia/weight loss
> Increased fatigue
> Acute confusion
> Signs of type 2 respiratory failure (drowsiness, confusion, cyanosis, flapping tremor, papilloedema)
> Signs of cor pulmonale (peripheral oedema, raised jugular venous pressure, hepatomegaly)
>
> *Source*: NICE (2010) and Bedside Clinical Guidelines Partnership (2010)

- What is the consistency? (e.g. liquid or semi-solid)
- Amount per day (e.g. teaspoon or ½ eggcupful)
- Is the patient pyrexial?
- Is haemoptysis present?

The assessment of circulation should include observation for signs of right ventricular failure (e.g. observe the peripheries for signs of oedema). Chest pain should be assessed using the PQRST tool (see Chapter 8 – Chest pain). Pleuritic pain is common and may hinder expectoration of secretions and restrict respiration. Sudden onset may indicate pulmonary embolus (see Chapter 8 – Chest pain). Box 7.8 provides a summary of the common presenting features of an exacerbation of COPD.

The assessment of anorexia and/or weight loss should include:

- Calculation of body mass index (BMI)
- Question the patient about any recent weight loss
- Ask about dietary intake
- Is the skin dry (indicating dehydration)?

Assessment of need for hospital admission

Many patients with exacerbation of COPD are treated safely and effectively with Hospital at Home and assisted-discharge schemes (NICE 2010). There is insufficient data available at the present time to make firm recommendations about patient selection for these schemes but NICE (2010) provide recommendations

Table 7.5 Factors to consider when deciding where to treat the patient. Reproduced with permission of National Clinical Guideline Centre. Chronic obstructive pulmonary disease: management of chronic obstructive pulmonary disease in adults in primary and secondary care. NICE (2010). London: National Clinical Guideline Centre. Available from: http://guidance.nice.org.uk/CG101/Guidance/pdf/English

Factor	Treat at home	Treat in hospital
Able to cope at home	Yes	No
Breathlessness	Mild	Severe
General condition	Good	Poor/deteriorating
Level of activity	Good	Poor/confined to bed
Cyanosis	No	Yes
Worsening peripheral oedema	No	Yes
Level of consciousness	Normal	Impaired
Already receiving LTOT	No	Yes
Social circumstances	Good	Living alone/not coping
Acute confusion	No	Yes
Rapid rate of onset	No	Yes
Significant comorbidity (particularly cardiac and insulin-dependent diabetes)	No	Yes
$SaO_2 < 90\%$	No	Yes
Changes on chest radiograph	No	Present
Arterial pH level	≥ 7.35	< 7.35
Arterial PaO_2	≥ 7 kPa	< 7 kPa

about what factors should be taken into consideration. Table 7.5 outlines the factors to consider when deciding whether to treat a patient at home or in hospital.

Immediate management

If the exacerbation is severe, it is important to document the patient's functional status before the exacerbation and the patient's ventilation and resuscitation status.

Ensure that the patient is sitting as upright as possible and is well supported by a backrest and pillows. Enable them to assume the position most comfortable to them. Constant reassurance and explanations are necessary especially if the patient is confused or agitated.

Oxygen therapy

If immediately available, check ABGs prior to the commencement of oxygen therapy. Oxygen should be given at 28% via a venturi mask (if no prior history of respiratory acidosis) to prevent life-threatening hypoxia. If there is a history of respiratory acidosis, give oxygen at 24% via venturi mask pending urgent ABGs. Aim to maintain SpO_2 at 88–92% initially, then follow BTS *Guideline for emergency oxygen use in adult patients* (BTS 2008). Alternatively, give oxygen to the pre-determined SpO_2 levels specified by the patient's oxygen alert card using their own venturi mask (if they have one). Some patients with COPD will have been in respiratory failure for some time and may have become so accustomed to hypercapnia that their respiratory centre may have lost its normal sensitivity to changes in CO_2 levels. To maintain respiration these patients require low blood oxygen levels (i.e. a 'hypoxic drive'). Giving these patients too much oxygen could reduce the hypoxic drive to breathe. It is therefore important to obtain arterial blood gases as soon as possible on air and continue with 24–28% oxygen therapy via venturi mask to maintain SpO_2 at 88–92%. Venturi masks (high flow devices) should be used if possible as an accurate concentration of oxygen can be given. With nasal cannulae concentration can be variable; they are therefore more suitable when the patient's condition has been stabilised.

Bronchodilators

Beta₂-agonists

Give salbutamol 2.5–5 mg or terbutaline 5–10 mg via air-driven nebuliser on admission and, thereafter, 4–6 hourly. Both may be given more frequently if required. Nebulised bronchodilators should be continued until the patient's clinical condition improves. It is important when prescribing and supervising nebulised therapy that health professionals have the required knowledge and can ensure that the correct system is used to deliver the drug using the correct driving gas, with an adequate flow rate. Knowledge of the fill volume and residual volume of the nebuliser is essential (BTS 1997a; European Respiratory Society 2001). Air is the preferred driving gas for nebulised therapy for COPD patients due to the risk of hypercapnia and acidosis. If oxygen therapy is needed during the duration of treatment it should be administered simultaneously by nasal cannulae.

Anticholinergics

Ipratropium bromide 250–500 µg can be added and given at 6-hourly intervals. Ipratropium bromide can lead to pupillary dilation and occasionally glaucoma; these complications are reduced if a mouthpiece is utilised on the nebuliser equipment instead of a mask. Studies suggest that ipratropium bromide is as efficacious as beta₂-agonists in treating patients with COPD (Tashkin et al. 1994).

Methylxanthines

If the patient is not responding to treatment, consider an intravenous infusion of aminophylline (0.5 mg/kg/h for adult non-smokers or ex-smokers and 0.9 mg/kg/h for adult smokers). Loading dose should only be given if the patient has not received oral theophylline within the last 24 hours. If loading dose is given, monitor heart rate throughout infusion and check serum potassium 1–2 hours after dose. Theophylline levels should be checked 4–6 hours after starting infusion and again after 24 hours. Always check in *British National Formulary* for list of interactions as several medications increase or decrease theophylline concentrations.

Antibiotics

Antibiotics should be used to treat exacerbations with a history of more purulent sputum (NICE 2010). Patients without more purulent sputum do not need antibiotic therapy unless there is consolidation on chest radiograph or clinical signs of pneumonia (NICE 2010). Local guidelines on prescribing antibiotic therapy should always be taken into account.

Systemic corticosteroids

NICE (2010) recommends oral corticosteroids for exacerbation of COPD in the absence of significant contraindications. Use a 7 to 14-day course of oral prednisolone 30 mg/day. If already on a maintenance dose, increase the daily dose by 30 mg for 7–14 days. There is no advantage to continuing longer than 14 days and all patients should have clear instructions about why, when and how to stop their corticosteroid treatment. Osteoporosis prophylaxis should be considered in patients having frequent rescue courses of oral corticosteroids.

Relief of chest pain

Avoid medications that cause respiratory depression. Give a non-opiate analgesic 4–6 hourly. Prophylactic subcutaneous heparin is recommended in patients with acute on chronic respiratory failure due to their higher risk of pulmonary embolism (BTS 1997b).

Treatment of right ventricular failure

Oral diuretics are indicated if there is evidence of peripheral oedema but they must be used carefully to avoid hypotension.

Respiratory stimulants

Respiratory stimulants are not recommended for the treatment of exacerbation of COPD and doxapram is only recommended for use when non-invasive ventilation is either unavailable or not recommended (GOLD 2010; NICE 2010).

Non-invasive positive pressure ventilation

Non-invasive positive pressure ventilation (NIPPV) has been found to improve respiratory acidosis (increase pH and decrease $PaCO_2$), decrease respiratory rate, severity of breathlessness and length of hospital stay (Elliot 2002; GOLD 2010). It is the treatment of choice for treating persistent hypercapnic ventilatory failure during exacerbations despite optimal medical therapy (NICE 2010) and has been found to be more effective and less expensive compared to standard therapy alone (Keenan et al. 2000; Plant et al. 2003). It is usually delivered via a mask that covers the nose, but a full face mask can be used.

Invasive ventilation and intensive care

Patients who are not suitable for NIPPV or who fail to respond may require invasive mechanical ventilation and admission to intensive care. Assessment for suitability for intubation and ventilation should include functional status, BMI, oxygen requirement when stable, co-morbidities and previous admissions to intensive care and not age and FEV_1 alone (NICE 2010).

Coping and breathing strategies

It is important to address the psychological factors (i.e. fear and anxiety) that may be exaggerating the patient's sensation and perception of dyspnoea (American Thoracic Society 1999). In addition to the provision of reassurance and explanations about their treatment and investigations, simple relaxation techniques and control strategies can be used to help reduce the amount of distress felt by the patient:

- Relaxation techniques – include the systematic tensing and relaxing of different parts of the body. Patients with COPD invariably overuse and tense the muscles in the upper body, therefore suggest that they drop their shoulders, while gently pressing on them if necessary. Advise the patient to close their eyes and repeat a word such as 'calm'.
- Body positioning – the head-down and leaning forward position has been found to reduce dyspnoea. This position is thought to allow the abdominal contents to push up the diaphragm, increasing its resting length and consequently its ability to generate force (Sharp et al. 1980). Patients with COPD usually find the best body position to relieve breathlessness themselves.
- Pursed-lip breathing – instruct the patient to inhale through the nose and to purse their lips (like they are going to whistle) and exhale slowly. Pursed-lip breathing is often adopted spontaneously and is thought to reduce respiratory rate, which may reduce dynamic hyperinflation and improve V/Q match (Casaburi et al. 1997).

Diagnostic investigations

Arterial blood gases

Arterial blood gases (ABGs) measure the degree of respiratory failure and should be taken before the initiation of oxygen therapy. However, this is often not possible, as the patient requires oxygen immediately or may have been given oxygen prior to assessment. Ensure that the percentage of inspired oxygen is recorded at the time that ABGs are taken, and that ABGs are checked 30–60 minutes following initiation or any change in delivery.

Oxygen saturation (SpO$_2$) (see Respiratory failure)

SpO$_2$ only measures the degree of oxygenation and does not provide any information about the state of ventilation or CO_2 retention. Therefore, while SpO$_2$ monitoring may reduce the need for painful ABG measurements in some cases, it should not replace ABG sampling for patients with COPD.

Chest X-ray

A chest X-ray cannot diagnose COPD but can exclude other pathologies including pneumonia, pneumothorax, left ventricular failure, right ventricular failure, pulmonary oedema, lung cancer (of which there is an increased incidence in COPD; Skillrid et al. 1986), pleural effusion and upper respiratory airway obstruction. When cor pulmonale is present, the hilar vasculature may become more prominent and cardiomegaly will be evident on the X-ray.

A plain posterior–anterior chest X-ray may be normal in mild COPD but, with progressive disease, hyperinflation will be shown by the presence of increased lung volumes and a low, flat diaphragm.

Blood investigations

Take blood samples for:

- full blood count – to assess for anaemia and raised white cell count
- haematocrit – to assess polycythaemia (haematocrit >47% in women, >52% in men)
- electrolytes – to monitor hypokalaemia and/or hyponatraemia which may occur in patients treated with diuretics and hypokalaemia which may occur when high doses of short-acting beta-agonists are given
- blood cultures if sputum is purulent and pyrexia is present
- ESR and CRP should also be obtained if infection is suspected

Peak expiratory flow

Peak expiratory flow (PEF) is not recommended for routine monitoring in exacerbation of COPD (NICE 2010).

Sputum sample collection

Routine culture of non-purulent sputum is unhelpful. Oral antibiotics are only indicated if there are signs of infection (e.g. purulent sputum, increased shortness of breath and/or increase in sputum volume).

ECG

To diagnose right ventricular hypertrophy, identify arrhythmias (e.g. atrial fibrillation) or co-existing coronary heart disease.

Discharge planning

Following hospital admission for an exacerbation of COPD, 30% of patients are likely to be readmitted within 3 months (Roberts et al. 2002). Advance discharge planning is recommended for all patients to ensure that patients have been re-established on their optimal maintenance bronchodilator therapy, that they understand the correct use of medications including oxygen therapy, and that the patient, family and carers are confident that the patient can manage successfully. Follow-up appointments and home care should be arranged before discharge. Spirometry should be measured and oximetry and/or arterial blood gases should be satisfactory prior to discharge.

Any interaction with healthcare professionals is also an opportunity to check inhaler technique, repeat advice to stop smoking, advise prophylactic influenza vaccination and review home medication. If the patient is still hypoxic when clinically stable, referral should be considered for assessment for long-term oxygen therapy (LTOT). Ideally all patients who have been admitted to hospital should be reviewed within 6 weeks following an exacerbation (NICE 2010).

C: ASTHMA
(Susan Hope)

Introduction

Asthma is one of the most common chronic diseases affecting people of all ages. It is described by the Global Initiative for Asthma (GINA) as a serious global health problem, affecting an estimated 300 million people (Beasley 2004; GINA 2009).

Uncontrolled asthma can cause severe limitations on daily life and is sometimes fatal (GINA 2009). Asthma can change over time and can be intermittent, mild, moderate, severe or life threatening. Patients at any level of severity can experience acute severe exacerbations. Many deaths from asthma are preventable, but delay in initiating treatment can be fatal.

There is no precise universally agreed definition of asthma but GINA (2009) gives an operational description:

> Asthma is a chronic inflammatory disorder of the airways in which many cells and cellular elements play a role. The chronic inflammation is associated with airway hyper-responsiveness that leads to recurrent episodes of wheezing, breathlessness, chest tightness and coughing, particularly at night or in the early morning. These episodes are usually associated with widespread, but variable, airflow obstruction within the lung that is often reversible either spontaneously or with treatment.
>
> GINA (2009)

Types and causes of asthma

- Childhood/young adult asthma. This is allergic or atopic asthma (extrinsic) characterised by an allergic response to identifiable specific triggers. Atopy involves a specific immunoglobulin E mediated reaction and is associated with a genetic predisposition to asthma, hayfever, eczema and urticarial.
- Late-onset asthma. Usually older adults, non-atopic (intrinsic) and often with more persistent symptoms.
- Occupational asthma. This is due to exposure to a specific agent or chemical in the workplace; it can be atopic or non-atopic.
- Aspirin-sensitive asthma. A small number of people have symptoms due to aspirin or other non-steroidal anti-inflammatory drugs (NSAIDs).
- Exercise-induced asthma. This is a common cause of asthma symptoms and may be the only cause in some people, usually children.
- Cough variant asthma. For some people cough is the only symptom and may precede airflow obstruction.
- Brittle asthma. There are two types:
  o Chaotic uncontrolled asthma with variable peak flow
  o Sudden severe deterioration from a stable baseline

Pathophysiology

As a result of inflammation, the airways become hyper-responsive and narrow easily in response to a wide range of stimuli. This may result in coughing, wheezing, chest tightness and shortness of breath. These symptoms are often worse at night. Narrowing of the airways is usually reversible but, in some patients with chronic asthma, the inflammation may lead to irreversible airflow obstruction. Characteristic pathological features include the presence in the airway of inflammatory cells, plasma exudation, oedema, smooth muscle hypertrophy, mucous plugging and shedding of epithelium. These changes may be present even in patients with mild asthma when they have few presenting features (BTS 1997c).

Mechanisms of inflammation

One of the most important advances in the management of asthma has been the recognition that asthma is an inflammatory disease rather than a disease characterised by altered smooth muscle function. Although the actual mechanisms causing airways inflammation are still not fully understood, it is thought that there is a genetic predisposition (host factor) that interacts with environmental factors (Holgate 1993). As well as a genetic predisposition to atopy or airway hyper-responsiveness, other host factors such as sex and obesity have been identified (GINA 2009). Environmental factors such as indoor and outdoor allergens, air pollution, tobacco smoke and infections are important triggers of asthma symptoms. Other triggers such as occupational sensitizers can be a host factor as well as a cause of asthma symptoms.

The inflammatory cells (e.g. activated mast cells, macrophages, eosinophils and T-helper lymphocytes) release multiple inflammatory mediators (including histamine, leukotrienes, prostaglandins and bradykinin). Inflammatory mediators result in bronchoconstriction, mucus secretion, exudation of plasma and airway hyper-responsiveness. Multiple intracellular messengers called cytokines (e.g. interleukin-1, interleukin-5) are responsible for co-ordinating, amplifying and perpetuating the inflammatory response and attracting additional inflammatory cells. Structural changes (i.e. airway remodelling) may occur with subepithelial fibrosis (i.e. basement membrane thickening), airway smooth muscle hyperplasia and new vessel formation. These changes may underlie irreversible airflow obstruction (Barnes & Godfrey 2000).

Presenting features

Exacerbations of asthma are episodes of progressive increase in shortness of breath, cough, wheezing or chest tightness or a combination of these symptoms. There is usually a progressive onset but some patients present more acutely. Exacerbations are characterised by decreases in expiratory airflow that can be measured by measurement of peak expiratory flow (PEF) or forced expiratory flow in one second (FEV_1). Box 7.9 describes the levels of severity of acute asthma.

All initial contact personnel should be aware that asthma patients complaining of respiratory symptoms may be at risk and should have immediate access to a doctor or trained asthma nurse (BTS/SIGN 2011). Any patients with features of acute severe or life-threatening asthma should be referred to hospital. However, other factors should be considered such as failure to respond to treatment, social circumstances or concomitant disease, psychological problems, physical disability or learning difficulties, previous near-fatal or brittle asthma, exacerbation despite adequate dose of steroid tablets pre-presentation, presentation at night or pregnancy (BTS/SIGN 2011; GINA 2009).

Box 7.9   Levels of severity of acute asthma

Features of near fatal asthma
- Elevated $PaCO_2$ plus/or requiring mechanical ventilation with raised inflation pressures

Features of life-threatening asthma
Any one of the following in a patient with severe asthma:

- Altered consciousness
- Exhaustion
- Arrhythmia
- Hypotension
- Cyanosis
- Silent chest
- Poor respiratory effort
- SpO_2 <92%
- PaO_2 <8 kPa
- $PaCO_2$ 4.6–6 kPa (normal)
- PEF <33% best or predicted

Features of acute, severe asthma
Any one of:
- Peak expiratory flow (PEF) 33–50% of predicted or best
- Unable to complete sentences in one breath
- Respirations ≥25 breaths per minute
- Pulse ≥110 bpm

Moderate asthma exacerbation
- Increasing symptoms
- PEF >50–75% best or predicted
- No features of acute severe asthma

Brittle asthma
- Type 1: wide PEF variability (>40% diurnal variation for >50% of the time over a period >150 days) despite intense therapy
- Type 2: sudden severe attacks on a background of apparently well-controlled asthma

Source: British Guideline on the Management of Asthma. Reproduced with permission from the British Thoracic Society/Scottish Intercollegiate Guidelines Network (2011)

Initial assessment

In addition to the usual ABCDE assessment, the initial assessment should include assessing the severity of the exacerbation, which will determine the treatment, and should focus on PEF measurement, pulse oximetry, respiratory rate, pulse rate, ability to talk in sentences, respiratory effort and alertness (Figure 7.1). Arterial blood gases (ABGs) should be measured if oxygen saturation is less than 92% or if the patient has any life-threatening features.

PEF is the simplest test of lung function and can be measured on simple portable devices in hospital and at home. It is measured as the maximum expiratory flow achieved during forced expiration – usually within the first few milliseconds of the expiratory effort. It is a very effort-dependent, but reproducible, test that mainly reflects large airway obstruction. Measurements are most easily interpreted when expressed as percentages of the predicted normal value (see Figure 7.1) or of the best obtainable value for the individual with optimal treatment. PEF must be interpreted in the light of other features of severity and the patient's history, particularly previous admissions to hospital, attendance at the emergency department or assessment unit, and current treatment, especially corticosteroids.

Immediate management and investigations

The immediate management of acute severe asthma is outlined in Figure 7.1. As discussed above, the only immediate investigations needed before treatment are PEF and pulse oximetry. If PaO_2 <92% arterial blood gases should be measured. Arterial blood gases showing a normal or raised $PaCO_2$ and severe hypoxia (PaO_2 < 8 kPa and a low pH) indicate a life-threatening attack.

Oxygen

Supplementary oxygen should be given to all hypoxaemic patients to maintain oxygen saturations (SpO_2) of 94–98% using a medium concentration mask, venturi mask or nasal cannulae (BTS 2008). Unlike patients with COPD, hypercapnea is not a risk with higher concentrations of oxygen and if present would indicate the development of near-fatal asthma.

Short-acting B₂ agonist bronchodilators (SABA)

Inhaled B₂ agonists should be used as early as possible, either via a metered dose inhaler (MDI) and large volume spacer (4–6 puffs, each inhaled separately; this dose can be repeated at 10- to 20-minute intervals) or by an oxygen-driven nebuliser (salbutamol 5 mg or terbutaline 10 mg) when available. A flow rate of 6 litres is required to drive most nebulisers (BTS/SIGN 2011). In severe asthma (PEF or FEV_1 < 50% and asthma that is poorly responsive to an initial bolus dose of B₂ agonist) consider continuous nebulisation using an appropriate nebuliser system (BTS/SIGN 2011).

Ipratropium bromide

Nebulised ipratropium bromide (0.5 mg 4–6 hourly) should be added to SABA treatment for patients with acute severe asthma or life-threatening asthma, or those with a poor initial response to SABA alone (GINA 2009; BTS/SIGN 2011).

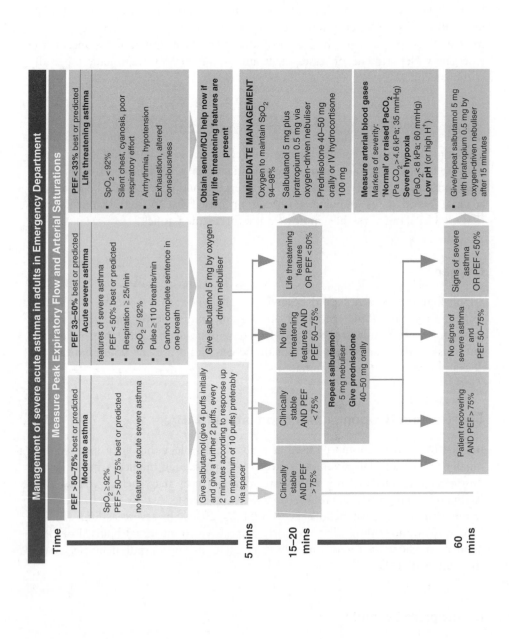

Management of severe acute asthma in adults in Emergency Department

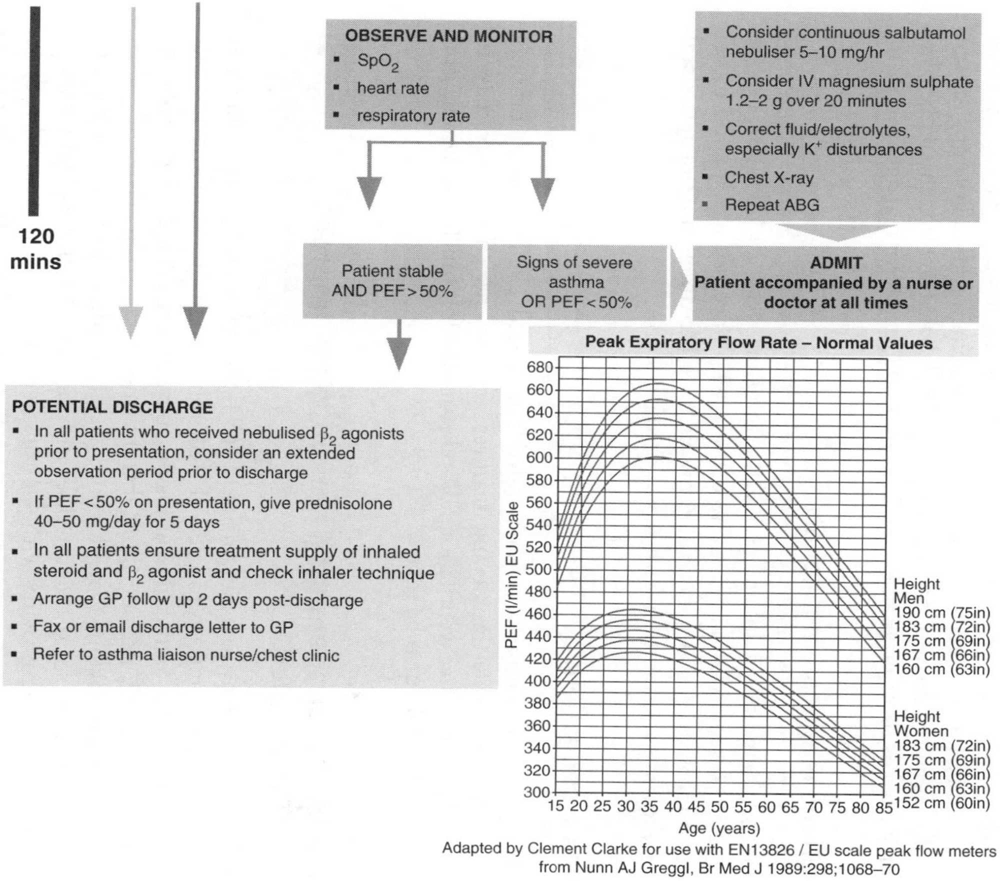

120 mins
OBSERVE AND MONITOR
SpO2
heart rate
respiratory rate
Consider continuous salbutamol nebuliser 5–10 mg/hr
Consider IV magnesium sulphate 1.2–2 g over 20 minutes
Correct fluid/electrolytes, especially K+ disturbances
Chest X-ray
Repeat ABG
Patient stable AND PEF > 50%
Signs of severe asthma OR PEF < 50%
ADMIT
Patient accompanied by a nurse or doctor at all times
POTENTIAL DISCHARGE
In all patients who received nebulised β2 agonists prior to presentation, consider an extended observation period prior to discharge
If PEF < 50% on presentation, give prednisolone 40–50 mg/day for 5 days
In all patients ensure treatment supply of inhaled steroid and β2 agonist and check inhaler technique
Arrange GP follow up 2 days post-discharge
Fax or email discharge letter to GP
Refer to asthma liaison nurse/chest clinic
Peak Expiratory Flow Rate – Normal Values
PEF (l/min) EU Scale
Age (years)
Height Men
190 cm (75in)
183 cm (72in)
175 cm (69in)
167 cm (66in)
160 cm (63in)
Height Women
183 cm (72in)
175 cm (69in)
167 cm (66in)
160 cm (63in)
152 cm (60in)
Adapted by Clement Clarke for use with EN13826 / EU scale peak flow meters from Nunn AJ Greggl, Br Med J 1989:298;1068–70

Figure 7.1 Immediate management of acute severe asthma in adults in the emergency department. Reproduced from the *British Guideline on the Management of Asthma* (2011) British Thoracic Society & Scottish Intercollegiate Guidelines Network. Reproduced with permission from the BTS. www.brit-thoracic.org.uk/clinical-information/asthma/asthma-guidelines.aspx.

Systemic glucocorticosteroids

Steroid tablets (prednisolone 40–50 mg daily) should be given as early as possible in acute exacerbation. They reduce mortality, speed resolution of exacerbation and reduce relapse and readmission (Rowe et al. 2001; BTS/SIGN 2011). Parenteral hydrocortisone 400 mg daily (100 mg 6-hourly) can be given but the oral route is as effective, less invasive and less expensive (Harrison et al. 1986). Oral prednisolone should be continued daily for at least 5 days or until recovery and can be stopped abruptly. Doses do not need to be tapered unless patients are on maintenance steroid therapy or oral steroids have been required for three or more weeks. Inhaled steroids should be continued or started as soon as possible and form part of a long-term management plan.

Intravenous magnesium sulphate

Intravenous magnesium sulphate (1.1–2.0 g infusion over 20 minutes) can be considered in patients with acute severe asthma who have not had a good initial response to inhaled bronchodilator therapy or have life-threatening or near-fatal asthma, following consultation with senior medical staff.

Further investigations

Chest X-ray is not routinely recommended but would exclude pneumothorax and consolidation. If life-threatening features are present, chest X-ray may be required prior to invasive ventilation. Blood samples for full blood count, urea and electrolytes should also be taken.

Subsequent management if patient is not improving after 15–30 minutes

Continue oxygen therapy to maintain SpO2 at 94–98%. Give nebulised salbutamol 5 mg or terbutaline 10 mg up to every 15–30 minutes and ipratropium bromide 0.5 mg every 4 hours. Salbutamol infusion may be considered in patients not improving (GINA 2009; Bedside Clinical Guidelines Partnership 2010).

Intravenous aminophylline (5 mg/kg body weight loading dose over 20 minutes unless on maintenance oral therapy, then infusion of 0.5–0.7 mg/kg/h) may be given in patients not improving with life-threatening or with near-fatal asthma, only after consultation with a senior clinician (BTS/SIGN 2011) If the patient is on oral aminophylline or theophylline, blood levels should be checked before the infusion is commenced and daily while the infusion continues.

Patients with life-threatening features

Patients should be considered for transfer to intensive care if they continue to deteriorate and develop the following:

- Falling PEF, worsening or persisting hypoxia, or hypercapnia
- Exhaustion, feeble respirations, confusion or drowsiness
- Coma or respiratory arrest

All patients transferred to an intensive care unit should be accompanied by a doctor suitably equipped and prepared to intubate if necessary, as the procedure is very difficult in this type of patient. Although non-invasive ventilation is well established in the management of type 2 respiratory failure in extrapulmonary and restrictive disorders and exacerbations of COPD, it is not recommended to replace intubation in these very unstable patients at the present time (BTS/SIGN 2011).

Ongoing assessment

Once treatment has begun, monitor the patient continuously to check their response. Monitoring should include:

- record PEF 15–30 minutes after starting treatment and chart PEF before and after nebulised beta agonists
- record oxygen saturations by pulse oximetry; continue oxygen therapy, and titrate to maintain saturations at 94–98%
- measure or repeat ABGs within one hour of starting treatment if:
    o the initial PO_2 was below 8 kPa (unless the arterial oxygen saturation was above 92%)
    o the initial PCO_2 was normal or raised
    o the patient's condition deteriorates
- record the heart rate
- measure the serum theophylline concentration if aminophylline is continued for more than 24 hours (aim at a concentration of 55–110 mmol/L)
- measure serum potassium and blood glucose concentrations

Certain treatments are considered to be unhelpful in the initial stabilisation of asthma and include:

- any form of sedation
- antibiotics (should only be given if bacterial infection is present)
- percussive physiotherapy

Inappropriate prescriptions of beta-blockers and NSAIDs can prove fatal in asthma. All patients should be asked about past reactions to these agents (BTS/SIGN 2011).

Nursing management and preparation for discharge home

All interactions with health professionals are an opportunity for patient education. As asthma is a chronic disease, the long-term management must focus on prevention of further exacerbations. This necessitates a move towards encouraging patients to take more responsibility for managing their own condition in partnership with health professionals. Self-management plans can range from simple instruction to complex plans including how to adjust treatment according to changes in peak flow or symptoms (Gibson et al. 1995, 1998; Partridge 1995; Gibson & Charpin 2000). Evidence suggests that self-management or individualised action plans have been particularly effective in those who have had recent exacerbations and have been shown to reduce emergency department attendances and hospitalisations in people with severe asthma (Yoon et al. 1993; Osman et al. 2002; BTS/SIGN 2011). Before discharging a patient following acute exacerbation, ensure that they have had:

- their inhaler technique checked, corrected if necessary and recorded
- a PEF of 75% of predicted or best
- advice re compliance with usual medication
- a discharge letter for their GP and practice nurse
- a PEF meter and PEF or symptom diary
- a written management plan of what to do if their asthma deteriorates
- a written plan of their current treatment including oral and inhaled steroids
- the reasons for their exacerbation and referral identified

It is essential that the patient's primary care practice is informed within 24 hours of discharge, ideally directly to a named individual responsible for asthma care within the practice by means of fax or email.

Patients who have needed admission to hospital for severe asthma should be followed up by a respiratory specialist for at least one year, and patients who have had near-fatal asthma or brittle asthma should be under specialist supervision indefinitely (BTS/SIGN 2011).

D: PNEUMONIA
(Michelle Garner)

Introduction

Pneumonia is a condition whereby the gas exchange regions of the lungs (the lung parenchyma) become inflamed as a result of infection with an invading organism. Pneumonia is therefore an infection of the lower respiratory tract.

Causes

Pneumonia can be either community-acquired (community-acquired pneumonia; CAP) or hospital-acquired (that which develops 2 or more days after admission to hospital). CAP is typically a primary infection or an infection occurring with another disease such as COPD. CAP is most commonly caused by *Streptococcus pneumoniae*. Hospital-acquired pneumonia is a secondary infection, most often the result of Gram-negative organisms such as *Pseudomonas aeruginosa* or *Escherichia coli* (Bourke 2003).

The remainder of this section is concerned with the initial assessment and management of patients who present with CAP.

Since 1997, the UK has seen a rise in hospital admissions due to CAP. The proportion of adult patients with CAP requiring hospital admission is reported to be between 22% and 42% (BTS 2009); 5% of these patients go on to require management in intensive care. Mortality in patients hospitalised with CAP ranges from 5.7% to 14.0%; however, mortality in cases of severe CAP admitted to intensive care is over 30% (BTS 2009) possibly as a result of severe forms of pneumonia rapidly deteriorating into multiple organ failure. With such a significant mortality rate, pre-hospital assessment to establish the severity of the illness is a crucial first step in determining risk and identifying those patients who should be managed in hospital.

Pathophysiology and presenting features

Patients may have a recent history of upper respiratory tract infection. Symptoms often develop suddenly and patients present with cough, purulent sputum, fever, pleuritic pain and dyspnoea. Elderly patients may present with non-specific symptoms, complicated by the presence of other conditions and may be a result of aspiration (BTS 2009). Those most at risk are young children and the elderly (over 70 years of age).

In pneumonia, consolidation occurs in either a single lobe or across multiple lobes. The invading organism (bacteria) stimulates an inflammatory response leading to the accumulation of fluid. This creates an environment in which the bacteria multiply. White blood cells migrate to the area; however the alveoli fill with fluid, white cells, red blood cells and fibrin which inhibit gas exchange and can lead to respiratory failure. Inflammation of the pleural membranes causes pain on respiration (Campbell 2006).

Initial assessment

Initial assessment focuses on the identification and correction of life-threatening and potentially life-threatening conditions using the ABCDE approach.

It is important to obtain a chest X-ray as soon as possible to confirm or refute the diagnosis. This will permit the goal of antibiotic therapy within 4 hours of hospital admission (BTS 2009) to be achieved. If the chest X-ray is equivocal, CT lung scan is indicated. Oxygen saturations should be recorded and ABGs obtained in order to determine the need for oxygen therapy.

Assessment of the severity of the pneumonia is crucial in determining whether the patient requires admission to critical care. A number of features are associated with greater risk of mortality (see Box 7.10). If any of these features are present, the patient requires a high level of monitoring within a critical care area. The CURB 65 score is a severity assessment tool which should be used in conjunction with clinical

Box 7.10   Features of severe pneumonia

Respiratory rate 30 breaths per minute or more
Systolic BP < 90 mmHg
Diastolic BP < 60 mmHg
Age 60 years or above
Underlying disease
Acute confusion
Multiple lobe involvement
Serum urea > 7 mmol/L
PO_2 8 kPa or less
Raised white cell count
Bacteraemia

Source: Bourke (2003)

judgement in the assessment of all patients with suspected CAP (BTS 2009) to enable patients to be stratified according to their level of risk. Patients are scored one point for each of the following: Confusion, Urea > 7 mmol/L, Respiratory rate > 30/min, low systolic Blood pressure < 90 mmHg or diastolic < 60 mmHg blood pressure, age > 65 years. Patients scoring 3, 4 or 5 are at high risk of death and warrant admission to a critical care unit.

Immediate management

Assist the patient into a comfortable position to aid breathing. Record temperature, peripheral pulse, and respiratory rate, depth and pattern as well as blood pressure. Look for any signs of cyanosis or respiratory distress. Give sufficient oxygen to maintain $PO_2 > 8$ kPa or SpO_2 94–98% in patients without pre-existing COPD. In patients with hypercapnic respiratory failure, oxygen should be given at 24–28% to maintain SpO_2 88–92% without causing a fall in $pH < 7.35$ (BTS 2009). In patients with an elevated pCO_2 and respiratory acidosis, mechanical ventilation is indicated. Take blood samples for FBC, WCC, C-reactive protein (CRP), plus urea and electrolytes, microscopy culture and sensitivity (preferably before antibiotic therapy is commenced). Send sputum samples for microscopy, culture and sensitivity. A urine sample should be sent for pneumococcal antigen testing. If pleural effusion is present, aspiration will be required with sampling for microscopy, culture and sensitivity. Listen to the chest; localised crackles, dullness or bronchial breathing are indications of pneumonia. If the patient has experienced rigors or has a very high fever, suspect sepsis. Give simple (non-drowsy) analgesia for pleuritic pain. Ensure that the patient has intravenous access and commence intravenous fluids to maintain hydration. Chest physiotherapy may be indicated, particularly in patients with underlying lung disease. If the patient is immobile, low molecular weight heparin should be given as prophylaxis against venous thromboembolism. Consider anti-embolism stockings.

The initial prescription of broad spectrum antibiotics is only indicated when a diagnosis of CAP has been confirmed by chest X-ray. IV antibiotics are indicated in patients with high severity pneumonia, in less severe cases oral antibiotics are recommended (BTS 2009). Once a specific pathogen is identified, narrow spectrum antibiotics should be given, however, in up to two thirds of patients, an organism will not be identified (BTS 2009).

Ongoing assessment and nursing management

Stable patients should have their temperature, pulse, blood pressure, respiratory rate and SpO_2 measured twice daily. Gradual mobilisation should begin as soon as possible in order to avoid complications associated with prolonged immobility. Attention to diet and adequate nutrition and hydration are important. Most patients will begin to improve within 2–3 days; however, there are a number of complications which may occur, which should be investigated by repeat chest X-ray, FBC, WCC and CRP. Complications include pleural effusion and empyema leading to persistent pyrexia, lung abscess, metastatic infection and septicaemia.

E: SPONTANEOUS PNEUMOTHORAX
(Ian Wood)

A pneumothorax is a condition in which air enters the space between the visceral and parietal pleurae. It is more common in previously fit and well young adults (often tall, athletic men) as well as older people with emphysema.

Pathophysiology

In normal respiration, as the chest expands the negative pressure in the potential space between the visceral pleura (attached to the lung surface) and parietal pleura (attached to the inside of the chest wall) ensures that the lungs expand. As they expand the negative pressure inside draws air into the lung for gaseous exchange. When the visceral pleura loses its integrity (often as a result of a ruptured bulla), air is able to leak from the lung into the space between the pleurae. In so doing, the negative pressure between the two layers is lost and the lung does not inflate as the chest expands. Consequently, the affected lung collapses and is unable to function effectively. If the air leak stops, a simple pneumothorax develops. If, however, the leak continues, air will leak into the pleural space, increasing the pressure within it. This pressure can continue to build until it is sufficient to compress the mediastinal contents, thereby making expansion of the unaffected lung more difficult, and impairing venous return and cardiac function. This condition is known as a tension pneumothorax. If untreated, the increasing pressure within the chest will cause cardiac arrest (see Chapter 4 – Cardiac arrest).

Box 7.11   Features of spontaneous pneumothorax

Dyspnoea (degree depends on size of pneumothorax)
Tachypnoea
Use of accessory muscles
Pain on inspiration
Reduced breath sounds on the affected side
Asymmetrical chest expansion (reduced on the affected side)
Resonance on percussion of the affected side
Restlessness or confusion

Box 7.12   Features of tension pneumothorax

Signs of increasing respiratory distress
Increased respiratory rate and effort
Tachycardia
Sweating
Inability to speak
Reduced/absent breath sounds on the affected side on auscultation
Inequality of chest movement/expansion
Hyperresonance of the chest on percussion
Distended neck veins
Cyanosis (late sign)
Tracheal deviation (late sign)

Source: Moulton & Yates (2006) and ALSG (2010)

Presenting features

Pneumothorax usually occurs in two groups of patient (Moulton & Yates 2006):

- young adults, usually male, who are previously fit and healthy
- older patients with emphysema

Features (see Box 7.11) may be difficult to detect if the pneumothorax is small or when emphysema is present.

Tension pneumothorax is an immediately life-threatening condition that requires immediate management (see Box 7.12 for presenting features).

Initial assessment

Assessment centres on the ABCDE approach already described. Patients who are younger and previously healthy will tolerate a relatively large pneumothorax whereas an older patient with emphysema is likely to be symptomatic with a relatively small air leak. It is important to make regular, accurate assessments of the patient's breathing for developing tension pneumothorax.

Immediate management and investigations

A simple pneumothorax is usually confirmed on chest X-ray (anterior–posterior and lateral films will be needed). The results of the X-ray will guide the treatment required (ALSG 2010). Patients who exhibit signs of developing a tension pneumothorax should NOT be X-rayed but should have a needle chest decompression (thoracocentesis) performed immediately after securing intravenous access. The latter is necessary because pneumothoraces can involve haemothorax if vessels have been damaged by the air leak from the lung. After needle decompression, an underwater seal chest drain should be inserted as definitive treatment. Chest X-ray is performed once the chest drain has been inserted.

Simple pneumothoraces in asymptomatic patients can be treated with analgesia (e.g. NSAIDs), observation and reassurance (Moulton & Yates 1999). Patients with larger pneumothoraces will require treatment with a chest drain and admission to hospital.

F: ACUTE HEART FAILURE
(Michelle Garner)

Introduction

Heart failure is a complex syndrome with many causes and a wide range of clinical symptoms. Heart failure typically occurs because of loss or dysfunction of myocardial muscle, usually with left ventricular dilatation or hypertrophy (or both) (Lindenfeld et al. 2010). Acute heart failure (AHF) is defined as the sudden onset or worsening of the symptoms of heart failure and typically presents with sudden development of pulmonary congestion (a medical emergency), though it may also present as worsening symptoms of chronic heart failure (decompensation) (Dickstein et al. 2008).

Causes of acute heart failure are outlined in Box 7.13.

Pathophysiology

When the heart starts to fail, the volume of blood in the left ventricle rises, cardiac output falls and a number of compensatory mechanisms are stimulated in an attempt to maintain an adequate circulation. Unfortunately, many of these mechanisms actually make the condition worse. In response to the increased volume of blood in the ventricle, the ventricle dilates. As the size of the ventricle increases, more tension is required to expel blood. This process increases ventricular oxygen requirements and further impairs contractility, which contributes to additional deterioration in the function of the ventricle (Julian et al. 1998). Components of the neuroendocrine system are also stimulated. Activation of the sympathetic nervous system increases heart rate and contractility and causes vasoconstriction of arteries and veins. These responses help to maintain blood pressure

---

Box 7.13   Causes of acute heart failure

Coronary heart disease: acute coronary syndrome, right ventricular MI, mechanical complications post MI
Cardiomyopathy: including postpartum and acute myocarditis
Valve disease
Hypertension
Tachyarrhythmia (e.g. atrial fibrillation, ventricular arrhythmia)
Circulatory failure; including septicaemia, thyrotoxicosis, pulmonary embolism, cardiac tamponade
Decompensation of chronic heart failure: due to lack of adherence to treatment plan, volume overload, infection (pneumonia typically), cerebrovascular disorder, surgery, renal dysfunction, asthma/COPD, drug or alcohol abuse

Source: Dickstein et al. (2008)

---

but also increase the workload of the heart. Stimulation of the renin–angiotensin–aldosterone system causes vasoconstriction, which increases vascular resistance. It also triggers the secretion of aldosterone which causes sodium and water retention, thus increasing blood volume and escalating congestion of blood within the left ventricle (Julian et al. 1998).

As congestion in the left side of the heart increases, pressure in the left ventricle, left atrium, pulmonary veins and capillaries rises. When the pressure within the pulmonary capillaries exceeds the osmotic pressure exerted by plasma proteins, fluid leaks into the interstitial tissues (interstitial oedema). If the capillary and interstitial pressures exceed the intra-alveolar air pressure, fluid leaks into the alveoli (alveolar pulmonary oedema) (Kumar 1997). This fluid reduces the compliance of the lungs, making breathing more difficult and interfering with oxygen and carbon dioxide exchange.

Presenting features

Patients with acute heart failure will typically present in one of six ways (see Table 7.6). The presenting features of acute heart failure result from pulmonary congestion and reduced cardiac output. The reduced lung compliance that accompanies interstitial oedema causes dyspnoea, particularly on exertion, orthopnoea and an inability to tolerate lying in a recumbent position. On auscultation, crackles will be heard in the dependent parts of the lung. Alveolar pulmonary oedema causes the patient to expectorate frothy, pink sputum as the fluid invades the large airways (Laurent-Bopp 2000). Mucous production is increased, leading to a cough and wheeze (Jowett & Thompson 2007). Impaired gas exchange leads to tachypnoea and cyanosis due to hypoxaemia. Reduced cardiac output causes the heart rate to rise. Pulsus alternans (an alternating pulse strength) may be present and indicates altered left ventricular function (Laurent-Bopp 2000). In very severe cases, hypotension will develop, signifying the onset of cardiogenic shock (see Chapter 5 – Shock).

Table 7.6   Typical presentations of acute heart failure (Dickstein et al. 2008)

Clinical presentation	Typical signs
Worsening or decompensation of chronic heart failure	Peripheral oedema/congestion and pulmonary congestion
Pulmonary oedema	Respiratory distress, tachypnoea, orthopnoea, rales, $SpO_2 < 90\%$ on air
Hypertensive heart failure	Tachycardia, vasoconstriction, pulmonary congestion
Cardiogenic shock	Tissue hypoperfusion, systolic $BP < 90\,mmHg$, oliguria ($< 0.5\,mL/kg/h$)
Isolated right-sided heart failure	Low cardiac output syndrome without pulmonary congestion
Acute coronary syndrome with heart failure	Signs of pulmonary congestion, or hypoperfusion, often precipitated by an arrhythmia

Initial assessment

Acute heart failure is a medical emergency requiring immediate assessment and management. The aim of the assessment is to promptly recognise life-threatening features and to identify the underlying cause, so that appropriate treatment can be commenced. The assessment should follow the ABCDE principles outlined in Chapter 1 – Initial assessment. A focused history should be taken, alongside a physical examination that evaluates skin temperature, tissue perfusion and venous filling.

Position the patient close to resuscitation equipment and ensure that they are continuously observed. Obtain medical assistance immediately so that appropriate medications can be administered without delay. Continuously monitor SpO_2, respiratory rate, pattern of breathing and skin colour to identify the severity of respiratory distress and pulmonary oedema. ABGs should be obtained (note that SpO_2 monitoring is unreliable when cardiac output is low, vasoconstriction and/or shock are present). Monitor haemodynamic status for signs of cardiogenic shock. Check blood pressure and pulse at least every 15 minutes, and with any change in condition. Commence continuous cardiac monitoring of heart rate and rhythm to detect arrhythmias and record a 12-lead ECG to identify any underlying cause (e.g. acute coronary syndrome, arrhythmia). A chest X-ray will reveal the extent of pulmonary congestion and help to identify the presence of other conditions. In very severe cases, it will be necessary to insert a urinary catheter so that a precise, hourly record of urine output can be maintained. Secure intravenous access and obtain blood for full blood count, urea and electrolytes, glucose, lipids, renal, liver and thyroid function and cardiac troponin to identify or eliminate acute coronary syndrome as a cause.

Immediate management and investigations

The aims of initial management are to improve symptoms and stabilise the circulatory system by:

1   Improving tissue oxygenation
2   Relieving pulmonary congestion and volume overload
3   Improving haemodynamic status and improving organ perfusion
4   Treating the underlying cause

Millane et al. (2000) and Dickstein et al. (2008)

Initial measures to improve tissue oxygenation

Sit the patient upright and help them to maintain as comfortable a position as possible. Administer initial oxygen at 15 L/min via a reservoir mask. Exercise caution in patients with known COPD. Once the patient is stable, reduce oxygen and maintain SpO_2 at 94–98% (BTS 2008). Measure ABGs to accurately assess oxygenation and acid–base balance. Arrange an urgent chest X-ray to assess the extent of pulmonary oedema. Consider non-invasive ventilation (NIV) as soon as possible in patients with pulmonary oedema and hypertensive heart failure. Constant reassurance is essential as the patient will be frightened and may be agitated due to hypoxia. Maintain constant contact with the patient and provide reassurance and explanation regarding all treatment and investigations.

Initial measures to relieve pulmonary congestion and volume overload

Give a loop diuretic (e.g. furosemide 20–40 mg intravenously). Furosemide causes venodilation, thereby reducing the amount of blood returning to the heart (preload) and reducing venous congestion before its diuretic effect takes effect (Millane et al. 2000). As a diuretic, furosemide quickly promotes a large diuresis, thus reducing circulating blood volume and relieving venous congestion (Julian et al. 1998). Urine output should be monitored closely. Furosemide may also cause potassium depletion; therefore, monitor the serum potassium level closely.

Intravenous morphine 2.5–5.0 mg should be given as soon as possible to patients who are restless, short of breath, anxious or who have chest pain (Dickstein et al. 2008). Morphine will help to reduce anxiety and promote venodilation (reduce preload). Morphine also helps to reduce myocardial oxygen demand. An antiemetic should also be given to counteract any nausea. Respiratory rate should be monitored carefully. Morphine should be used with caution in patients who are hypotensive, bradycardic, in heart block or who have elevated CO_2.

Intravenous nitrates (for example, continuous infusion of nitroglycerine) are indicated for patients with a systolic BP > 110 mmHg and may be used cautiously in patients with a systolic BP > 90 mmHg. Nitrates act as vasodilators and, thereby, reduce blood pressure, left and right filling pressures and lower systemic vascular resistance; they also relieve shortness of breath (Dickstein et al. 2008). As an alternative to intravenous infusion, 2 puffs of GTN spray may be given every 5–10 minutes or 1–3 mg of buccal nitrate may be given (Dickstein et al. 2008).

Improve the haemodynamic status

The therapies described above should positively influence haemodynamic status by reducing venous congestion. If, however, blood pressure is low and the patient has signs of congestion or hypoperfusion (cold, clammy skin, liver impairment, renal impairment, impaired mental status), intravenous inotropes (e.g. dobutamine and/ or dopamine) may be commenced. Such inotropes may be an important bridge to definitive therapy such as circulatory support or transplantation (Dickstein et al. 2008). Where inotropes are indicated they should be commenced as soon as possible and reduced very gradually once the patient has stabilised. Both agents increase the risk of tachycardia and ventricular arrhythmias so close monitoring of heart rate and rhythm is required.

Treat the underlying cause

The specific treatment strategy will depend on the underlying condition (Dickstein et al. 2008). In many cases, the cause will be attributed to acute myocardial infarction. Cardiac echocardiography with Doppler should be performed as soon as possible as this is a useful means of evaluating cardiac function. If the ECG indicates acute myocardial infarction, treatment should not be delayed (see Chapter 8 – Chest pain). Similarly, if a mechanical complication is suspected, urgent referral to a cardiologist is necessary.

The patient's response to treatment should be prompt but, if this is not the case, respiratory function may deteriorate and respiratory arrest may occur. In some cases, endotracheal intubation and intermittent positive pressure ventilation will be necessary. In these cases, nurses have an important role to play in the safe transfer of the patient to the critical care unit.

Summary

This chapter has provided a comprehensive guide to the assessment and initial management of patients who present with the most common causes of shortness of breath. A vast number of disorders can actually cause the patient to experience shortness of breath, and these are listed in Box 7.14. The detailed description of the causes, pathophysiology, presenting features, immediate management and investigations for each of the most common disorders provides the reader with an understanding of how the breathless patient should be managed. The reader is

> **Box 7.14   Less common causes of shortness of breath**
>
> Diabetic ketoacidosis (See Chapter 6 – Altered consciousness)
> Anaphylaxis (see Chapter 5 – Shock)
> Anxiety, hyperventilation
> Anaemia
> Renal failure
> Fractured ribs/chest trauma
> Pneumothorax (see Chapter 4 – Cardiac arrest)
> Pleural effusion
> Lung cancer
> Smoke inhalation

directed to the sources of further reading at the end of the chapter for information on the continuing management of the patient with shortness of breath.

References

Adam S, Odell M & Welch J (2010) *Rapid Assessment of the Acutely Ill Patient*. Wiley-Blackwell: Chichester.

Advanced Life Support Group (ALSG) (2010) *Acute Medical Emergencies: The Practical Approach* (2nd edition). Oxford: Blackwell.

American Thoracic Society (1999) Dyspnea: Mechanisms, assessment and management: a consensus statement. *American Journal of Respiratory and Critical Care Medicine*, 159, 321–340.

Barker S & Shah N (1996) Effects of motion on the performance of pulse oximeters in volunteers. *Anaesthesiology*, 85(4), 1774–1781. Cited In: Lowton K (1999) Pulse oximeters for the detection of hypoxaemia. *Professional Nurse*, 14(5), 350.

Barnes P & Godfrey S (2000) *Asthma* (2nd edition). London: Martin Dunitz.

Beasley R (2004) *The Global Burden of Asthma Report Global Initiative for Asthma (GINA)*. Available from www.ginaasthma.org.

Bedside Clinical Guidelines Partnership (2010/2011) Medical Guidelines. *General Adult Medicine Issue 15 – Exacerbation of Chronic Obstructive Disease (COPD)*. University Hospital of North Staffordshire: Bedside Guidelines Partnership.

Bedside Clinical Guidelines Partnership (2010/2011) Medical Guidelines. *General Adult Medicine Issue 15 – Asthma*. University Hospital of North Staffordshire: Bedside Guidelines Partnership.

Borg A (1982) Psychophysical bases of perceived exertion. *Medicine and Science in Sport and Exercise*, 14(5), 377–381.

Bourke S (2003) *Lecture Notes on Respiratory Medicine* (6th edition). Oxford: Blackwell.

Bourke S & Brewis R (1998) *Respiratory Medicine* (5th edition). Oxford: Blackwell Science.

British Medical Association and the Royal Pharmaceutical Society of Great Britain (2011) *British National Formulary* London: BMJ Books and Pharmaceutical Press.

British Thoracic Society (1997a) Current best practice for nebuliser treatment. *Thorax*, 52, Supplement 2.

British Thoracic Society (1997b) Guidelines for the management of chronic obstructive pulmonary disease. *Thorax*, 52, Supplement 5.

British Thoracic Society (1997c) Asthma management guidelines. *Thorax*, 52, Supplement 1.

British Thoracic Society (2006) *The Burden of Lung Disease* (2nd edition). London: British Thoracic Society.

British Thoracic Society Emergency Oxygen Guideline Development Group (2008) Guideline for emergency oxygen use in adult patients. *Thorax*, 63, Supplement VI.

British Thoracic Society (2009) *Update of the Guidelines for the Management of Community Acquired Pneumonia in Adults*. London: British Thoracic Society.

British Thoracic Society/Scottish Intercollegiate Guidelines Network (2011) *British Guideline on the Management of Asthma: A national clinical guideline*. London: British Thoracic Society.

Bucher L & Melander S (1999) *Critical Care Nursing*. Philadelphia: W.B. Saunders.

Campbell J (2006) *Campbell's Pathophysiology Notes*. Carlisle: Lorimer.

Casaburi R, Porzasz J, Buens R et al. (1997) Physiological benefits of exercise training in rehabilitation of patients with severe COPD. *American Journal of Respiratory and Critical Care Medicine*, 155, 1541–1551.

Celli B, Benditt J & Albert R (1999) Chronic obstructive pulmonary disease. In Albert R, Spiro S & Jett J (eds) *Comprehensive Respiratory Medicine*. London: Moseby.

Cooper N, Forrest K & Cramp P (2006) *Essential Guide to Acute Care*. Oxford: Blackwell.

Copstead L-E & Banasik J (2000) *Pathophysiology: Biological and Behavioral Perspectives*. Philadelphia: W.B. Saunders.

Dickstein K, Cohen-Solal A, Filippatos G et al. (2008) European Society of Cardiology Guidelines for the diagnosis and treatment of acute and chronic heart failure. *European Heart Journal*, 29, 2388–2442.

Donaldson G, Seemungal T, Browmik A & Wedzicha J (2002) The relationship between exacerbation frequency and lung function decline in chronic obstructive pulmonary disease. *Thorax*, 57(10), 847–852.

Elliot M (2002) Non-invasive ventilation in chronic ventilatory failure due to chronic obstructive pulmonary disease. *European Respiratory Journal*, 20(3), 529–538.

Esmond G & Mikelsons C (2009) *Non-Invasive Respiratory Support Techniques: Oxygen therapy, non-invasive ventilation and CPAP*. Chichester: Wiley-Blackwell.

European Respiratory Society (2001) Guidelines on the use of nebulisers. *European Respiratory Journal*, 18, 228–242.

Field D (2000) Respiratory care. In Sheppard M, Wright M (2000) (eds) *Principles and Practice of High Dependency Nursing*. Edinburgh: Baillière Tindall/RCN.

Francis C (2006) *Respiratory Care*. Oxford: Blackwell.

Garcia-Aymerich J, Farrero E & Felez M (2003) Risk factors of readmission to hospital for a COPD exacerbation: A prospective study. *Thorax*, 58, 100–105.

Gibson P, Talbot P & Toneguzzi R (1995) Self-management autonomy, and quality of life in asthma. *Chest*, (107), 1003–1008.

Gibson P, Coughlan J & Wilson A (1998) Review: Limited asthma education reduces the number of visits to emergency departments but does not improve patient outcomes. *Evidence-Based Medicine*, July/August, 121.

Gibson P & Charpin D (2000) Educating adolescents about asthma. *Chest*, (118), 1514–1515.

Global Initiative for Asthma (GINA) (2009) *Global Strategy for Asthma Management and Prevention*. Available from: www.ginasthma.org.

GOLD (2010) Global Initiative for Chronic Obstructive Lung Disease: *Global Strategy for the Diagnosis, Management and Prevention of Chronic Obstructive Pulmonary Disease* updated 2010. Available from www.goldcopd.org.

Hansell A, Walk J & Soriano J (2003) What do chronic obstructive pulmonary disease patients die from? A multiple cause coding analysis. *European Respiratory Journal*, 22(5), 809–814.

Harrison B, Stokes T, Hart G, Vaughan D, Ali N & Robinson A (1986) Need for intravenous hydrocortisone in addition to oral prednisolone in patients admitted to hospital with severe asthma without ventilatory failure. *Lancet*, 1(8474), 181–184.

Healthcare Commission (2006) *Clearing the Air: A national study of chronic obstructive pulmonary disease*. London: Healthcare Commission.

Holgate S (1993) Asthma: Past, Present and Future. The 1992 Cournand Lecture. *European Respiratory Journal*, (6), 1507–1520.

Hurst J (2009) Clinical management of respiratory failure. In Esmond G & Mikelsons C (eds) *Non-Invasive Respiratory Support Techniques: Oxygen therapy, non-invasive ventilation and CPAP*. Chichester: Wiley-Blackwell.

Jowett N & Thompson D (2007) *Comprehensive Coronary Care* (4th edition). Edinburgh: Baillière Tindall/Elsevier.

Julian D, Cowan J & McClenachan J (1998) *Cardiology* (7th edition) London: W.B. Saunders.

Keenan S, Gregor J, Sibbald W. et al. (2000) Non-invasive positive pressure ventilation in the setting of severe, acute exacerbations of chronic obstructive pulmonary disease: More effective and less expensive. *Critical Care Medicine*, 28(6), 2094–2102.

Kumar A (1997) Chest X-ray. In Thompson P (ed.) *Coronary Care Manual*. London: Churchill Livingstone.

Laurent-Bopp D (2000) Heart failure. In Woods S, Froelicher E & Motzer S (eds) *Cardiac Nursing* (4th edition). Philadelphia: Lippincott.

Lewis A (1999) Respiratory Emergency! *Nursing*, 99, 62–64.

Lindenfeld J, Albert N, Boehmer J et al. (2010) Executive Summary: Heart Failure Society of America Comprehensive Heart Failure Practice Guideline. *Journal of Cardiac Failure*; 16, 475–539.

Lowton K (1999) Pulse oximeters for the detection of hypoxaemia. *Professional Nurse*, 14(5), 343–350.

Mahler D, Weinberg D, Wells C et al. (1984) The measurement of dyspnoea: Contents inter-observer agreement and physiological correlates of two new clinical indices. *Chest*, 85, 751–758.

Millane T, Jackson G, Gibbs C & Lip G (2000) ABC of heart failure: Acute and chronic management strategies. *BMJ*, 320, 559–562.

Moore T (2000) Supporting respiration. In Bassett C, Makin L (eds) *Caring for the Seriously Ill Patient*. London: Arnold.

Moulton C & Yates D (2006) *Lecture Notes on Emergency Medicine* (3rd edition). Oxford: Blackwell Science.

National Institute for Health and Clinical Excellence (2010) *Clinical guideline 101 Chronic Obstructive Pulmonary Disease: Management of chronic obstructive pulmonary disease in adults in primary and secondary care* London: NICE.

Office for National Statistics (2000) *Health Statistics Quarterly* (8). London: HMSO.

Osman L, Calder C, Godden D et al. (2002) A randomised trial of self-management planning for adult patients admitted to hospital with acute asthma *Thorax*, 57(10), 869–874.

Partridge M (1995) Asthma: Lessons from patient education. *Patient Education and Counselling* (26), 81–86.

Place B (2000) Pulse oximetry: Benefits and limitations. *Nursing Times*, 96(26), 42–44.

Plant P, Owen J & Parrott S (2003) Cost effectiveness of ward based non-invasive ventilation for acute exacerbations of chronic obstructive pulmonary disease: Economic analysis of randomised controlled trial. *BMJ*, 326(7396), 956.

Roberts C, Lowe D & Bucknall C (2002) Clinical audit indicators of outcome following admission to hospital with acute exacerbation of chronic obstructive pulmonary disease. *Thorax*, 57(2), 137–141.

Rowe B, Spooner C & Ducharme F (2001) Early emergency department treatment of acute asthma with systemic corticosteroids (Cochrane Review). *Cochrane Library, Issue 3.* Oxford: Update software.

Seemungal T, Donaldson G & Paul E (1998) Effect of exacerbation on quality of life in patients with chronic obstructive pulmonary disease. *American Journal of Respiratory and Critical Care Medicine*, 151(5 Pt1), 1418–1422.

Sharp JT, Drutz WS, Moisan T, Foster J & Machnach W (1980) Postural relief of dyspnea in severe chronic obstructive pulmonary disease. *American Review of Respiratory Diseases*, 122(2), 201–211.

Skillrid D, Offord K & Miller R (1986) Higher risk of lung cancer in chronic pulmonary disease: A prospective matched case-controlled study. *Annuls of International Medicine*, 105, 503–507.

Soler-Cataluna J, Martinez-Garcia M & Roman Sanchez P (2005) Severe acute exacerbations and mortality in patients with chronic obstructive pulmonary disease. *Thorax*, 60(11), 925–931.

Tashkin D, Detels R, Simmons M et al. (1994) The UCLA population studies of chronic obstructive respiratory disease 6. Impact of air pollution and smoking on annual change in forced expiratory volume in one second. *American Journal of Respiratory and Critical Care Medicine*, 149, 1209–1217.

Thelan L, Urden L, Lough M & Stacy K (1998) *Critical Care Nursing: Diagnosis and Management* (3rd edition). St. Louis: Mosby.

Woodruff D (1999) How to ward off complications of mechanical ventilation. *Nursing*, 29(11), 35–39.

Yoon R, McKenzie D & Bauman A (1993) Controlled trial evaluation of an asthma education programme for adults. *Thorax*, 48, 110–116.

Further reading

British Thoracic Society Emergency Oxygen Guideline Development Group (2008) Guideline for emergency oxygen use in adult patients. *Thorax*, 63, Supplement VI.

British Thoracic Society (2009) *Update of the Guidelines for the Management of Community Acquired Pneumonia in Adults*. London: British Thoracic Society.

British Thoracic Society/Scottish Intercollegiate Guidelines Network (2011) *British Guideline on the Management of Asthma. A national clinical guideline*. London: British Thoracic Society.

Dickstein K, Cohen-Solal A, Filippatos G et al. (2008b) European Society of Cardiology Guidelines for the diagnosis and treatment of acute and chronic heart failure. *European Heart Journal*, 29, 2388–2442.

GOLD (2010) Global Initiative for Chronic Obstructive Lung Disease: Global Strategy for the Diagnosis, Management and Prevention of Chronic Obstructive Pulmonary Disease. Updated 2010. www.goldcopd.org.

National Institute for Health and Clinical Excellence (2010) Clinical guideline 101 *Chronic Obstructive Pulmonary Disease: Management of chronic obstructive pulmonary disease in adults in primary and secondary care*. London: NICE.

Jessup M, Abraham W, Casey T et al. (2009) Focused Update: ACCF/AHA Guidelines for the Diagnosis and Management of Heart Failure in Adults. *Circulation*, 119, 1977–2016.

For further information on any lung disorders. British Lung Foundation, 78 Hatton Garden, London EC1N 8LD. Tel: 020 7831 5831. http://www.blf@britishlungfoundation.com

8 Chest Pain

Michelle Garner

Aims

This chapter will:

- describe a systematic approach to the initial assessment and management of patients with chest pain
- describe the presenting features, pathophysiology, investigations and management of patients who present with the most common causes of chest pain

---

Introduction

Between 20% and 40% of the UK population will experience chest pain at some time in their lives. People experiencing chest pain make approximately 700,000 visits (5%) to emergency departments each year. Chest pain accounts for up to 25% of emergency admissions to hospital each year (NICE 2010a).

A number of potentially life-threatening and non-life-threatening conditions may cause the patient to experience chest pain (Table 8.1) and may give rise to specific presenting features (Table 8.2).

Patients presenting with chest pain can be categorised into one of three groups:

1 Acute coronary syndrome (ACS) comprising one of the following:
   o ST elevation myocardial infarction (STEMI)
   o Non-ST elevation myocardial infarction (NSTEMI)
   o Unstable angina
2 Stable angina
3 Non-cardiac chest pain

Initial Management of Acute Medical Patients: A Guide for Nurses and Healthcare Practitioners,
Second Edition. Edited by Ian Wood and Michelle Garner.
© 2012 John Wiley & Sons, Ltd. Published 2012 by John Wiley & Sons, Ltd.

Table 8.1   The causes of chest pain

	Cardiac	Pulmonary	Gastrointestinal	Musculoskeletal and other
Most common causes of chest pain				
Life-threatening causes	Acute coronary syndrome: MI or unstable angina	Pulmonary embolism		
Non-life-threatening causes	Stable angina		Oesophagitis Gastro-oesophageal reflux Hiatus hernia	Costochondritis
Less common causes of chest pain				
Life-threatening causes	Dissecting thoracic aortic aneurysm Pericarditis Arrhythmia Aortic valve stenosis	Pneumothorax Severe chest infection	Peptic ulcer	
Non-life-threatening causes		Pleurisy		Rib fractures Osteoarthritis Cervical spondylosis Anxiety/depression

Initial assessment of patients with chest pain

The initial assessment of patients with chest pain uses the ABCDE principles (see Chapter 1 – Initial assessment). The priority is the identification of high-risk patients with potentially life-threatening conditions who require immediate treatment and the differentiation between cardiac and non-cardiac causes of chest pain. Consider the following.

Airway

- Is the patient's airway clear?

Breathing

- Is the respiratory rate elevated or depressed?
- Is the patient having difficulty breathing?

Table 8.2 Symptoms commonly associated with chest pain due to a specific cause

Condition causing chest pain	Associated symptoms
Cardiac: Acute coronary syndrome: • STEMI • NSTEMI • Unstable angina	Pallor Diaphoresis Dyspnoea Pink frothy sputum Nausea and vomiting Weakness Dizziness
Cardiac arrhythmia Aortic valve stenosis	Palpitations Indigestion Syncope Shock
Dissecting thoracic aortic aneurysm	Tearing chest pain, typically in interscapular area, but may radiate to throat and/or both arms Pain more severe at onset Paralysis of limbs Unequal BP and pulse on each arm History of untreated hypertension Shock
Pericarditis	Pleuritic pain, worse on inspiration and relieved by sitting forwards
Pulmonary: Pulmonary embolism Pneumothorax Chest Infection	Collapse Signs of DVT Tachypnoea Dyspnoea Cough with/without haemoptysis Cyanosis Desaturation Shock Pleuritic chest pain
Gastrointestinal: Oesophageal spasm Gastro-oesophageal reflux Peptic ulcer Hiatus hernia	Vomiting Dyspepsia Dysphasia Regurgitation Bloating History of poor diet
Musculoskeletal: Costochondritis Rib fracture Osteoarthritis Cervical spondylosis	Limb numbness and weakness Limb tingling History of recent strenuous activity Precipitated by abrupt movement Pleuritic chest pain
Psychogenic: Anxiety Depression	Hyperventilation panic attacks, numbness, tingling dizziness light-headedness palpitations

- Is chest expansion equal?
- Is there peripheral or central cyanosis (indicating shock)?
- Is there a cough? Is sputum being produced? Is the sputum frothy and/or blood-stained (indicating pulmonary oedema)?
- Is the patient's trachea central? Deviation may indicate tension pneumothorax.
- Has the patient received an opioid analgesic, which may be causing respiratory depression? If so, administer naloxone 400 μg intravenously (BMA & RPSGB 2011).

Circulation

- Measure the heart rate (HR).
- Is the peripheral pulse strong, or thready and weak (indicating shock)?
- Is the HR regular or irregular (indicating an arrhythmia)?
- If the patient is on a cardiac monitor, what is the heart rhythm?
- What is the blood pressure? Is the systolic BP < 90 mmHg (hypotension) or > 140 mmHg (hypertension)?
- Is the patient's skin warm and dry (normal perfusion) or cool, clammy and wet (indicating shock)?
- What is the capillary refill time? > 3 seconds indicates poor peripheral perfusion.

Disability

- Assess the patient's consciousness level according to the AVPU scale. Have they received an opioid analgesic? If so, and they are P or U on the scale, administer naloxone as above.
- Assess the patient's pain. Use the PQRST mnemonic (Table 8.3) and differentiate between the chest pain caused by specific conditions (Table 8.2).
- Does the patient have any relevant prior history (e.g. myocardial infarction, angina, pulmonary embolism or aortic aneurysm)?
- Look for any other clinical signs or symptoms accompanying the pain (Table 8.2).

Exposure

- Undress the patient's chest initially and attach cardiac monitoring electrodes.
- Record their temperature.
- Check their capillary blood sugar. This is especially important in diabetic patients.
- Undress the patient fully.
- Observe for peripheral oedema, signs of deep vein thrombosis (DVT) and skin mottling.

Initial measures to stabilise the high risk patient

- Secure intravenous access.
- Commence continuous cardiac monitoring of heart rate and rhythm.
- Record a resting 12-lead ECG.

Table 8.3 Assessment of pain associated with myocardial infarction (from Thompson P 1997a; Del Bene & Vaughan 2000; Katz & Purcell 2006)

Characteristics of chest pain associated with MI	
P	Provokes	Chest discomfort occurs at rest, or with less physical exertion than usual angina. Not relieved by GTN or rest
Q	Quality	Aching, burning sensation. Gripping, tightening, crushing, constricting, oppressive. Typically described like a heavy weight on the chest
R	Radiation	Left arm to the elbow, both arms. Neck, lower jaw, upper jaw. Epigastrium, interscapular area
S	Site and severity	Central chest. Retrosternal. Severe: the worst pain possible. Highest score on a chest pain evaluation tool. Associated with apprehension and fear. Described as terrifying
T	Time	Prolonged, lasting more than 20 minutes

Atypical features of chest discomfort associated with MI
Pain presenting as lower jaw pain or epigastric pain
Pain isolated to interscapular area, shoulders or antecutibal fossa
May present as fatigue, faintness or syncope without pain

- Do not routinely administer oxygen, but do monitor oxygen saturation using pulse oximetry (target range 94–98%). For seriously ill patients who are hypoxaemic, administer 2–6 L/min via nasal cannulae or 5–10 L/min via simple face mask. If $SpO_2 < 85\%$, use reservoir mask at 15 L/min. Note the following:
    - In people with chronic obstructive pulmonary disease who are at risk of hypercapnic respiratory failure, the target SpO_2 is 88–92% until blood gas analysis is available.
    - If the patient is critically ill or in a peri-arrest condition, administer oxygen at 15 L/min via a reservoir mask/bag-valve mask (BTS 2008).
- Give 300 mg aspirin to chew, if acute coronary syndrome suspected.
- Pain relief (sublingual GTN and/or intravenous morphine 5–10 mg).
- Consider administering an anti-emetic (e.g. metoclopramide 10 mg IV).
- Access to immediate basic and advanced life support in case of cardiac arrest.

At this point, it should be possible to identify whether the pain is of cardiac origin or not so that further management can follow the appropriate pathway.

A: CHEST PAIN OF CARDIAC ORIGIN

Coronary heart disease (CHD) is the most common cause of premature death (in people aged under 75 years of age) in the UK (Allender et al. 2008). The British Heart Foundation has estimated that there are around 146,000 myocardial infarctions in the UK each year, 96,000 new cases of angina each year and that 2.5 million people in the UK have CHD (Allender et al. 2008).

The NICE (2010b) guideline for the assessment of acute chest pain of suspected cardiac origin makes the following recommendations:

- Determine whether the chest pain may be cardiac by assessing the history of the pain, the presence of cardiovascular risk factors, history of CHD and any previous investigations for chest pain.
- Assess for symptoms of acute coronary syndrome (ACS) which would include:
    - Chest pain lasting longer than 15 minutes or radiating to the back, neck or jaw
    - Chest pain with nausea/vomiting, sweating, breathlessness
    - Haemodynamic instability
    - New onset of pain or sudden worsening of previously stable angina
- If ACS is suspected, record a 12-lead ECG and begin treatment as soon as possible which should include pain relief, aspirin, and continuous cardiac and haemodynamic monitoring. Perform a brief physical examination to evaluate haemodynamic status and detect complications or signs of a non-cardiac cause (for example, dissecting thoracic aortic aneurysm or pulmonary embolism).

Acute coronary syndrome

The term 'acute coronary syndrome' (ACS) is now widely used to define the acute manifestations of CHD, namely unstable angina, ST elevation myocardial infarction (STEMI) and non-ST elevation myocardial infarction (NSTEMI) (NICE 2010b).

All three arise as a result of the same pathophysiological processes; however, the manifestation depends on a number of factors, including the severity of the coronary artery obstruction, the presence or absence of a collateral blood supply to the myocardium and the myocardial oxygen requirements within the area affected by the obstruction (Fox 2000). Only STEMI is treated with immediate reperfusion and thus requires prompt recognition and distinction from the other coronary syndromes.

Pathophysiology

Atherosclerosis, the underlying condition that gives rise to the symptoms of myocardial infarction (MI) or angina, begins as an accumulation of lipid-laden cells within the intima of the coronary arteries. A plaque develops as deposits of cholesterol, lipid, smooth muscle cells, inflammatory cells, fibrous tissue, fibrin and blood are deposited and covered by a fibrous cap. Such plaques are present in a large proportion of the adult population but do not necessarily cause symptoms (Weissberg 2000). Symptoms may develop if the plaque becomes so large that it restricts blood flow to an area of myocardium, with resultant angina on exertion (stable angina). If, however, the plaque ruptures, platelets rapidly accumulate at the site of rupture leading to the formation of a thrombus with possible occlusion of the coronary artery and the symptoms of MI or unstable angina (Weissberg 2000). In STEMI, the platelet core of the thrombus is stabilised by a mesh of cross-linked fibrin strands and trapped red blood cells, producing total occlusion of the artery by the thrombus (Katz & Purcell 2006). Typically, this results in a larger area of infarction. In unstable angina, an unstable plaque rupture leads to the formation of a platelet-rich thrombus. This thrombus does not fully occlude the vessel and causes resting ischaemia (unstable angina). It is common for a piece of the thrombus to break off and travel to a smaller, more distal vessel producing a small area of necrosis and causing the release of biomarkers such as troponin (NSTEMI) (Katz & Purcell 2006).

When the blood supply to myocardial cells is critically reduced or ceases completely, severe myocardial ischaemia occurs. In the absence of a collateral blood supply, myocardial cells will die if the ischaemia lasts for more than 15–30 minutes. The area of necrosis starts at the centre of the ischaemic zone and spreads outwards from the subendocardium (inner wall of the heart) towards the epicardium (outer wall of the heart) (Van de Werf et al. (2008). Unless reperfusion occurs in time to limit the necrosis, the area of infarction will involve the entire ischaemic zone and will become transmural (STEMI) (Fletcher 1997). Since all of the cells within the area of infarction are irreversibly damaged, the pumping function of the heart or the conduction of electrical impulses may be compromised, leading to acute heart failure and/or cardiac arrhythmias (see later).

In response to MI, the autonomic nervous system is stimulated, so that in addition to the typical chest pain that is experienced, several other symptoms arise including nausea, vomiting, burping, sweating and clamminess (Fletcher 1997). Different types of myocardial infarction lead to different types of autonomic nervous system response. With anterior MI, tachycardia and vasoconstriction lead to an increase in BP that may also be a consequence of left ventricular dysfunction. In an inferior MI, reflex bradycardia and vasodilation lead to a reduction in BP, and ischaemia of the sino-atrial and atrio-ventricular nodes may cause bradyarrhythmias (Fletcher 1997).

Presenting features of acute coronary syndrome

It is important to remember that, although 75–80% of all patients who present with MI experience some chest discomfort, a small percentage of patients experience no chest pain symptoms (Del Bene & Vaughan 2000). It is known that certain groups of people commonly present with atypical symptoms of MI. These groups include women, people with diabetes mellitus, older people and people from ethnic minorities (Department of Health 2000). As a consequence, all patients who present with chest discomfort require very careful, detailed assessment of their symptoms to differentiate between the symptoms of ACS and other conditions that can mimic ACS (e.g. pulmonary embolism and aortic dissection).

The priority in the initial assessment is to make a rapid diagnosis in order to identify those patients who will benefit from early intervention. Patients with STEMI must be identified quickly so that the appropriate reperfusion therapy can be commenced. Such an approach will reduce the patient's risk of disability or death both during and after hospitalisation (DH 2000). The nurse, therefore, has a fundamental role in the rapid assessment and identification of such patients. It is changes to the ST segment of the ECG which discriminates between STEMI where there is complete vessel occlusion (leading to ST elevation) and NSTEMI or unstable angina where the thrombus is non-occlusive or occurs in the presence of a good collateral circulation (leading to ST depression) (Webster & Hatchett 2007). The first part of this section will consider the presenting features and initial management of STEMI, before going on to consider NSTEMI/unstable angina and stable angina. Table 8.4 provides an overview of diagnostics for acute coronary syndromes.

Presenting features and diagnosis of STEMI

The diagnosis of STEMI is based on a universal definition (Thygesen et al. 2007) which includes: (1) a history of chest pain/discomfort; (2) persistent ST elevation or presumed new left bundle branch block; and (3) a rise in cardiac markers of necrosis (troponin I or T) (don't wait for blood results before initiating reperfusion) (see Box 8.1).

1. Evaluation of chest pain

When evaluating the patient's pain, reassurance and explanations will help to allay the patient's anxiety. Calm questioning and the use of a chest pain evaluation tool (such as the PQRST tool; see Table 8.3) will permit the rapid and detailed assessment of the patient's pain. At the same time, take a brief, targeted history. Obtain information about the patient's personal and family risk factors for coronary heart disease and information about any contra-indications to thrombolytic therapy. The emphasis should be on obtaining accurate information with the

Table 8.4 Diagnosis of acute coronary syndromes

Clinical syndrome	ECG features	Pathophysiology	Enzyme features	Indication for reperfusion
ST elevation myocardial infarction (STEMI)	ST elevation New bundle branch block ECG changes of posterior MI Evolution of Q waves	Abrupt occlusion of coronary artery by thrombus, leading to acute ischaemia and infarction usually resulting in Q wave MI	Troponin T elevated >2 times upper limit of CK-MB, CK	Requires immediate reperfusion
Non–ST elevation MI (NSTEMI)	ST depression T inversion Minor non-specific ECG changes	Partial coronary artery obstruction with distal ischaemia and therefore minor enzyme rise usually resulting in NSTEMI	Troponin T elevated <2 times elevation CK-MB, CK	No indication for immediate reperfusion
Unstable angina	Transient ST elevation ST depression T inversion Minor non-specific ECG changes Normal ECG	Non-occlusive coronary thrombus without enzyme rise	Troponin T within normal range CK-MB, CK<upper limit of normal	No indication for immediate reperfusion

> **Box 8.1   Universal definition of STEMI**
>
> Rise and/or fall of cardiac biomarkers (preferably troponin I or T) with at least one value above the 99th percentile of the upper reference limit, together with evidence of myocardial ischaemia with at least one of the following:
>
> - symptoms of ischaemia
> - ECG changes indicative of new ischaemia (new ST-T changes or new LBBB)
> - development of pathological Q wave changes in the ECG
> - imaging evidence of new loss of viable myocardium or new regional wall motion abnormality
>
> *Source*: Thygesen et al. (2007)

Table 8.5   Presenting features frequently associated with myocardial infarction (Fletcher 1997, Del Bene & Vaughan 2000)

Presenting features	Mechanism of action
Nausea and vomiting*	*Occur as a result of increased sympathetic nervous system activity and pain
Sweating*	
Shortness of breath*	
Pale*	
Anxious and distressed*	
Indigestion*	
Weakness*	
Light-headed*	
Hypertension*	
Cough – producing pink, frothy or blood stained sputum	Indicating acute left ventricular failure and pulmonary oedema
Hypotension, pallor and confusion	Indicating cardiogenic shock or arrhythmia
Dyspnoea and tachypnoea	Suggesting significant left ventricular dysfunction or arrhythmia
Loss of consciousness	Indicating hypotension due to arrhythmia or shock

minimum of delay and avoidance of repetition. This requires good teamwork and collaboration between ambulance, medical and nursing staff. In many hospitals, chest pain assessment proformas have been developed to aid this process.

Chest pain is often accompanied by a number of other symptoms (see Table 8.5) which may arise simply as a result of the pain itself or as a result of the compromising effects of the MI on the cardiovascular system.

2.   *ECG changes associated with STEMI*

A 12-lead ECG should be recorded immediately on arrival of medical assistance, be that in the community or in hospital. Accurate and immediate interpretation of the

Table 8.6 ECG changes indicating presence of STEMI (Thompson & Ilton 1997, Antman et al. 2004)

ECG change diagnostic of STEMI	Pathophysiology
ST-segment elevation In 2 or more contiguous leads: >1 mm in limb leads: II, III, AVF, I AVL >2 mm in chest leads: V1–V6 >1 mm in II, III, AVF & V4R Localised to area of infarction Typically accompanied by peaking of T waves, followed by T wave flattening and T wave inversion ST-elevation gradually lowers as the T wave inverts	Occurs within 1–2 minutes of coronary occlusion. Indicates the early phase of myocardial injury. May be reversed by early reperfusion The number of leads involved indicates the extent of the injury The height of ST elevation tends to reflect the amount of injury
Tall peaked T waves Localised to the area of infarction	Represents the hyper-acute phase of infarction and can occur before ST elevation
Deep T wave inversion Localised to the area of infarction	Part of the sequence of changes indicating MI. Occurs in both STEMI and NSTEMI. Usually resolves after weeks/months
Development of abnormal Q waves Q waves>0.04 seconds in duration (1 small square) and more than 25% of the height of the R wave In 2 or more contiguous leads: limb leads: II, III, AVF, I AVL chest leads: V1–V6 New or presumed new LBBB Note: In the presence of RBBB the diagnosis of STEMI is still possible	Indicate myocardial cell death and transmural myocardial infarction. Begin to develop 2–12 hours after the onset of symptoms. Usually persist but can occasionally return to normal after 3 years Diagnosis of MI in the setting of LBBB is very difficult, as the presence of ST elevation, Q waves and T wave inversion is obscured. Therefore, presume LBBB is a result of STEMI
Other ECG changes: **ST-segment depression** Flat, horizontal or downsloping of the junction of the ST segment with the QRS (ST depression confined to V1–V4 without ST elevation indicates posterior wall MI)	When present in 2 or more leads without ST elevation, represents myocardial ischaemia. When present alongside ST elevation, may represent a reciprocal change

ECG is essential and should be carried out by appropriately trained professionals. The aim is to differentiate between those patients with a diagnostic ECG who require immediate evaluation regarding their suitability for reperfusion therapy, and patients whose ECG is not diagnostic. The first stage of ECG interpretation involves identifying any changes indicating STEMI or other acute coronary syndrome (Table 8.6).

The 12-lead ECG is central to the diagnosis of STEMI and other acute coronary syndromes. The ECG is often abnormal even in the first few minutes of STEMI. The classical changes of ST-segment elevation and/or abnormal Q waves or left bundle branch block (LBBB) indicate the presence of STEMI and identify those patients who will benefit from reperfusion. Where these features are not present, repeated ECG recordings are required and comparisons should be made with

Table 8.7 Classification of site of myocardial infarction (Thompson & Ilton 1997; Antman et al. 2004)

Site of infarct	ECG leads involved
Inferior wall of left ventricle	II, III, AVF
Right ventricle	$V4_R$ (V4 lead placed on the right side of the chest, in the 5th intercostal space on the mid-clavicular line)
Anterior wall of left ventricle	V2, V3, V4
Lateral wall of left ventricle	I, AVL, V5, V6
Antero-lateral walls of left ventricle	I, AVL, V2–V6
Posterior wall of left ventricle	Tall R wave & ST-depression in V1 ST depression V1–V4

previous records where possible. Use of posterior leads (V7–V8) or right ventricular lead ($V4_R$) may help to identify infarction involving territory not covered by the standard 12-lead ECG (Van de Werf et al. 2008). Patients with equivocal ECG changes will require evaluation by a cardiologist.

Two-dimensional echocardiography may be indicated if the diagnosis of STEMI is unclear from the ECG. It should not, however, delay the initiation of treatment. Echocardiography will identify wall motion abnormalities (due to ischaemia and infarction) and help to rule out other causes of chest pain. It will also help to identify abnormalities in left ventricular function, measured as the ejection fraction, and will thus identify patients who may benefit from treatment with ACE inhibitors (Katz & Purcell 2006; Van de Werf et al. 2008).

Once STEMI has been confirmed on the ECG, the next stage of the interpretation involves classifying the infarction according to its location within the heart (see Table 8.7). MI usually involves the walls of the left ventricle and is classified as being anterior, posterior or lateral (Del Bene & Vaughan 2000). MI may also involve the right ventricle. Significant right ventricular infarctions almost always occur in the presence of an inferior MI (Anderson et al. 1987). Therefore, evidence of right ventricular infarction (ST elevation of 1 mm or more in $V4_R$, which may resolve within 10 hours of symptom onset) (Robalino et al. 1989) should be sought in all patients with acute inferior MI (Figure 8.1).

The location of the MI can have a significant impact on the patient's prognosis. Infarcts involving the anterior wall of the left ventricle may severely affect the function of the left ventricle, resulting in complications such as acute left ventricular failure and cardiogenic shock (Del Bene & Vaughan 2000) (see Chapter 5 – Shock and Chapter 7 – Shortness of breath). Anterior infarcts may cause extensive damage to the interventricular septum and the bundle branch system leading to conduction disturbances (e.g. bundle branch block) and/or rhythm disturbances (e.g. heart block). These may require temporary and, sometimes, permanent cardiac pacing (Thompson 1997) (see Chapter 4 – Cardiac arrest). In the majority of cases,

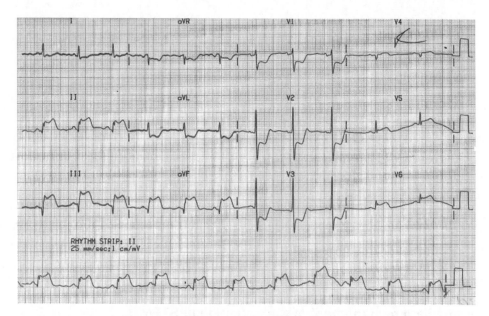

Figure 8.1   STEMI: inferior–posterior MI with lateral involvement.
Note: ST-segment elevation >1 mm in leads II, III and AVF, abnormal Q waves in III and AVF indicating acute inferior MI. ST-segment elevation of nearly 1 mm in V4$_R$ indicating possible acute right ventricular MI. ST elevation >2 mm in V6 indicating lateral wall involvement. ST-segment depression in V1–V3. Tall R waves V1, V2 indicating posterior wall MI.
Note: V4$_R$ replaces the standard V4 lead.

anterior MI is accompanied by sinus tachycardia due to sympathetic nervous system stimulation (Del Bene & Vaughan 2000).

Patients with inferior MI (Figure 8.1) often develop cardiac rhythm disturbances due to ischaemia or necrosis of the atrioventricular node. This may lead to heart block, which may require temporary cardiac pacing if the patient becomes symptomatic (Thompson 1997) (see Chapter 4 – Cardiac arrest). Inferior MI is often accompanied by sinus bradycardia and hypotension due to activation of the parasympathetic nervous system (Del Bene & Vaughan 2000). Up to 50% of all patients with inferior MI will also have ECG evidence of right ventricular involvement; although only 10–15% will develop significant right ventricular infarction leading to haemodynamic abnormalities (Ryan et al. 1999) (see Chapter 5 – Shock). When right ventricular MI does accompany inferior MI, mortality is significantly higher than for inferior MI alone (Zehender et al. 1993). It is, therefore, essential that, as part of the continuing assessment, the nurse maintains continuous close observation of the patient's heart rate and rhythm, and circulatory and respiratory function for signs of shock.

3. Serum markers of myocardial damage

The cardiac troponins (I and T) are specific markers of myocardial damage. They are sensitive enough to detect NSTEMI. Levels of troponin start to increase after 3–6 hours from pain onset (Antman et al. 2004). Both troponin I and T offer the same prognostic significance and are equally sensitive and specific (Katz & Purcell 2006). They can be available as a rapid assay (within 1 hour) and should be recorded on admission and again 10–12 hours later (Katz & Purcell 2006). Blood samples should be taken for cardiac markers along with other routine haematological and biochemical tests (e.g. full blood count, urea and electrolytes, glucose and lipid profile) as soon as the patient has been stabilised. The specific markers measured, the methods of analysis used and the length of time taken to receive results will vary according to local hospital policy.

For patients with a definite STEMI, the initial assessment, physical examination and ECG should be completed within 20 minutes of their arrival in hospital (Del Bene & Vaughan 2000). This will help to ensure the commencement of reperfusion therapy to eligible patients within 30 minutes of their arrival (door-to-needle time) as recommended (DH 2000). Thrombolysis should be commenced immediately before transferring the patient to the coronary care unit (or equivalent) for continuing management (DH 2000). This will help to avoid any unnecessary delays.

Immediate management of the patient with STEMI

1   Relief of pain, breathlessness and anxiety
2   Treatment of potentially life-threatening ventricular arrhythmias
3   Reduction of the size of the infarct and reperfusion of the affected coronary artery
4   Early detection/prevention of complications

1. *Relief of pain, breathlessness and anxiety*

Patients with ACS are not normally hypoxaemic; therefore, routine oxygen use is not recommended (BTS 2008). Oxygen should only be given if the patient is hypoxaemic or has symptoms of heart failure, shock or continuing myocardial ischaemia (BMA & RPSGB 2011). Continuous SpO_2 monitoring is essential. Observe the patient for signs of hypoxaemia (e.g. shortness of breath, $SpO_2 < 94\%$ or cyanosis). This may indicate the presence of a complication (e.g. left ventricular failure and pulmonary oedema) which will require immediate medical intervention and, in some cases, non-invasive or invasive ventilation.

Once the patient has undergone initial assessment, they should be given pain relief as soon as possible. Pain causes sympathetic activation (Van de Werf et al. 2008) which increases myocardial oxygen demand by increasing the heart rate and blood pressure. It can, therefore, increase the area of infarction (Ryan et al. 1999).

Gain intravenous access or, if already in situ, ensure the patency of the cannula before commencing any drug therapy. Check which drugs (if any) the patient has already received. To relieve chest pain and reduce the patient's anxiety, give an opioid analgesic. Morphine is usually the drug of choice and should be administered by slow (1–2 mg/minute) intravenous injection of 5–10 mg, followed by further doses of 2 mg at intervals of 5–15 minutes. In frail or elderly patients, reduce the dose by half (BMA & RPSGB 2011). As opiates can cause respiratory depression, hypotension and bradycardia, monitor blood pressure, heart rate and respiratory rate continuously. If the respiratory rate drops significantly, administer intravenous naloxone 400 μg to reverse the effects, and repeat at intervals of 2–3 minutes to a maximum of 10 mg if necessary (BMA & RPSGB 2011). Remember that, once reversed by naloxone, the analgesic effects of morphine will be lost. Hypotension and bradycardia may be treated with atropine 0.5–1 mg intravenously to a total of 2 mg (Van de Werf et al. 2008). To combat any pre-existing or concomitant nausea and vomiting, administer an anti-emetic such as metoclopramide 10 mg IV over 1–2 minutes or cyclizine 50 mg if left ventricular function is not compromised (BMA & RPSGB 2011).

The patient will need reassurance and information about their condition and the treatment that they are receiving. The administration of an opioid will help to relieve anxiety. In some cases a tranquilliser may be necessary (Van de Werf et al. 2008). Family and relatives will also need reassurance.

2.   Detection of potentially life-threatening ventricular arrhythmias (VF or VT)

Ensure that the patient is monitored continuously via a cardiac monitor connected to a central monitoring station. Resuscitation equipment should be easily accessible. Nurses should be trained in advanced life support so that when VF or pulseless VT are recognised and loss of consciousness confirmed, defibrillation can be performed within 15 seconds (Thompson & Morgan 1997) (See Chapter 4 – Cardiac arrest).

Primary VF may occur within the first 48 hours of AMI, though the risk is highest in the first 4 hours (Campbell et al. 1981). Primary VF is not associated with heart failure or cardiogenic shock (Volpi et al. 1990). A number of factors may precipitate VF and these include increased sympathetic nervous system activity (e.g. during pain), hypokalaemia, hypomagnesaemia, acidosis and reperfusion of the ischaemic myocardium (Norderhaug & von der Lippe 1983; Higham et al. 1993; Campbell 1994). For this reason, check the serum electrolyte levels on admission and maintain the serum potassium at > 4.0 mmol/L. The use of prophylactic antiarrhythmic agents is not recommended in the routine management of STEMI, or for the treatment of non-sustained VT, ventricular ectopic beats or accelerated idioventricular rhythm (Ryan et al. 1999).

Secondary VF or VT that occurs after 48 hours post-MI requires careful evaluation regarding the cause. VF or VT that occurs in association with heart failure or cardiogenic shock has a poor prognosis (Ryan et al. 1999).

3.   Reperfusion of coronary arteries and reduction of infarct size

Anti-platelet therapy. Chewable aspirin (150–300 mg) should be given to all patients with STEMI, unless contra-indicated (i.e. hypersensitivity, active gastro-intestinal bleeding, clotting disorder or severe hepatic disease). This is followed by a daily dose of 75–150 mg aspirin for life. Other non-steroidal anti-inflammatory drugs should not be given (due to increased risk of death and serious complications such as cardiac rupture and re-infarction) (Van de Werf et al. 2008). The initial dose of aspirin should be chewed to promote its rapid absorption (Ryan et al. 1999). Aspirin causes an anti-thrombotic effect by inhibiting platelet aggregation and is important in reducing coronary re-occlusion and ischaemia after thrombolytic therapy (Roux et al. 1992). The main side effects of aspirin are dose-related and include gastrointestinal bleeding.

Clopidogrel is used as an additional anti-platelet therapy in patients undergoing PCI (percutaneous coronary intervention) and in those receiving thrombolytic therapy (during the acute phase and continued for a 4-week period). A loading dose of 300 mg is given, followed by a daily dose of 75 mg. Patients over 75 years of age start with 75 mg (BMA & RPSGB 2011; Van de Werf et al. 2008).

Reperfusion therapy. The primary goal of reperfusion therapy is the restoration of normal blood flow through the affected coronary artery (Robinson & Timmis 2000). For patients who present with signs and symptoms of STEMI within 12 hours from onset of symptoms, early reperfusion by either primary PCI or thrombolysis is indicated. Primary PCI may also be considered for patients with clinical or ECG evidence of ongoing ischaemia, even if their symptoms started more than 12 hours ago (Van de Werf et al. 2008).

Primary PCI (angioplasty with or without stenting) is the preferred method of reperfusion where it can be performed by an experienced team as soon as possible after first medical contact with the patient (Van de Werf et al. 2008). This treatment is, therefore, only available in hospitals offering a 24-hour PCI service and is not currently available across the whole of the UK. Primary PCI results in lower mortality rates and better coronary artery patency while avoiding the bleeding risks of thrombolytic therapy. Long delay times for primary PCI are, however, related to worse outcome. It is therefore recommended that primary PCI is performed within 2 hours of first medical contact. Primary PCI is also recommended for patients who are not eligible for thrombolytic therapy (for example, due to the presence of contra-indications) and for patients in shock.

Rescue PCI (PCI on an artery which remains occluded despite thrombolytic therapy) is indicated in patients with clinical signs and insufficient ST segment resolution (less than 50% resolution of ST elevation in the leads with the highest ST elevation 60–90 minutes after the start of thrombolytic therapy) if it can be performed within 12 hours of symptom onset (Van de Werf et al. 2008). Rescue PCI has been found to reduce the incidence of heart failure and to reduce mortality compared with conservative treatment, though there is an increased risk of stroke and bleeding complications (Van de Werf et al. 2008).

Thrombolytic therapy. The most widely used and best-tested method of reperfusion is the administration of thrombolytic therapy. As the benefits of thrombolytic therapy are time related, the earlier treatment is begun, the better the outcome for the patient in terms of mortality and morbidity reduction. Pre-hospital thrombolysis should be initiated to eligible patients, providing it is the most appropriate

Table 8.8 Indications for thrombolytic therapy (Antman et al. 2004)

ECG	ST ↑ >1 mm in 2 or more contiguous leads (2 mm in anteroseptal leads)
	ST ↓ confined to V1–V4 (suggesting posterior wall infarction due to occlusion of circumflex artery)
	Hyperacute T waves before ST elevation indicates early sign of injury therefore repeat ECG every 15 minutes
	Left bundle branch block – new or presumed new
Chest pain	Typical cardiac pain and accompanying symptoms
	<12 hours since onset of symptoms
	>12 hours since onset if ongoing ischaemic symptoms and ST elevation in more than 2 contiguous leads

treatment (Van de Werf et al. 2008). While benefit is greatest when treatment is started within the first 3 hours of symptom onset, patients still benefit when treatment is given up to 12 hours after onset (FTT Collaborative Group 1994). As many patients suffering STEMI find it difficult to identify the precise time that their symptoms started, it is important to obtain a detailed history regarding their symptoms. The time of symptom onset should be taken as 'the beginning of the continuous, persistent discomfort that brought the patient to hospital' (Ryan et al. 1999). The indications for thrombolytic therapy are listed in Table 8.8.

Thrombolytic agents currently used in the UK include streptokinase, which is administered as an intravenous infusion over 60 minutes, t-PA (Actilyse), which is given as an accelerated infusion over 90 minutes, r-PA (Reteplase) which is given as two intravenous bolus doses 30 minutes apart. TNK t-PA (Tenecteplase) may be given by a single bolus, weight-adjusted injection and is associated with a significantly lower rate of non-cerebral bleeding and has become the agent of choice, though it is recommended to be given within 6 hours of symptom onset (BMA & RPSGB 2011). With the exception of streptokinase, current thrombolytic agents act as plasminogen activators by enzymatically converting plasminogen to plasmin, which degrades the fibrin within the blood clot and causes the thrombus to break up (BMA & RPSGB 2011). Administration of streptokinase causes a non-specific fibrinolytic state, resulting in the systemic breakdown of the coagulation system. Patients treated with streptokinase develop anti-streptococcal antibodies, which can inactivate the drug if subsequent treatment is needed. Streptokinase should, therefore, only be administered once (NICE 2002).

Antithrombin therapy. In 25% of patients, reperfusion following thrombolytic therapy will be incomplete or a thrombus will re-occur (Katz & Purcell 2006). Antithrombin therapy (with heparin) is, therefore, recommended with all thrombolytic agents. Heparin is consequently given to enhance vessel patency and prevent re-thrombosis (Katz & Purcell 2006).

Alteplase, reteplase or tenecteplase should be accompanied by an intravenous bolus of enoxaparin followed by a subcutaneous dose. Ideally, enoxaparin should be administered 15 minutes before and 30 minutes after the start of thrombolytic therapy. Subcutaneous enoxaparin is then continued at 1 mg/kg every 12 hours for up to 8 days (BMA & RPSGB 2011). Patients over 75 years of age should start with a reduced first subcutaneous dose (no intravenous dose) and continue with 750 μg/kg every 12 hours for up to 8 days (BMA & RPSGB 2011). If enoxaparin is not available a weight-adjusted bolus of intravenous heparin followed by a weight-adjusted intravenous infusion is indicated (with close aPTT control after 3 hours) for a maximum of 2 days (BMA & RPSGB 2011; Van de Werf et al. 2008). For patients receiving streptokinase, an intravenous bolus of fondaparinux followed by a subcutaneous dose 24 hours later is recommended, or alternatively, intravenous enoxaparin followed by a subcutaneous bolus 15 minutes later. If unavailable, intravenous heparin (weight-adjusted) followed by a weight-adjusted heparin infusion should be given (Van de Werf et al. 2008).

The complications associated with thrombolytic therapy relate largely to bleeding problems and, in particular, to haemorrhagic stroke (which occurs in 0.5–1% of patients and is associated with high mortality and disability in survivors). The risk of haemorrhagic stroke increases with age and blood pressure (NICE 2002). Other complications include allergic reactions (with streptokinase) and cardiac arrhythmias. Because of the large number of risks, and in order to reduce the likelihood of complications, there are a large number of contra-indications to thrombolytic therapy against which the patient must be assessed before a decision regarding their suitability for therapy can be made (Table 8.9). In most hospitals, proformas (which include indications for thrombolytic therapy, contra-indications and cautions) have been developed to assist nurses and doctors to obtain relevant information and to hasten the assessment process. The aim is to ensure that thrombolytic therapy is commenced within 30 minutes of the patient's arrival at hospital (door-to-needle time) (DH 2000).

Thrombolytic therapy restores blood flow in 60–80% of cases (GUSTO Angiographic Investigators 1993; Cannon et al. 1994), although normal blood flow only returns in 30–55% of cases and in 5–10% re-occlusion of the artery occurs. If there is evidence of persistent occlusion or reinfarction with recurrence of ST elevation, PCI is recommended. If PCI is not available a second administration of thrombolytic agent (not streptokinase if previously given) may be considered providing the infarct is large and there is not a high risk of bleeding (Van de Werf et al. 2008).

Success of thrombolytic therapy is measured by repeat ECG 60–90 minutes after treatment. Resolution of ST segment elevation of more than 50%, typical reperfusion arrhythmia and relief of chest pain all indicate successful reperfusion (Van de Werf et al. 2008). The European Society of Cardiology (Van de Werf et al. 2008) recommends that all patients who have been successfully thrombolysed undergo coronary angiography within 3–24 hours unless there are contra-indications.

For patients who present with STEMI after 12 hours of symptom onset, or in whom reperfusion therapy is not given, aspirin, clopidogrel and an antithrombin agent should be given as soon as possible (Van de Werf et al. 2008). Providing there

Table 8.9 Absolute and relative contra-indications to thrombolytic therapy (Van de Werf et al. 2008)

Absolute contra-indications	Previous haemorrhagic stroke or stroke of unknown origin
	Ischaemic stroke in preceding 6 months
	Central nervous system trauma or neoplasms
	Known bleeding disorder
	Non-compressible punctures
	Aortic dissection
	Recent major trauma/surgery/head injury within preceding 3 weeks
Relative contra-indications	Refractory hypertension (>180/110 mmHg)
	Transient ischaemic attack in preceding 6 months
	Current use of oral anticoagulants
	Prolonged CPR >0 minutes, surgery, trauma or head injury in last 3 weeks
	Advanced liver disease
	Infective endocarditis
	Active peptic ulcer
	Pregnancy or 1 week postpartum

Note: Diabetic retinopathy and successful resuscitation are *not* contraindications to thrombolytic therapy.

are no contra-indications, such patients should undergo coronary angiography before discharge from hospital.

Anti-ischaemic therapy

Beta-blockers. Long-term oral beta-blockers should be given to all patients who present with STEMI, to reduce morbidity and mortality (Van de Werf et al. 2008). They are, however, contra-indicated by the presence of asthma, pulmonary oedema, hypotension, bradycardia or heart block. When given early (within 12 hours of the MI), beta-blockers reduce the workload of the heart by reducing contractility and heart rate. They have an important role in reducing the size of the MI, the incidence of ischaemic chest pain and ventricular arrhythmias (Antman et al. 2004). It is recommended that beta-blockers are started once the patient has been stabilised.

Angiotensin converting enzyme inhibitors. Angiotensin converting enzyme (ACE) inhibitors should be started within 24 hours in all patients with an impaired ejection fraction or symptoms of heart failure in the early stage of STEMI (Van de Werf et al. 2008), unless contra-indicated by the presence of hypotension, renal failure or previous complications with ACE inhibitors (Van de Werf et al. 2008). ACE inhibitors reduce the incidence of ischaemia and left ventricular dysfunction. Treatment should be reviewed after 4–6 weeks, but may continue indefinitely in patients with symptomatic heart failure (DH 2000).

4. Early detection or prevention of complications

Patients who are admitted with STEMI are at risk from a number of life-threatening complications. The nurse must, therefore, be aware of these complications, and ensure that patients are monitored (for arrhythmias and ST segment changes) continuously for the first 24 hours at least and until event free for 12–24 hours. It is recommended that such patients are managed within a defined coronary care unit (or equivalent) which offers a quiet environment with facilities for continuous cardiac and haemodynamic monitoring, and which is staffed by experienced personnel trained in advanced life support.

Recurrent chest pain (ischaemia or pericarditis). The most common causes of post-infarct chest pain are ischaemia and pericarditis. Pain in the first 12 hours is often related to the original infarction (Antman et al. 2004); pericarditis is more typical after 24 hours. If the patient experiences additional pain, record an ECG and look for signs of pericarditis (concave upward ST elevation in most leads) or ischaemia (ST elevation or ST depression, inverted T waves becoming upright) (Antman et al. 2004). Assess the patient's chest pain and symptoms. The chest pain of pericarditis is usually pleuritic in nature, made worse by lying down, radiates to the left shoulder and is often accompanied by a pericardial friction rub. Pericarditis is usually successfully treated with aspirin. Non-steroidal anti-inflammatory drugs (NSAIDs) may be considered but not for extended periods because they affect platelet function (Antman et al. 2004). If the chest pain is similar to the initial pain experienced by the patient and occurs at rest, or on minimal exertion, suspect reinfarction (Antman et al. 2004). Cardiac markers should be repeated and immediate referral made to a cardiologist for urgent coronary angiography.

Cardiac rupture. Rupture of the left ventricular free wall is usually preceded by chest pain, and ST and T wave changes on the ECG. It may occur within 24 hours of symptom onset or between 3–5 days after STEMI and leads rapidly to shock, cardiac tamponade and pulseless electrical activity on the ECG (for treatment, see Chapter 4 – Cardiac arrest). Cardiac rupture occurs most commonly in patients with anterior MI, the elderly, women and people experiencing their first MI (Antman et al. 2004).

Heart failure and shock in STEMI. Heart failure usually occurs due to myocardial damage, but can also be due to arrhythmia or mechanical complications (involving the mitral valve or a ventricular septal defect, for example). Heart failure represents a poor prognosis for the patient and usually occurs when a large area of left ventricle has infarcted. If more than 40% of the left ventricle has been damaged, cardiogenic shock may develop. This is associated with a very poor prognosis (see

Chapter 5 – Shock). In heart failure, reduction in the contractility of the left ventricle causes pressure within the ventricle to rise, and stroke volume and cardiac output to fall. The increased pressure is transmitted to the left atrium and pulmonary veins leading to the development of pulmonary oedema (Fletcher 1997) (see Chapter 7 – Shortness of breath). Continuous monitoring of BP is essential, as hypotension (systolic BP < 90 mmHg) indicates a low cardiac output and cardiogenic shock (see Chapter 5 – Shock). In some patients, heart failure may occur due to myocardial stunning (the myocardium is reperfused but with delayed contractile recovery) or hypoperfused viable myocardium. In these cases, identification of the problem is crucial and revascularisation is warranted (Van de Werf et al. 2008).

Mild heart failure is treated with oxygen therapy (with continuous SpO$_2$ monitoring) and a loop diuretic (e.g. furosemide 20–40 mg given slowly IV and repeated every 1–4 hours) (Van de Werf et al. 2008). Diuretics are used to reduce the amount of blood returning to the heart (preload). Intravenous nitrates (e.g. GTN) are indicated in the absence of hypotension as they promote venodilation and reduce preload. They also promote coronary vasodilation and thus reduce coronary ischaemia. ACE inhibitors should be started within 24 hours of STEMI, as previously stated. The use of an ACE inhibitor to promote vasodilation (reduce afterload) prevents worsening of left ventricular function, provided there is no evidence of renal dysfunction or hypotension (Antman et al. 2004).

Severe heart failure (pulmonary oedema and shock) may occur due to extensive myocardial damage or because of mechanical complications such as ventricular septal defect, mitral valve regurgitation, papillary muscle rupture or left ventricular aneurysm. All of these lead to sudden or progressive deterioration in the patient's condition. If the patient is hypotensive and/or pulmonary oedema develops post STEMI, urgent referral to a cardiologist is required so that the cause can be identified and appropriate treatment commenced.

Severe heart failure requires treatment with oxygen, which should be monitored by arterial blood gas (ABG) sampling. Non-invasive ventilation should be considered for acute pulmonary oedema and mechanical ventilation may be necessary for patients with inadequate oxygenation or hypercapnia (as determined by arterial blood gases) (Van de Werf et al. 2008). Providing the patient is not hypotensive, intravenous nitrates should be commenced. Inotropes may be necessary if BP is low.

Cardiogenic shock is diagnosed when other causes of hypotension have been excluded (for example, vasovagal, hypovolaemia, tamponade, pharmacological side effects, arrhythmias or electrolyte disturbance; Van de Werf et al. 2008) (see Chapter 5 – Shock, for management of cardiogenic shock).

Right ventricular infarction may manifest as cardiogenic shock; however, the pathophysiology is very different to shock caused by left ventricular damage (see Chapter 5 – Shock). In patients with inferior MI accompanied by hypotension, clear lung fields and raised jugular venous pressure, right ventricular MI should be suspected. Diagnosis can be made by recording lead V4$_R$ in all cases of inferior MI with shock, diagnosis may also be confirmed by echocardiography. The aim of treatment is to maintain right ventricular preload, therefore avoid nitrates, diuretics, opioids and ACE inhibitors. Rapid intravenous infusion is necessary, typically of 0.5–1.0 litres of 0.9% saline to resolve hypotension. If BP does not return to normal, inotropic support with intravenous dobutamine is required (Van de Werf et al. 2008).

STEMI in diabetic patients.   Mortality for diabetic patients experiencing an MI is twice that of non-diabetic patients. Evidence has shown that diabetic patients tend not to receive the same extensive treatment, their symptoms are often atypical and they frequently have heart failure (Van de Werf et al. 2008). All standard treatment is recommended including thrombolytic therapy in patients with diabetic retinopathy. Higher glucose levels are associated with worse outcome; therefore, strict glycaemic control to maintain blood glucose at normal levels using insulin infusion is recommended. Care must be taken to avoid hypoglycaemia as this may induce ischaemia and affect outcome (Van de Werf et al. 2008).

Management of dyslipidaemia.   Long-term statins have been proven to reduce mortality in patients with CHD. Current targets are for total cholesterol of 4.5 mmol/L and LDL cholesterol of 2.5 mmol/L. Recent evidence supports the use of intensive statin regimens for patients with established CHD (Graham et al. 2007). As well as lowering cholesterol, statins have been found to stabilise mild to moderate-sized plaques, making them less likely to rupture. They also have anti-inflammatory and antithrombotic properties providing additional benefits (Katz & Purcell 2006). Maintenance of a low-fat diet is a basic requirement for any patient who has survived STEMI. The nurse is in a unique position to educate the patient about diet and healthy lifestyle, even during the acute phase of their illness.

Cardiac arrhythmias.   Disturbances in the cardiac rhythm are very common after STEMI and only require treatment if they are life-threatening, cause symptoms or increase the workload of the heart (Thompson 1997). Nurses should be skilled in the recognition and management of the following arrhythmias that commonly accompany STEMI.

Atrial fibrillation.   Atrial fibrillation (AF) complicates 10–20% of STEMIs (Van de Werf et al. 2008), usually occurs in the first 24 hours after STEMI and is often a temporary arrhythmia. It is associated with large (anterior) infarcts, acute heart failure and older patients. Patients who develop AF may become symptomatic because of a rapid ventricular rate or because of the loss of atrial contraction. Signs of haemodynamic compromise (e.g. hypotension, breathlessness, chest pain) indicate the need for rapid treatment with cardioversion. Intravenous beta-blockers or amiodarone may be utilised (see Chapter 4 – Cardiac arrest).

Bradycardia.   Sinus bradycardia is common early in the course of STEMI and complicates 9–25% of patients. It often accompanies inferior MI and requires treatment with 500 µg intravenous atropine if the patient develops symptoms such as a heart rate less than 50 bpm, hypotension, chest pain, ventricular escape (late) beats or ventricular ectopic (early) beats. Profound bradycardia due to a significant pause in electrical activity may occur following successful reperfusion of the right coronary artery (Antman et al. 2004) (see Chapter 4 – Cardiac arrest).

Atrioventricular block. This comprises first-degree AV block, second-degree AV block (Mobitz type I and type II) and third-degree AV block (complete heart block or CHB). AV block is associated with a higher mortality as it often occurs as a result of extensive myocardial damage (anterior MI). When AV block occurs following inferior MI, it is usually due to localised AV node ischaemia with a narrow QRS escape rhythm and often does not require treatment with a temporary pacemaker. AV block accompanying anterior MI is associated with a much poorer prognosis, typically with a wide and unstable QRS escape rhythm due to extensive myocardial necrosis. This requires treatment with a temporary transvenous pacemaker which in some cases will need to be followed by a permanent pacemaker (Van de Werf et al. 2008) (see Chapter 4 – Cardiac arrest).

Ongoing assessment and management (first 24 hours)

The ongoing assessment and management of the patient with STEMI focuses on the need to reduce the workload of the heart and to ensure the effective detection and relief of pain. During the initial 24 hours, ensure that the patient is kept under constant observation. Continuous cardiac monitoring (preferably through a centralised monitoring system) will permit the rapid identification of any change in heart rate or rhythm, and also prompt the recording of a repeat 12-lead ECG if changes in QRS, ST-segment and T waves are noted. Ensure that the patient has complete bed rest for at least 12 hours, after which time, if the infarct is uncomplicated, the patient may sit out of bed and care for their own personal needs. During this time, continuously observe the patient for any complications following reperfusion therapy (e.g. bleeding or intracranial haemorrhage), life-threatening arrhythmias (e.g. VF/VT, profound bradycardia or AV block), mechanical complications and/or acute heart failure. Be alert to the greater risks associated with certain patient groups such as those with diabetes, the elderly and those with large or previous infarcts. Assess for signs of haemodynamic compromise by regular BP recording (the frequency depends on the individual patient's condition) and oxygen saturation monitoring. Be aware of the particular needs of the patient's family and ensure that they are included in the plan of care.

NSTEMI and unstable angina

Presenting features

Most patients with acute coronary syndrome present with either NSTEMI or unstable angina (Jowett & Thompson 2007). These are unstable conditions which place the patient at high risk of further symptoms and may progress to either STEMI or death in up to 10% of cases (Collinson et al. 2000). Unstable angina is defined as angina at rest which lasts for more than 20 minutes, worsening angina and angina which occurs more than 24 hours after MI (Webster & Hatchett 2007). In NSTEMI, patients present with all the symptoms of an MI; however, the ECG can be normal (though it is usually abnormal). Sufficient myocardial damage occurs to cause an increase in biochemical markers of myocardial damage (Webster & Hatchett 2007). In both conditions, patients present with the same range of symptoms as those experiencing STEMI; however, neither condition requires immediate reperfusion therapy. The ECG in NSTEMI or unstable angina may reveal regional ST segment depression or deep T wave inversion. Even in the absence of ST-segment changes, suspect NSTEMI or unstable angina if there are other changes in the resting 12-lead ECG, particularly T wave changes.

Immediate management

The immediate management of both NSTEMI and unstable angina is the same. All forms of ACS are caused by the rupture of an atherosclerotic plaque with the development of a thrombus which either completely or incompletely occludes the artery. The actions of platelets and thrombin are key to the development of the thrombus. Drug therapy for unstable angina and NSTEMI is, therefore, targeted at this process. The aim of the initial management is to relieve pain and symptoms during the acute attack and to stabilise the plaque. Bed rest is crucial during episodes of pain in order to reduce myocardial oxygen demand. As in the case of STEMI, a quiet, restful environment is important as well as the provision of information to both the patient and their family to help reduce anxiety. Continuous cardiac monitoring is recommended alongside regular assessment of haemodynamic stability.

Once the patient is stable, a full clinical history should be taken including age, previous myocardial infarction and previous PCI or coronary artery bypass grafting (CABG). This should be followed by a physical examination (including measurement of blood pressure and heart rate) and blood tests (such as troponin I or T, creatinine, glucose and haemoglobin).

A formal risk assessment must be completed in order to assess the individual's risk of adverse events and to predict 6-month mortality. NICE (2010c) recommends the use of the Global Registry of Acute Cardiac Events (GRACE) risk scoring system. The results of the risk assessment will ensure that current evidence-based guidelines are followed. Webster and Hatchett (2007) have usefully identified those features which define the risk of a further cardiac event (such as MI) (Table 8.10).

Pain relief

For relief of pain, sublingual GTN may be given. If ineffective, intravenous or buccal nitrate may be used. Nitrates relieve cardiac ischaemic pain by dilating the coronary arteries and are, therefore, effective in patients with unstable angina. Nitrates also dilate peripheral arteries and large veins which may benefit the patient. They can, however, cause bradycardia or significant hypotension with

Table 8.10   Features defining risk of further acute event (Webster & Hatchett 2007)

High risk	Medium risk	Low risk
Age over 70 years	History of MI and/or left ventricular failure	No high-risk features
ST depression on 1st ECG	Recurrent ischaemia	Normal ECG
Refractory angina	Already taking aspirin	Clinically stable
Haemodynamic instability	Mildly raised troponin	No past history of CHD
Markedly raised troponin		Troponin not raised

reflex tachycardia (Ryan et al. 1999). Therefore, monitor the patient's BP and HR closely during and after nitrate therapy. Do not give nitrates to patients with a systolic BP less than 90 mmHg, a bradycardia less than 50 bpm, a tachycardia or a suspected right ventricular MI (Ryan et al. 1999). If the pain does not respond to nitrates, give intravenous morphine. Oxygen may be administered to patients who are hypoxaemic or in whom there is haemodynamic compromise.

Anti-platelet therapy

Aspirin 300 mg should be given to chew immediately, unless contra-indicated. In addition to aspirin, in patients with a predicted 6-month mortality of more than 1.5% and patients who may undergo PCI within 24 hours (with no contra-indications to clopidogrel), a loading dose of 300 mg clopidogrel should be given. NICE (2010c) recommend that treatment with clopidogrel in combination with low-dose aspirin should be continued for 12 months after the most recent acute episode of non-ST segment elevation ACS. Thereafter, low-dose aspirin should be taken indefinitely. NICE (2010c) also recommend intravenous eptifibatide or tirofiban as part of the early management for patients with predicted 6-month mortality above 3.0%, and who are scheduled to undergo angiography within 96 hours of hospital admission. Eptifibatide and tirofiban are glycoprotein IIb/IIIa inhibitors. These drugs prevent platelet aggregation by blocking the binding of fibrinogen to receptors on platelets. They help to prevent early myocardial infarction in patients with unstable angina or non-ST segment elevation myocardial infarction (BMA & RPSGB 2011c).

Antithrombin therapy

NICE (2010c) suggests the administration of intravenous fondaparinux to patients who do not have a high bleeding risk, unless coronary angiography is planned within 24 hours of admission. Fondaparinux is a synthetic pentasaccharide which mimics the effects of heparin (Katz & Purcell 2006). For patients who are likely to undergo coronary angiography within 24 hours or in patients with significant renal impairment, intravenous unfractionated heparin should be used instead (NICE 2010c).

Coronary angiography (with PCI if indicated)

Coronary angiography should be performed as soon as possible on patients who are unstable or at high risk (of MI). Patients with an intermediate or higher risk of adverse cardiovascular events (predicted 6-month mortality above 3.0%) should undergo angiography within 96 hours. Patients with a low risk of adverse cardiovascular events (predicted 6-month mortality 3.0% or less) do not need early angiography. However, if they develop further ischaemia, angiography is indicated. Depending on the results of angiography, revascularisation by PCI or CABG may be indicated (NICE 2010c).

Other routine investigations and treatments

Echocardiography should be performed to assess left ventricular function in all patients with MI and is also recommended in patients with unstable angina (NICE 2010c). Low-risk patients may undergo an exercise stress test prior to discharge in order to detect inducible ischaemia.

All patients with MI should be started on beta-blockers an ACE inhibitor and a statin (see STEMI) for control of angina and for secondary prevention purposes. Calcium channel blockers may also be used, particularly in patients who cannot tolerate beta-blockers.

Ongoing assessment and management

Most patients' symptoms will be under control within 24 hours. During this time, they should be constantly monitored for further pain and signs of any complications such as heart failure. Repeat ECG and serum markers should be taken in the event of further symptoms. Referral to a cardiologist is recommended for any patient with unstable angina or NSTEMI.

Early advice to reduce cardiovascular risk is crucial to the management of ACS. Information regarding smoking cessation, diet and weight loss, exercise and medication should be given. Patients with NSTEMI and unstable angina should, alongside patients with STEMI, be offered the opportunity to attend cardiac rehabilitation classes. Low-risk patients with no further symptoms after 12 hours may be discharged from hospital. Investigations (non-cardiovascular) may be indicated if the diagnosis is uncertain (Jowett & Thompson 2007).

Stable angina

Causes and pathophysiology

The cause of stable angina is similar to that of ACS. Angina is a symptom of the presence of coronary atherosclerosis and typically occurs when blood flow to an area of myocardium is restricted (usually during times of increased demand such as exercise, exertion or emotional stress) resulting in reduced nutrient and oxygen supply to the myocardium and leading to ischaemia. It may be precipitated by cold weather or eating. Stable angina is not associated with myocardial necrosis. A diagnosis of angina is more likely when the following are present:

- older patients
- male
- cardiovascular risk factors such as diabetes, smoking, hypertension, dyslipidaemia, family history of CHD, other cardiovascular disease

Presenting features

Typical angina pain is described as a constricting discomfort in the chest, arms, shoulders, neck or jaw. It usually occurs during physical exertion and is relieved by rest (or sublingual GTN) within 2–10 minutes. A diagnosis of stable angina is unlikely if the chest pain is very prolonged, unrelated to breathing, caused by breathing in or is associated with dizziness, tingling, palpitations or swallowing (NICE 2010b).

Immediate management and investigations

Stable angina is not in itself life-threatening; however, it is associated with an increased risk of MI and sudden death (Webster & Hatchett 2007). It may provoke feelings of fear and anxiety and patients require a full explanation of the treatment and investigations, backed up by the provision of written information. A resting ECG may be normal when the patient is pain free; however, during pain, ST depression and/or flattening or inversion of the T wave may be present (Webster & Hatchett 2007). A detailed clinical assessment should include a full cardiovascular risk profile to detect the presence of risk factors and estimate the cardiovascular event risk. Blood tests to check for anaemia, thyroid dysfunction, diabetes mellitus and dyslipidaemia are usually performed. Prognosis is usually assessed by means of an exercise tolerance test. In patients identified as high risk or where diagnosis is unclear, coronary angiography is indicated (Scottish Intercollegiate Guidelines Network 2007).

Sublingual GTN is provided for the immediate relief of anginal symptoms and is recommended to be taken before exertion. Beta-blockers are used as first-line treatment with the addition of a calcium channel blocker if angina is not controlled. In terms of secondary prevention, long-term aspirin and statins are indicated to help prevent new events and should be used in combination with lifestyle measures (such as smoking cessation) to control risk (NICE 2006). ACE inhibitors may also be considered. Revascularisation (to relieve symptoms) by CABG or PCI may be considered (SIGN 2007).

Nursing management

Provision of evidence-based care, supported by relevant written information, is paramount. The process of lifestyle change will begin in hospital and nurses are well placed to assist the patient to begin to address modifiable risk factors such as smoking, diet and weight control.

B: NON-CARDIAC CHEST PAIN

For the majority of patients who present with chest pain, the cause will be non-cardiac, often due to a non-life-threatening respiratory, gastrointestinal, musculo-skeletal or anxiety-related cause (Chambers et al. 1999). Nurses need to be able to distinguish between different causes of chest pain in a patient group that will include people with co-existing CHD and people with more than one non-cardiac cause for their pain (Chambers et al. 1999). This assessment is particularly difficult in patients who are very anxious, patients who are perceived to be at high risk of CHD or patients with an abnormal ECG (Dowling 1997). Patients with chest pain should have a thorough assessment of their pain and symptoms utilising the PQRST principles (Table 8.3). This should also comprise an assessment of risk factors for CHD so that those at risk can be identified and referred to appropriate personnel for further evaluation. The features, assessment and treatment of the most common non-cardiac causes of chest pain are summarised in Table 8.11.

The remainder of this section will focus on pulmonary embolism, a potentially life-threatening cause of chest pain.

Pulmonary embolism

Causes

In most cases pulmonary embolism (PE) is caused by a thrombus, which travels from its site of origin, usually a DVT, to the pulmonary vasculature, where it obstructs pulmonary blood flow (Timmis et al. 1997). In around 70% of cases of PE, DVT can be found in the lower limbs (Torbicki et al. 2008). Alternatively, the thrombus may originate within the right atrium or may be the result of injected drug misuse or an infected vascular access site (Lea & Zierler 2000). PE may also occur as a result of air, amniotic or fat embolism (Timmis et al. 1997), although such causes are rare. Acute PE has a mortality rate of between 7 and 11% (Torbicki et al. 2008). A number of risk factors for the development of PE have been identified; those that indicate the greatest risk of developing PE are listed in Box 8.2.

Pathophysiology

The physiological effects of PE are mainly haemodynamic and only become apparent when more than 30–50% of the pulmonary circulation is occluded (Torbicki et al. 2008). The occlusion may be due to a single large embolism or multiple emboli which cause a sudden increase in pulmonary vascular resistance, raising the afterload of the right ventricle (the pressure which the right ventricle must overcome in order to pump blood through the lungs) and leading to acute right ventricular failure. As a result, the right ventricle pumps less blood to the left side of the heart (lowered left ventricular preload), causing cardiac output and blood pressure to drop (Lea & Zierler 2000), leading to systemic hypotension, syncope,

Table 8.11 Evaluation of non-cardiac chest pain

Source of chest pain	Assessment of chest pain	Associated features	Assessment and investigations	Initial treatment for chest pain
Respiratory: Pneumonia (see Chapter 7–SOB)	Pleuritic chest pain, worse on deep inspiration. Induced by coughing.	Fever, sputum, dyspnoea, cough	Temperature, pulse, respiratory rate. Chest X-ray. Sputum culture.	Simple oral analgesia Steam inhalation
Pneumothorax (See Chapter 7 – Shortness of breath)	Pleuritic chest pain.	Sudden onset of dyspnoea Signs of tension pneumothorax (see Chapter 4 – Cardiac arrest)	Chest X-ray and examination ABGs	Simple oral analgesia
Musculo-skeletal:	Brief duration (<1 minute) to constant pain lasting days Precipitated by abrupt movement or application of pressure to the chest wall Induced by exercise and subsides slowly	History of recent strenuous activity	Physical examination History	Simple oral analgesia Non-steroidal anti-inflammatory drug (NSAID) Heat
Costochondritis	Sharp, pleuritic pain localised to costochondrial or costosternal junctions	Localised swelling		
Cervical & upper thoracic osteoarthritis	Chest pain worse when bending or moving, coughing or sneezing. Pain can be traced to an initiating event	Numbness, tingling, weakness, stiffness, vertigo, parasthesia		

(continued)

Table 8.11 (cont'd)

Source of chest pain	Assessment of chest pain	Associated features	Assessment and investigations	Initial treatment for chest pain
Gastro-intestinal: Dyspepsia	Chest pain typically described as heartburn, warmth, fullness, pressure, gnawing Provoked by food, especially hot or cold food, large meals or eating after moving from a recumbent position Pain usually sub-sternal, may extend to the left or right of the chest and the jaw Pain lasts for hours, disturbs sleep and is precipitated by swallowing, exercise and/or emotion Often relieved by GTN (though not quickly).	Dysphagia, oesophageal reflux, belching, regurgitation of stomach contents, epigastric pain	Take full history Endoscopy in any patient with chronic gastrointestinal bleeding, progressive unintentional weight loss, progressive difficulty swallowing, persistent vomiting, iron deficiency anaemia, epigastric mass or suspicious barium meal Endoscopy in patients over 55 yrs of age with unexplained and persistent recent onset dyspepsia	Proton pump inhibitor or testing & treatment for *Helicobacter pylori* Advice to avoid precipitants Advice on healthy eating, weight reduction & smoking cessation
Psychological causes: Anxiety	Pain in infra-mammary region, near to the apex of the heart Pain dull and aching or sharp and stabbing Pain lasts seconds to hours Not caused by exertion Related to emotional strain	Numbness, dizziness, light-headedness, weakness, headache, palpitations, depression, fatigue Hyperventilation, shortness of breath Panic attack	Ask about panic attacks History of unexplained medical symptoms History of recent upsetting events	Investigation Reassurance Provide positive explanation about cause of pain

Source: Becker (2000), Chambers et al. (1999), Dowling (1997), NICE (2004, 2007)

Box 8.2   Major risk factors for the development of PE (British Thoracic Society 2003)

Surgery
- Major abdominal/pelvic surgery
- Hip/knee replacement
- Postoperative intensive care

Obstetrics
- Late pregnancy
- Caesarian section
- Puerperium

Lower limb problems
- Fracture
- Varicose veins

Malignancy
- Abdominal/pelvic
- Advanced/metastatic

Reduced mobility
- Hospitalisation
- Institutional care

Miscellaneous
- Previous proven venous thromboembolism (VTE)

shock and, possibly, sudden death (Torbicki et al. 2008). In patients who survive the initial embolic event, compensatory mechanisms lead to an increase in heart rate, myocardial contractility and systemic vasoconstriction which together help to restore or maintain cardiac output. However, these mechanisms may not be sufficient to maintain right ventricular function beyond 24–48 hours and the right ventricle may subsequently fail either as a result of decompensation or from the occurrence of further emboli (Torbicki 2008).

In terms of the respiratory effects of PE, for adequate gas exchange to occur, ventilation (V) and perfusion (Q) must be equal. The reduction in lung perfusion that accompanies PE leads to a reduction in arterial oxygen levels (PaO_2) resulting in hypoxaemia (Torbicki et al. 2008). In order to increase arterial oxygen levels, the respiratory rate increases. This increase causes too much carbon dioxide to be exhaled with the result that $PaCO_2$ falls. The low $PaCO_2$ then stimulates further bronchoconstriction and vasoconstriction which exacerbates the ventilation/perfusion (V/Q) mismatch (Lea & Zierler 2000). In some patients, the situation is worsened by the presence of a patent foramen ovale. Blood is shunted from right atrium to left atrium (bypassing the lungs), which may lead to severe hypoxaemia and an increased risk of emboli and stroke (Kasper et al. 1992).

In patients with smaller, more distal PE where haemodynamic function is not compromised, pulmonary infarction may occur, leading to areas of alveolar haemorrhage, haemoptysis, pleuritis and mild pleural effusion. Gas exchange may be mildly disturbed (Torbicki et al. 2008).

Box 8.3   Presenting features of pulmonary embolism

1 **Circulatory collapse (usually due to extensive vascular obstruction)**
  - Hypotension and/or loss of consciousness
  - Faintness on sitting up
  - Central chest tightness
  - Tachypnoea
  - Tachycardia
  - Signs of right ventricular failure (elevated JVP)
  - ECG changes (of right ventricular strain)
  - Chest X-ray may be normal
  - ABGs show marked hypoxia and hypocapnia (due to hyperventilation)
2 **Pulmonary haemorrhage (usually due to more distal pulmonary emboli)**
  - Pleuritic pain and/or haemoptysis
  - Chest X-ray may show changes at the site of pleuritic pain which resolve rapidly
  - ECG often normal
  - ABGs may be normal
3 **Isolated dyspnoea (usually due to a central embolus)**
  - Acute shortness of breath with no other symptoms
  - ABGs show hypoxia
  - Risk factor(s) for thromboembolism

Presenting features and diagnosis of pulmonary embolism

The features of PE vary considerably. The most common symptoms are listed in Box 8.3. Dyspnoea, pleuritic chest pain and tachypnoea occur most frequently (Torbicki 2008). Haemoptysis may also be present. Syncope is rare but indicates severe haemodynamic deterioration. In the most severe cases, hypotension and shock will be present. Isolated, sudden-onset dyspnoea is usually indicative of a central PE with haemodynamic compromise. In patients with existing heart failure or chronic lung disease, worsening dyspnoea may be the only clinical sign.

In the assessment of the patient presenting with suspected PE, it is important to accurately establish two things: first, the likelihood that the patient has had a PE; and, second, the severity of the PE.

PE is difficult to diagnose due to the limited sensitivity and specificity of the various signs and symptoms experienced by the patient (Torbicki et al. 2008). Assessment for the presence of any predisposing factors for venous thromboembolism and evaluation of the patient's presenting signs and symptoms are crucial in determining the probability of PE. Two scoring systems have been developed to classify patients according to their probability of having a PE. Both are based on the presence or absence of clinical signs (Figure 8.2). The result can then be used to determine the patient's management.

The severity of the PE is determined by assessment of the patient's risk of early mortality (Torbicki et al. 2008). The level of risk is determined by the presence or absence of specific clinical markers including shock, hypotension, signs of right ventricular dysfunction and raised troponin. High-risk patients are those with a

Revised Geneva Score (Le Gal et al 2006) :

Variable	Points
Predisposing factors	
Age > 65 years	+1
Previous DVT or PE	+3
Surgery or fracture within 1 month	+2
Active malignancy	+2
Symptoms	
Unilateral lower limb pain	+3
Haemoptysis	+2
Clinical signs	
Heart rate	
75–94 beats/min	+3
≥95 beats/min	+5
Pain on lower limb deep vein at palpation and unilateral oedema	+4

Clinical probability (3 levels)	Total
Low	0–3
Intermediate	4–10
High	≥11

Wells Score (Wells et al 2000):

Variable	Points
Predisposing factors	
Previous DVT or PE	+1.5
Recent surgery or immobilization	+1.5
Cancer	+1
Symptoms	
Haemoptysis	+1
Clinical signs	
Heart rate	
>100 beats/min	+1.5
Clinical signs of DVT	+3
Clinical judgement	
Alternative diagnosis less likely than PE	+3

Clinical probability (3 levels)	Total
Low	0–1
Intermediate	2–6
High	≥7

Clinical probability (2 levels)	Total
PE unlikely	0–4
PE likely	>4

Figure 8.2 Clinical prediction rules for pulmonary embolism: the Revised Geneva Score and the Wells Score. From Torbicki et al. (2008) Guidelines on the diagnosis and management of acute pulmonary embolism. *European Heart Journal* 29, 2276–2315. By permission of the European Society of Cardiology.

high probability of having had a PE, who require PE-specific treatment (typically presenting with shock or hypotension). Patients in the non-high-risk group can be further stratified as either intermediate- or low-risk PE. In low-risk groups, all markers are negative. In intermediate-risk groups, one marker of right ventricular dysfunction or myocardial injury is present (Torbicki et al. 2008). Such differentiation is important in determining further investigations and immediate management.

For patients with high-risk PE, immediate echocardiography should be performed in order to diagnose PE and exclude other causes of the symptoms (including tamponade, acute valvular dysfunction, cardiogenic shock and aortic dissection). Echocardiography will reveal pulmonary hypertension and signs of right ventricular overload. If available, transthoracic echocardiography may be useful in visualising the embolus within the pulmonary artery. Once the patient is stable, diagnosis may be confirmed by computed tomography (CT) scanning (Torbicki et al. 2008).

For patients with non-high risk and low probability of PE, the first-line test is plasma D-dimer measurement which will reduce the need for unnecessary imaging and will exclude PE in up to 30% of patients. If the patient has been assessed as having a high probability of PE, D-dimer is not necessary. For these patients, and those with a positive D-dimer, CT angiography by multi-detector CT scan (MDCT) is indicated. Single-detector CT scanning (SDCT) may be used; however, it is less sensitive and must be combined with venous ultrasound. A negative MDCT can safely exclude PE (Torbicki et al. 2008).

Other investigations may include measurement of brain natriuretic peptide (BNP), a substance which is released into the blood when myocardial cells have been stretched more than usual (for example, due to excessive right ventricular stretching as occurs with right ventricular failure). The level of BNP may be associated with the degree of right ventricular dysfunction (Torbicki 2008). Troponin I and T become elevated due to myocardial injury (as a result of PE) and may be associated with poorer prognosis (Becattini et al. 2007). The 12-lead ECG may indicate signs of right ventricular strain, such as new complete or partial right bundle branch block, or the classic S1Q3T3 (an S wave in lead I, Q wave in lead III and an inverted T wave in lead III) (Timmis et al. 1997). Importantly, the ECG may be useful in ruling out other causes of chest pain such as acute coronary syndrome. Jugular vein distension is also an indicator of right ventricular dysfunction; however, other causes (such as cardiac tamponade) must be ruled out (Torbicki 2008). Chest X-ray is useful to exclude other disorders as it is often normal in PE. In an acutely breathless and hypoxic patient, a normal chest X-ray is highly indicative of PE.

Immediate management

The immediate management of patients with possible massive PE is outlined in Figure 8.3. In general terms, management of PE involves:

- effective relief of pain and anxiety
- provision of supplemental oxygen for hypoxaemia

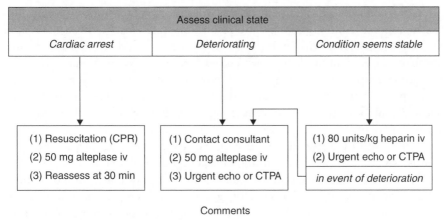

Comments

1   Massive PE is highly likely if:

- collapse/hypotension, and
- unexplained hypoxia, and
- engorged neck veins, and
- right ventricular gallop (often)

2   In stable patients where massive PE has been confirmed, iv dose of alteplase is 100 mg in 90 min (i.e. accelerated myocardial infarction regimen).

3   Thrombolysis is followed by unfractionated heparin after 3 hours, preferably weight adjusted.

4   A few units have facilities for clot fragmentation via pulmonary artery catheter. Elsewhere, contraindications to thrombolysis should be ignored in life threatening PE.

5   'Blue light' patients with out-of-hospital cardiac arrest due to PE rarely recover.

Figure 8.3   Management of probable massive pulmonary embolism (BTS 2003). Reproduced from British Thoracic Society guidelines for the management of suspected acute pulmonary embolism (2003). British Thoracic Society Standards of Care Committee PE Guideline Development Group, *Thorax*, 58, 470–484. With permission from BMJ Publishing Group Ltd.

- monitoring and maintenance of haemodynamic function
- dissolution of the blood clot

Use the ABCDE framework to prioritise the initial management and to differentiate high-risk patients from those at intermediate or low risk of early mortality from PE. Position the patient appropriately. If normotensive, help the patient to sit upright to assist breathing. If they are hypotensive (systolic blood pressure <90 mmHg), the semi-recumbent or recumbent position is preferred. Record the respiratory rate (>20 breaths/min indicates tachypnoea). Observe skin colour for cyanosis and monitor oxygen saturation. Many patients with PE will not be hypoxaemic and will not, therefore, require oxygen therapy (BTS 2008). Oxygen may be given to maintain SpO_2 at 94–98% by nasal cannulae at 2–6 L/min or by simple face mask at 5–10 L/min. For patients with high-risk PE (with hypotension or signs of shock), administer oxygen through a non-rebreathe reservoir mask at 15 L/min. Obtain arterial blood gases (ABG) to monitor hypoxaemia and hypocapnia (which occurs due to hyperventilation). Give appropriate intravenous opiate analgesia to relieve chest pain. As this can cause hypotension and respiratory depression, monitor blood pressure and respiratory rate closely. Given the risk of cardiac arrest associated with high-risk PE, the patient should be nursed in an area where they can be continuously observed, with resuscitation equipment close by. Take blood samples to establish the pre-treatment clotting screen including activated partial thromboplastin time (aPTT), prothrombin time, fibrinogen and platelets. Full blood count, urea and electrolytes should be routinely obtained in the critically ill patient.

In patients with high-risk PE, continuous cardiac monitoring of heart rate and rhythm is essential. In patients with hypotension, a central venous line should be inserted to monitor right atrial pressure and to allow the administration of intravenous fluids and drugs (Riedel 2001). Avoid aggressive fluid replacement as this may be detrimental (increasing the workload of the right ventricle); therefore, plasma expanders should be used cautiously. Positive inotropes may be used to support the blood pressure (for example, intravenous adrenaline, noradrenaline or dobutamine, providing blood pressure, heart rate and rhythm are monitored continuously) (Torbicki 2008).

The patient and their family will be extremely anxious, given the presenting features of PE. Ensure that detailed explanations about the nature and purpose of any investigations and treatment are given and that questions are answered openly and honestly.

Thrombolytic therapy

Thrombolytic therapy, in the form of intravenous alteplase 100 mg over 90 minutes should be given immediately to high-risk patients without contra-indications, who present with shock or persistent hypotension (BTS 2003). Thrombolysis may be indicated in some patients with intermediate risk, but should not be given to low-risk patients (Torbicki 2008). If the patient experiences a cardiac arrest prior to commencement of thrombolysis, a bolus dose of 50 mg alteplase should be given. If thrombolysis is contra-indicated or has failed to improve the blood pressure, surgical embolectomy (if available) is indicated; alternatively, catheter embolectomy may be used to fragment the embolus.

Because of the risk of bleeding after thrombolytic therapy, closely observe blood pressure and heart rate during and after the infusion and also check any venous or arterial puncture sites.

Anticoagulation

Heparin has been shown to reduce mortality and morbidity from PE by preventing the redevelopment of the thrombus and the development of new thrombi. This allows the body's natural mechanisms to dissolve the emboli that have already occurred (Riedel 2001). Heparin should be continued for at least 5 days (Torbicki et al. 2008).

Commence heparin as soon as possible in patients in whom PE is suspected. For high-risk patients, weight-adjusted intravenous unfractionated heparin is preferred. To be effective, unfractionated heparin must be maintained at a therapeutic level (aPTT 1.5–2.5 times the patient's pre-treatment level or the laboratory control level).

Measure aPTT 4–6 hours after commencing heparin and 3 hours after any change in heparin dosage (Torbicki et al. 2008). In most cases, a heparin regime will specify the amount required for any given aPTT. If the aPTT is not maintained within the desired range, the patient will be at risk of further thromboembolism (Riedel 2001). Heparin is associated with complications (e.g. haemorrhage and thrombocytopenia) although the former is more likely to occur in patients with a pre-existing bleeding disorder or risk factor (Riedel 2001).

For non-high-risk patients with stable blood pressure and without severe renal dysfunction, weight-adjusted subcutaneous low molecular weight heparin or fondaparinux should be commenced. In patients with severe renal dysfunction or high risk of bleeding, give an intravenous infusion of unfractionated heparin with an aPTT target range of 1.5–2.5 times normal.

Oral anticoagulation

Long-term oral anticoagulation is needed to prevent recurrent venous thromboembolism. Warfarin should be started with heparin therapy, and the two treatments should be given together for at least 5 days before heparin is discontinued. It is essential that a therapeutic dose of warfarin is administered. This is determined by the international normalised ratio (INR), which is a measure of the prothrombin time. The aim should be to maintain the INR within the range 2.0–3.0. Once the INR is within this range for at least 2 consecutive days, the heparin can be discontinued.

Nursing management

Patients with low-risk PE may be discharged early, providing appropriate outpatient management of the anticoagulation can be provided. High-risk patients will require initial monitoring of haemodynamic and respiratory function. Ongoing management includes applying compression stockings to the lower limbs, ensuring adequate hydration and commencing early ambulation once the patient is stable in order to prevent the occurrence of DVT. Vigilance is necessary in order to detect any bleeding complications or signs of recurrence of DVT or PE. Information about anticoagulation therapy, risks and complications should be given, along with advice on reducing the risk of DVT.

Summary

This chapter has considered in detail the initial assessment and management of patients who present with chest pain. Chest pain is a common complaint, which usually arises because of a disorder of the cardiac, respiratory, musculo-skeletal or gastrointestinal systems or may be related to a psychological disorder. Nurses require skill in differentiating between the different life-threatening causes of chest pain and this chapter has provided a detailed guide to that assessment. The initial management of patients with the most common, life-threatening disorders has been discussed in detail and the reader is encouraged to refer to the recommended further reading at the end of the chapter for information on the continuing management of such patients (beyond their first 24 hours in hospital).

References

Allender S, Peto V, Scarborough P, Kaur A & Rayner M (2008) *Coronary Heart Disease Statistics* (16th edition). London: British Heart Foundation.

Anderson H, Falk E & Nielsen D (1987) Right ventricular infarction: Frequency, size and topography in coronary heart disease: a prospective study comprising 107 consecutive autopsies from a coronary care unit. *Journal of the American College of Cardiology*, 10, 1223–1232 cited by Ryan T et al.. on behalf of the Committee on Management of Acute Myocardial Infarction (1999) 1999 update: American College of Cardiology/American Heart Association guidelines for the management of patients with acute myocardial infarction. *Journal of the American College of Cardiology*, 34, 890–911.

Antman E, Anbe D, Armstrong P et al. (2004) American College of Cardiology/American Heart Association Guidelines for the Management of Patients with ST-Elevation Myocardial Infarction. A Report of the American College of Cardiology/American Heart Association Task Force on Practice Guidelines (Committee to Revise the 1999 Guidelines for the Management of Patients With Acute Myocardial Infarction). *Journal of the American College of Cardiology*. 110(9), e82–e293.

Becattini C, Vedovati MC & Agnelli G (2007) Prognostic value of troponins in acute pulmonary embolism: A meta-analysis. *Circulation*, 116, 427–433.

Becker R (2000) *Chest Pain*. Boston, MA: Butterworth Heinemann.

British Medical Association & Royal Pharmaceutical Society of Great Britain (2011) *British National Formulary 61*. London: BMJ Books & Pharmaceutical Press.

British Thoracic Society (2003) British Thoracic Society guidelines for the management of suspected pulmonary embolism. *Thorax*, 58, 470–484.

British Thoracic Society Emergency Oxygen Guideline Development Group (2008) Guideline for emergency oxygen use in adult patients. *Thorax*, 63. Supplement VI.

Campbell R (1994) Arrhythmias. In: Julian D & Braunwald E (eds) *Management of Acute Myocardial Infarction*. London: W.B. Saunders.

Campbell R, Murray A & Julian D (1981) Ventricular arrhythmias in first 12 hours of acute myocardial infarction: Natural history study. *British Heart Journal*, 46, 351–357.

Cannon C, McCabe C, Diver D et al. (1994) Comparison of front-loaded recombinant tissue-type plasminogen activator, anistreplase and combination thrombolytic therapy for acute myocardial infarction: Results of the TIMI 4 trial. *Journal of the American College of Cardiology*, 24, 1602–1610.

Chambers J, Bass C & Mayou R (1999) Non-cardiac chest pain: Assessment and management. *Heart*, 82, 656–657.

Collinson J, Flather M, Fox K et al. (2000) Clinical outcomes, risk stratification and practice patterns of unstable angina and myocardial infarction without ST elevation: Prospective Registry of Acute Ischaemic Syndromes in the UK (PRAIS-UK). *European Heart Journal*, 21, 1450–1457.

Del Bene S & Vaughan A (2000) Diagnosis and management of myocardial infarction. In: Woods S, Froelicher E & Motzer S (eds) *Cardiac Nursing* (4th edition). Philadelphia: Lippincott.

Department of Health (2000) *National Service Framework for Coronary Heart Disease.* London: DH.

Dowling J (1997) Other causes of chest pain. In: Thompson P (ed.) *Coronary Care Manual.* London: Churchill Livingstone.

Fibrinolytic Therapy Trialists (FTT) Collaborative Group (1994) Indications for fibrinolytic therapy in suspected acute myocardial infarction: Collaborative overview of early mortality and major morbidity results from all randomised trials of more than 1000 patients. *Lancet,* 343, 311–322.

Fletcher P (1997) Pathophysiology of myocardial infarction. In: Thompson P (ed.) *Coronary Care Manual.* London: Churchill Livingstone.

Fox K (2000) Acute coronary syndromes: presentation: clinical spectrum and management. *Heart,* 84, 93–100.

Graham L, Atar D, Borch-Johnsen K et al. (2007) European guidelines on cardiovascular disease prevention in clinical practice: Executive summary. *European Heart Journal,* 28(19), 2375–2414.

GUSTO Angiographic Investigators (1993) The comparative effects of tissue plasminogen activator, streptokinase, or both on coronary artery patency, ventricular function and survival after acute myocardial infarction. *New England Journal of Medicine,* 329, 1615–1622 cited by Robinson N & Timmis A (2000) Reperfusion in acute myocardial infarction. *BMJ,* 320, 1354–1355.

Higham P, Adams P, Murray A & Campbell R (1993) Plasma potassium, serum magnesium and ventricular fibrillation: A prospective study. *Quarterly Journal of Medicine,* 86, 609–617.

Jowett N & Thompson D (2007) *Comprehensive Coronary Care* (4th edition). London: Baillière Tindall.

Kasper W, Geibel A, Tiede N & Just H (1992) Patent foramen ovale in patients with haemodynamically significant pulmonary embolism. *Lancet,* 340, 561– 564.

Katz R & Purcell H (2006) *Acute Coronary Syndromes.* London: Elsevier.

Le Gal G, Righini M, Roy PM et al. (2006) Prediction of pulmonary embolism in the emergency department: The revised Geneva score. *Annals of Internal Medicine,* 144, 165–171.

Lea H & Zierler B (2000) Hematopoiesis and coagulation. In: Woods S, Froelicher E & Motzer S (eds) *Cardiac Nursing* (4th edition). Philadelphia: Lippincott.

National Institute for Health and Clinical Excellence (2002) *Guidance on the use of drugs for early thrombolysis in the treatment of acute myocardial infarction.* Technology Appraisal 52. London: NICE.

National Institute for Health and Clinical Excellence (2004) *Dyspepsia: Managing dyspepsia in primary care.* NICE Clinical Guideline CG17. London: NICE.

National Institute for Health and Clinical Excellence (2006) *Statins for the prevention of cardiovascular events.* NICE Technology Appraisal 94. London: NICE.

National Institute for Health and Clinical Excellence (2007) *Anxiety.* Clinical Guideline 22. London: NICE.

National Institute for Health and Clinical Excellence (2010a) *New NICE guidelines on diagnosis of chest pain set to save thousands of lives.* NICE Press Release 2010/035. London: NICE.

National Institute for Health and Clinical Excellence (2010b) *Chest Pain of Recent Onset.* NICE Clinical Guideline 95. London: NICE.

National Institute for Health and Clinical Excellence (2010c) *Unstable angina and NSTEMI: The early management of unstable angina and non-ST-segment-elevation myocardial.* Clinical Guideline 94. London: NICE.

Riedel M (2001) Emergency diagnosis of pulmonary embolism. *Heart*, 85, 607–609.

Robalino B, Whitlow P, Underwood D & Salcedo E (1989) Electrocardiographic manifestations of right ventricular infarction. *American Heart Journal*, 118, 138–144.

Robinson N & Timmis A (2000) Reperfusion in acute myocardial infarction. *BMJ*, 320, 1354–1355.

Roux S, Christeller S & Ludin E (1992) Effects of aspirin on coronary reocclusion and recurrent ischaemia after thrombolysis: A meta-analysis. *Journal of the American College of Cardiology*, 19, 671–677 cited by Ryan T et al. on behalf of the Committee on Management of Acute Myocardial Infarction (1999).

Ryan T, Antman E, Brooks N et al. on behalf of the Committee on Management of Acute Myocardial Infarction (1999) 1999 update: American College of Cardiology/American Heart Association guidelines for the management of patients with acute myocardial infarction. *Journal of the American College of Cardiology*, 34, 890–911.

Scottish Intercollegiate Guidelines Network (2007) *Management of Stable Angina. Guideline 96.* Edinburgh: SIGN.

Thompson P (1997) AMI: Management of cardiac arrhythmias. In: Thompson P (ed.) *Coronary Care Manual.* London: Churchill Livingstone.

Thompson P & Morgan J (1997) AMI: Emergency department care. In: Thompson P (ed.) *Coronary Care Manual.* London: Churchill Livingstone.

Thygesen K, Alpert JS, White HD on behalf of the joint SC/ACCF/AHA/WHF Task Force for the redefinition of myocardial infarction (2007) Universal definition of myocardial infarction. *Journal of the American College of Cardiology*, 50, 2173–2195.

Timmis A, Nathan A & Sullivan I (1997) *Essential Cardiology* (3rd edition). Oxford: Blackwell.

Torbicki A, Perrier A, Konstantinides S et al. (2008) Guidelines on the diagnosis and management of acute pulmonary embolism. *European Heart Journal*, 29, 2276–2315.

Van de Werf F, Bax J, Betriu A et al. (2008) Management of acute myocardial infarction in patients presenting with persistent ST-segment elevation. *European Heart Journal*, 29(23), 2909–2945.

Volpi A, Cavalli A, Santoro E & Tognoni G (1990) Incidence and prognosis of secondary ventricular fibrillation in acute myocardial infarction: Evidence for a protective effect of thrombolytic therapy. *Circulation*, 82, 1279–1288 cited by Ryan T et al. on behalf of the Committee on Management of Acute Myocardial Infarction (1999).

Webster R & Hatchett R (2007) Coronary heart disease: Stable angina and acute coronary syndromes. In: Hatchett D & Thompson D (eds) *Cardiac Nursing: A Comprehensive Guide* (2nd edition). London: Churchill Livingstone.

Weissberg P (2000) Atherogenesis: Current understanding of the causes of atheroma. *Heart*, 83, 247–252.

Wells P, Anderson D, Rodger M et al. (2000) Derivation of a simple clinical model to categorize patients' probability of pulmonary embolism: Increasing the model's utility with the SimpliRED D-dimer. *Thrombosis and Haemostasis*, 83, 416–420.

Zehender M, Kasper W, Kauder E et al. (1993) Right ventricular infarction as an independent predictor of prognosis after acute inferior myocardial infarction. *New England Journal of Medicine*, 328, 981–988 cited by Ryan T et al. on behalf of the Committee on Management of Acute Myocardial Infarction (1999).

Useful links and further reading

GRACE. Global Registry of Acute Coronary Events: an international database designed to track outcomes of patients presenting with acute coronary syndromes, including myocardial infarction or unstable angina. GRACE includes hospitals in North America, South America, Europe, Asia, Australia and New Zealand. www.outcomes-umassmed.org/grace. Click on the quick link to the web version of the risk score calculator.

British Thoracic Society Emergency Oxygen Use in Adult Patients, guideline, appendices and additional information. www.brit-thoracic.org.uk/clinical-information/emergency-oxygen/emergency-oxygen-use-in-adult-patients.aspx.

National Institute for Health and Clinical Excellence (2004) *Dyspepsia: Managing dyspepsia in primary care*. NICE Clinical Guideline CG17. NICE, London.

National Institute for Health and Clinical Excellence (2007) *Anxiety*. Clinical Guideline 22. NICE, London.

National Institute for Health and Clinical Excellence (2010a) *Chest Pain of Recent Onset*. NICE Clinical Guideline 95. NICE, London.

National Institute for Health and Clinical Excellence (2010b) *Unstable angina and NSTEMI. The early management of unstable angina and non-ST-segment-elevation myocardial*. Clinical Guideline 94. NICE, London.

Torbicki A, Perrier A, Konstantinides S et al. (2008) Guidelines on the diagnosis and management of acute pulmonary embolism. *European Heart Journal*, 29, 2276–2315.

Van de Werf F, Bax J, Betriu A et al. (2008) Management of acute myocardial infarction in patients presenting with persistent ST-segment elevation. *European Heart Journal*, 29(23), 2909–2945.

9 Abdominal Pain and Upper Gastrointestinal Bleeding

Toni Jordan, Ruth Harris
and Terry Wardle

Aims

This chapter will:

- provide a framework for the accurate assessment of the acutely ill medical patient with abdominal pain and/or upper gastrointestinal bleeding
- describe the initial management and investigations of these patients
- describe the specific management of three of the most common conditions
- provide brief details of some of the less common conditions

---

Introduction

Patients with abdominal pain and/or upper gastrointestinal bleeding may present with a variety of clinical features (Box 9.1). Some of these features are specific to gastrointestinal disorders while others are common to a range of conditions. It is important for the clinician to recognise this and to facilitate effective assessment and management.

Box 9.1   Common presenting features associated with abdominal pain and gastrointestinal bleeding

Haematemesis	Constipation
Melaena	Weight loss
Vomiting	Anorexia
Tachypnoea	Dysphagia
Tachycardia	Dysuria/frequency
Diarrhoea	Pyrexia
Hypotension	

Initial Management of Acute Medical Patients: A Guide for Nurses and Healthcare Practitioners,
Second Edition. Edited by Ian Wood and Michelle Garner.
© 2012 John Wiley & Sons, Ltd. Published 2012 by John Wiley & Sons, Ltd.

Pathophysiology of abdominal pain

Abdominal pain may arise from within the peritoneal cavity, the retroperitoneum, from within the pelvis or from the abdominal wall. There are three main mechanisms of abdominal pain:

- Visceral pain
- Parietal or somatic pain
- Referred pain

Visceral pain

Visceral pain is characterised by inflammation, ischaemia, distension or neoplasm of either the wall of a hollow viscus or the capsule of a solid intra-abdominal organ. The pain, mediated by autonomic nerves, usually perceived in the midline, is poorly demarcated and does not correspond to the site of the affected viscus or organ. Visceral pain is often described as cramp-like or colicky, gnawing or burning in nature, and associated with autonomic features like nausea, vomiting, pallor and sweating. The pain is usually localised to one of three regions depending on the embryonic origin of the involved organ or viscus.

1 Foregut structures produce pain in the epigastrum
   - Stomach
   - Liver
   - Gall bladder
   - Pancreas
   - Proximal duodenum
2 Midgut structures produce pain around the umbilicus
   - Distal duodenum
   - Small intestine
   - Appendix
   - Ascending and proximal transverse colon
3 Hindgut structures produce pain in the hypochondrium and lower back
   - Descending colon
   - Bladder
   - Ureters
   - Pelvic organs

Parietal or somatic pain

Parietal or somatic pain is caused by inflammation of the parietal peritoneum. Pain is more localised to the structure from which the pain originates. It is characteristically sharp in nature, aggravated by movement, coughing and sometimes breathing.

Referred pain

Referred pain is localised to a site distant from the structure that is the source of the pain. The affected structure and the site of referred pain are of a common embryonic origin and thus share common neuronal pathways. For example, pain from subphrenic irritation of the diaphragm may be felt in the shoulder tip, the supraclavicular area or the side of the neck. The neuronal pathways from all of these areas are derived from the fourth cervical segment.

Initial assessment

The initial assessment of the patient presenting with abdominal pain and/or upper gastrointestinal bleeding can be divided into primary and secondary phases. In the primary assessment, life-threatening conditions are identified and treated, while in the secondary assessment, a detailed history and thorough examination are completed. Following completion of the secondary assessment, further investigations can be arranged and additional treatment established.

Primary assessment

The aim of the primary assessment is to identify and treat the patient presenting with a life-threatening cause of acute abdominal pain and/or upper gastrointestinal haemorrhage.

Box 9.2 lists the life-threatening conditions that may be present in the patient with abdominal pain.

The components of the primary ABCDE assessment are outlined in Chapter 1 (Initial Assessment). However, the following section emphasises issues pertinent to abdominal pain and upper gastrointestinal bleeding.

Airway

The airway is at risk in any patient who is vomiting. This risk is increased in those who have a reduced level of consciousness. Endotracheal intubation should be considered in all patients with a reduced level of consciousness who are unable to

---

Box 9.2 Life-threatening conditions associated with abdominal pain

Acute pancreatitis
Gastrointestinal haemorrhage
Septicaemia (e.g. following perforation of colon) (see Chapter 5 – Shock)
Leaking abdominal aortic aneurysm
Acute myocardial infarction (see Chapter 8 – Chest pain)
Diabetic ketoacidosis (see Chapter 6 – Altered consciousness)
Small bowel infarction (mesenteric artery occlusion)
Ectopic pregnancy
Splenic rupture

protect their own airway (Glasgow coma score < 8/15). In addition, anaesthetic help should be sought in any patient who is hypoxaemic with the potential for airway compromise (e.g. haematemesis). Pass a large-bore nasogastric tube to drain fluid and air from the stomach and to reduce the risk of aspiration in patients suspected of having obstruction of either the gastric outflow or small bowel.

Breathing

A patient with severe abdominal pain may exhibit dyspnoea because of splinting of chest movement or the diaphragm. Likewise, pain can cause tachypnoea from activation of the sympathetic nervous system. Cardiorespiratory conditions in which dyspnoea is common may either present with abdominal pain (e.g. acute myocardial infarction, pneumonia) or may co-exist (e.g. chronic obstructive pulmonary disease).

Remember that tachypnoea can be due to non-'B' causes, for example, haemorrhagic shock, brainstem stroke. In addition, Kussmaul's respiration (i.e. deep sighing breathing) is a manifestation of a metabolic acidosis (e.g. diabetic ketoacidosis, which can present with abdominal pain).

Circulation

Circulatory assessment in patients with abdominal pain and, in particular, where there is evidence of upper gastrointestinal bleeding, is important to diagnose shock; for example, hypovolaemic shock due to haemorrhage, septic shock secondary to ascending cholangitis, toxic shock associated with small bowel infarction and severe colitis. In patients presenting with abdominal pain, shock may be multifactorial due to a critical reduction in preload or afterload or both, or pump failure:

- Preload reduction occurs in hypovolaemia. The cause of hypovolaemia may be overt (e.g. haematemesis, diarrhoea) or covert (e.g. intra-abdominal haemorrhage from a leaking aortic aneurysm)
- Afterload reduction (reduced systolic vascular resistance) occurs with vasodilatation (e.g. in sepsis/toxic shock)
- Pump failure due to negative inotropes e.g. acidosis, inflammatory compounds

The treatment of shock is outlined in Chapter 5 but, in addition, consider the following measures for patients with abdominal pain and/or upper gastrointestinal bleeding:

- Insert a 14 G cannula and start controlled fluid resuscitation
- Through a second 14 G cannula, take blood for:
  o full blood count (FBC) – a raised white cell count is commonly found in this group of patients but does not necessarily mean an infective cause of the abdominal pain (e.g. patients with diabetic ketoacidosis often complain of abdominal pain and have a neutrophil leucocytosis in the absence of infection)

- o urea, electrolytes and creatinine – electrolyte disturbance and renal failure may occur secondary to diarrhoea and/or vomiting. A raised urea level is common following upper gastrointestinal haemorrhage due to protein absorption or 'pre-renal failure'
- o glucose – hypoglycaemia can mimic shock. If not already done, do a rapid stick test (e.g. BM stix) in addition to sending a sample to the laboratory
- o amylase – a normal amylase does not exclude acute pancreatitis and a raised amylase may occur in a variety of other conditions including cholecystitis, perforated peptic ulcer and diabetic ketoacidosis
- o blood group±cross match
- o clotting studies – if the patient is taking anticoagulants or liver disease is suspected
- o liver enzymes (often referred to as liver function tests; LFTs). These indicate structural integrity of the liver. Tests of liver function include prothrombin time, albumen and bilirubin. All of these tests should be requested in patients who are jaundiced or if hepatobiliary disease is suspected
- o calcium – features of hypercalcaemia include abdominal pain, vomiting, constipation, polyuria, confusion and coma
- o blood cultures – if the patient is pyrexial or sepsis is suspected
- o sickle cell screen for patients of Afro-Caribbean descent
- o β-HCG in all females of child-bearing age

Although the results of some of these investigations may not affect immediate management, it often saves time to obtain all the relevant blood investigations during the initial assessment.

Hypovolaemia resulting from bleeding (e.g. from the gastrointestinal tract or from an aneurysm) requires replacement with blood. While waiting for blood, 2 litres of warm crystalloid can be given intravenously. If there is no improvement in the respiratory rate, pulse and blood pressure, 'O' negative blood should be given until cross-matched blood is available. The aim of fluid resuscitation is to maintain a systolic blood pressure of approximately 100 mmHg (i.e. 'controlled hypotension'). Blood pressure at higher levels may encourage continued bleeding by disturbing clots that have formed in conditions such as bleeding oesophageal varices or leaking aortic aneurysm.

If either septic or toxic shock is suspected, consider:

- intravenous fluids
- a broad-spectrum antibiotic initially (e.g. Tazocin 4.5 g TDS) and alter appropriately when the results of cultures are known
- inotropes. In sepsis, peripheral vasodilatation results in reduced systemic vascular resistance and, if hypotension remains despite adequate fluid replacement, a vasoconstrictor such as noradrenaline (norepinephrine) may be required. This is given by intravenous infusion via a central venous catheter and the dose adjusted according to response. Side effects include hypertension, arrhythmias and peripheral ischaemia

> **Box 9.3   High-risk patients with upper gastrointestinal bleeding**
>
> High-risk patients are patients with three or more of the following criteria:
>
> - Age >60 years
> - Fresh haematemesis with melaena – twice the mortality of either alone
> - Non-steroidal anti-inflammatory drug (NSAID) intake
> - Continued bleeding, or a rebleed in hospital
> - Heart failure
> - Chronic airflow limitation
> - Chronic liver disease
> - Onset of bleeding in a patient already in hospital for another reason
> - Pulse >100 bpm – suggests the need for transfusion
> - Systolic BP <100 mmHg – but it may be preserved until very late in young patients
> - Postural drop in systolic BP >15 mmHg on sitting up
> - Endoscopic stigmata present:
>   - active arterial bleeding (80% risk of rebleed)
>   - visible vessel in the ulcer bare (50% risk of rebleed)
>   - fresh adherent clot or oozing (30% risk of rebleed) or
>   - black dots on the ulcer base (5% risk of rebleed)
> - Endoscopic evidence of oesophageal varices or portal hypertensive gastropathy

Consider calling the surgical team if any of the following are suspected:

- hypovolaemic shock not responding to fluid resuscitation
- peritonitis (generalised or local)
- perforation of a viscus
- bowel obstruction
- pancreatitis
- leaking abdominal aortic aneurysm
- bowel infarction or ischaemia
- upper gastrointestinal bleeding in a high-risk patient (see Box 9.3)
- lower gastrointestinal bleeding

Disability

Level of consciousness may be depressed secondary to shock. Remember to check plasma glucose if not performed in 'C'.

External

Clues include rash. Remember to check the patient's temperature. Hypothermia may be associated with sepsis and pancreatitis.

In the majority of medical patients presenting with abdominal pain and/or upper gastrointestinal bleeding, the primary assessment is often completed within minutes.

Box 9.4 lists some of the many conditions that can present with abdominal pain. As soon as any immediately life-threatening conditions have been treated or

Box 9.4   Conditions that can present with acute abdominal pain and/or upper GI bleeding that are not necessarily immediately life-threatening

Intra-abdominal conditions
Gastroenteritis
Acute appendicitis
Acute cholecystitis, gall bladder and biliary tract disease
Peptic ulcer disease
Intestinal obstruction
Pseudo-obstruction
Acute pancreatitis
Perforated viscus
Neoplastic disease
Diverticular disease
Infarction of bowel or spleen
Inflammatory bowel disease
Primary infective peritonitis
Tense ascites

Urological conditions
Lower urinary tract infection/pyelonephritis
Ureteric/renal colic
Acute urinary retention
Testicular torsion
Acute epididymitis

Gynaecological and obstetric conditions
Miscarriage
Pelvic inflammatory disease
Ovarian disease: ovarian torsion, haemorrhage into an ovarian cyst
Ectopic pregnancy
Retained products of conception
Labour
Abruption of placenta

Toxins/poisoning
Certain foods
Alcohol
Iron
Lead
Aspirin

Cardio-respiratory conditions
Myocardial infarction
Basal pneumonia
Pulmonary embolus

Other conditions
Diabetic ketoacidosis
Sickle cell crisis
Addisonian crisis
Hypercalcaemia
Herpes zoster

Non-specific abdominal pain

excluded and the patient's vital signs stabilised, a relevant history should be obtained and an appropriate examination completed, i.e. the secondary assessment.

Secondary assessment

The aim of the secondary assessment is to identify all conditions not detected in the primary assessment. This is achieved by seeking corroborative evidence for a provisional diagnosis through the history of the presenting complaint and physical examination. Following the secondary assessment, further investigations may be requested and an appropriate initial management plan established.

History

Obtaining a clear history, particularly of the presenting problem, is extremely important. If the patient is not able to give this, gather a corroborative history from relatives or carers, the patient's general practitioner and/or ambulance personnel. In addition to the elements of history taking outlined in Chapter 1, the following approach can be used.

In secondary assessment of abdominal pain, it is important to gather information regarding all clinical features. Box 9.5 indicates the key elements of a medical history. for which 'PHRASED' is a useful mnemonic.

Presenting features (P) and associated history (H)

Abdominal pain

It is important to assess the patient's pain effectively. The PQRST mnemonic is recommended and comprises the following.

Provoking/relieving factors. A patient with peritonitis will find movement, coughing and deep inspiration painful. Vomiting may provide transient relief of pain in small intestinal obstruction.

Quality (duration and character). Pain can be constant (e.g. in bowel infarction) or intermittent (e.g. gastroenteritis). An obstructed viscus usually results in colicky

---

Box 9.5   Essential elements of a medical history (PHRASED)

Presenting features
Associated **H**istory of presenting complaint
Relevant past medical and surgical history
Allergies
Systems review
Essential social and family history
Drugs

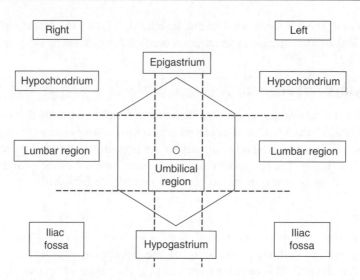

Figure 9.1 Areas of the abdomen.

pain (present all the time but with fluctuating intensity). Patients often find it difficult to describe the character of pain and different terms can mean different things to different people. However, sharp pain usually indicates somatic pain. Visceral pain is more likely to be poorly localised and described as a dull ache.

Radiation.   Abdominal pain may radiate to the patient's back (e.g. pain from a leaking abdominal aortic aneurysm). Upper abdominal pain radiating to the back is suggestive of pancreatitis. Hypogastric pain radiating to the patient's back and thighs suggests large bowel pathology.

Site and severity.   (See Figure 9.1.) An ill-defined site suggests visceral pain early in a disease process or a metabolic, toxic or psychological cause. Migration of pain is characteristic of an inflamed viscus. Examples of this would be migration from the peri-umbilical region to the right iliac fossa in acute appendicitis or from the epigastrium to the right hypochondrium in cholecystitis.

Time and treatment.   Sudden onset of severe pain is characteristic of a vascular problem (e.g. leaking abdominal aortic aneurysm). Pain from pancreatitis may develop relatively rapidly, but over minutes rather than seconds. Diverticulitis or appendicitis tends to progress more slowly, over hours or days.

Other pain measurement tools can be used to supplement this assessment.

Haematemesis (vomiting of blood)

Haematemesis is a feature of oesophageal, gastric and duodenal pathology, especially inflammatory, ulcerative and neoplastic disease. Vomiting a small amount of bright red blood after repeated retching is suggestive of a Mallory–Weiss tear.

In contrast, haematemesis can be copious with ruptured oesophageal varices. A brown fluid ('coffee ground') vomit without any other symptoms or signs is unlikely to be due to a significant gastrointestinal bleed.

Melaena (passage of black, tarry stool per rectum)

Melaena is altered blood and this implies bleeding proximal to the splenic flexure of the colon. Ingestion of iron supplements, that may have been obtained 'over the counter', often results in black stool.

Vomiting

Vomiting is a common, non-specific presenting feature. A careful history will identify clues as to the cause. Faeculent vomiting indicates intestinal obstruction. In contrast 'faecal' vomiting indicates a gastrocolic fistula.

Diarrhoea

Diarrhoea is another non-specific feature that can be a manifestation of many conditions including gastroenteritis, drug treatment, pneumonia and thyrotoxicosis. Diarrhoea with blood or mucus can be a symptom of inflammatory bowel disease, ischaemic bowel, malignancy or certain infections (e.g. Campylobacter, Shigella, Salmonella, E. coli and amoebiasis).

Constipation

Absolute constipation with abdominal pain and vomiting is indicative of intestinal obstruction.

Weight loss with anorexia

Weight loss and anorexia commonly occur with malignant disease, but can be associated with extensive inflammation.

Dysphagia

Preceding dysphagia may indicate an underlying oesophageal malignancy.

Trauma

Splenic rupture characterised by shock, left shoulder tip pain with abdominal tenderness and distension can occur after blunt abdominal trauma.

Relevant past medical and surgical history (R)

Has the patient had any episodes similar to the present problem? In addition, ask about the results of previous investigations, treatment and the response. Collect details of any prior abdominal surgery and other conditions such as:

- diabetes mellitus
- cardiovascular disease
- cerebrovascular disease
- respiratory conditions
- infections (e.g. tuberculosis)
- psychiatric illness

Allergies (A)

Note any adverse reactions or allergies to medications, topical antiseptics and cleansing agents (e.g. iodine) or wound dressings.

Systems review (S)

Particular attention should be paid to the following systems.

Respiratory system

A recent cough productive of purulent sputum could indicate a basal pneumonia that might be presenting as abdominal pain. Any history of haemoptysis needs further investigation in its own right. However, the combination of upper abdominal pain and haemoptysis might occur in a pulmonary embolus.

Cardiovascular system

Preceding chest pain on exertion could suggest that the patient's upper abdominal pain is resulting from an inferior myocardial infarction.

Urinary system

Dysuria and frequency of micturition may suggest a urological cause for the abdominal pain, but remember that an inflamed appendix or a colonic diverticulum abutting the ureter or bladder can cause urinary symptoms.

From women, obtain a gynaecological history including details of menstrual pattern and contraception. Remember the possibility of ectopic pregnancy, especially in the female patient of child-bearing age presenting with unexplained hypovolaemia even in the absence of abdominal pain.

Essential family and social history (E)

Ask the patient if any of their family has gastrointestinal disorders (e.g. inflammatory bowel disease, carcinoma) or any relevant inherited conditions (e.g. sickle cell disease, acute intermittent porphyria).

Social history in respect of abdominal pain should specifically include details of smoking habits, detailed alcohol history and contact with other people with similar symptoms.

Drugs (D)

Record details of all the patient's medications, including the dose and dosing schedule. Ask about and record the patient's use of 'over-the-counter' medications.

The use of NSAIDs (including aspirin) and warfarin should be specifically questioned in patients presenting with upper gastrointestinal bleeding. Previous treatment with glucocorticoids is particularly important to note as the clinical and laboratory responses to inflammation or perforation of an abdominal viscus may be masked. Also, patients who have been taking long-term gluco-corticoids may have adrenal suppression and, on admission, the dose of glucocorticoids should be, at least, doubled to mimic the usual stress response to acute illness.

Physical examination

The physical examination comprises general observation, inspection, palpation, percussion and auscultation.

General observation

Patients with visceral pain (e.g. ureteric colic) tend to roll around in the bed while patients with generalised peritonitis tend to lie still and have rapid, shallow respiration. While looking at the patient's face, ask the patient to cough. An observation of abdominal pain, flinching or a protective movement of hands towards the abdomen suggests peritonitis.

Inspection

Asking the patient to take a deep breath may reveal organomegaly or masses in the abdomen. Inspect the mouth for telangiectasia (permanent dilatation of groups of superficial blood vessels), perioral pigmentation and pigmentation on the buccal mucosa (Addison's disease). Inspect the sclera for signs of jaundice and the conjunctiva of the lower eyelid for pallor that may indicate anaemia. Box 9.6 gives details of the characteristic signs of chronic liver disease.

Dry skin with reduced skin turgor implies chronic dehydration due to extracellular fluid loss, which can occur in gastroenteritis or intestinal obstruction.

The clinical features outlined in Box 9.7 may also be observed in relation to their respective disorders.

Box 9.6   Characteristic features of chronic liver disease

- Palmar erythema
- Dupuytren's contracture
- Leuconychia (white fingernails)
- Clubbing of the fingernails
- Spider naevi
- Abnormal veins around the umbilicus (in portal hypertension the direction of flow of these veins below the umbilicus is downward; dilated veins can also occur around the umbilicus in inferior vena caval obstruction where the direction of flow below the umbilicus is upwards)
- Loss of body hair
- Gynaecomastia
- Testicular atrophy
- Ascites
- Signs of encephalopathy (e.g. liver flap)

Box 9.7   Presenting features associated with their respective disorders

- Pigmented scars and palmar creases associated with Addison's disease
- Visible pulsation of an abdominal aortic aneurysm may be seen
- Visible peristalsis implies bowel obstruction
- An everted umbilicus occurs with gross ascites
- Bluish discoloration around the umbilicus (Cullen's sign) can occur when blood is in the peritoneal cavity (e.g. in acute pancreatitis or ruptured ectopic pregnancy)
- Discoloration in the flanks (Grey Turner's sign) is occasionally seen in haemorrhagic pancreatitis and in other causes of retroperitoneal haemorrhage (e.g. leaking abdominal aortic aneurysm)
- Erythema nodosum (painful, red nodular lesions on the anterior shins, thighs or fore-arms) is associated with inflammatory bowel disease
- Hernial orifices should be carefully examined. A small, incarcerated femoral hernia can be missed easily.
- Look for lymphadenopathy. Virchow's node is an enlarged left supraclavicular lymph node associated with cancer of the stomach. Troisier's sign describes enlargement of left supraclavicular nodes due to metastases from carcinoma of stomach or lung.

Palpation

It is important that the examiner's hands should be warm for the patient's comfort. Furthermore, cold hands might cause the patient to flinch or grimace and thereby make it difficult to assess areas for tenderness.

To examine the patient's abdomen, the examiner should either kneel or sit. In either of these positions, the examining hand is more relaxed and in more contact with the patient than if the examiner is standing. Therefore, more information can be obtained. During palpation, the hand should be flat on the abdomen. Avoid forceful palpation, either kneading with the knuckles or digging with fingertips, as this may cause pain. Examination should start in an area away from pain.

Palpate each area sequentially while continuously looking at patient's face for any evidence of pain, tenderness or guarding (tensing of abdominal muscles because of either actual or anticipated pain). Localised tenderness suggests an inflammatory source of the patient's pain. Rebound tenderness (pain is greater when removing hand pressure) is a sign of local peritoneal inflammation, but if this becomes generalised, rigidity will occur.

Feel for organomegaly and masses. A central, large pulsatile mass is likely to be an aortic aneurysm, but this will not be felt if the aneurysm has ruptured.

Percussion

This can be used to confirm organomegaly (of liver, spleen or bladder) and ascites which can be manifested as dullness (horseshoe or shifting) and a fluid thrill.

Auscultation

Bowel sounds are non-specific. Classically, they are high-pitched in obstruction and absent when there is a perforated viscus with peritonitis. However, it is important to realise that bowel sounds may be normal even in cases of serious intra-abdominal pathology.

The physical examination is usually concluded by examination of the hernial orifices and external genitalia, checking for lymphadenopathy and performing a digital rectal examination. This is mandatory for patients who present with abdominal pain and/or gastrointestinal bleeding. Any perianal disease (which may indicate Crohn's disease), the colour of the stool and presence of blood and/or mucus should be noted. The finding of melaena on digital rectal examination confirms a gastrointestinal bleed proximal to the splenic flexure.

Elderly patients

The elderly have less physiological reserve; combined with reduced cardiovascular compliance this means that they do not tolerate even small changes in blood volume. This is often exacerbated by concomitant drug therapy, especially diuretics. In comparison with younger patients, fever, tachycardia and leucocytosis are less common in inflammatory conditions such as appendicitis. Pain tends to be less predominant and delayed presentation is more common. The presence of co-existent conditions is likely to lead to a variety of symptoms and signs.

Immediate management and investigations

In the initial management of acutely ill medical patients presenting with abdominal pain and/or upper gastrointestinal bleeding, the following should be considered:

1   Fluid resuscitation
2   Analgesia
3   Antibiotics
4   Control of vomiting

Fluid resuscitation

During the primary assessment, patients with circulatory failure will have been identified and resuscitated with appropriate intravenous fluids. Careful fluid balance is mandatory in any patient who is seriously ill; this involves urinary catheterisation and documentation of hourly urine output and 'vital' signs, and co-operation and communication between the medical and nursing staff. Fluid and electrolytes need to be replaced with an appropriate crystalloid. This is particularly important for patients who might need urgent surgery. For elderly patients (or those with cardiac disease) who are at risk of the complications of fluid overload, consider central venous pressure monitoring.

Analgesia

Adequate analgesia is paramount in any patient presenting with acute abdominal pain. Opioid analgesia is often required and should be given by slow intravenous injection and titrated against the patient's pain (e.g. morphine, initially 5–10 mg, given at a rate of 1 mg/min, with further doses as required). Appropriate analgesia will facilitate clinical examination.

Antibiotics

Antibiotics should be used when there is evidence – or high clinical suspicion – of infection. Blood cultures and other appropriate cultures should be taken before giving antibiotics. The antibiotic choice should be tailored to the most likely organism(s) causing the sepsis. Consult local hospital guidelines for the prescription of antibiotics.

Control of vomiting

An anti-emetic (e.g. metoclopramide) should be prescribed if the patient is or has been vomiting or following opioid analgesia. A large-bore nasogastric tube should be passed if any of the following are suspected:

- gastric outflow obstruction
- small bowel obstruction
- perforation of viscus
- pancreatitis
- persistent vomiting despite the use of anti-emetic medication

Investigations

During the primary and secondary assessments, a range of investigations may be considered depending upon findings. Appropriate investigations may include:

- blood tests
- urine tests
- electrocardiogram (ECG)
- radiological investigations

Blood tests

In addition to the blood investigations outlined above, arterial blood gases should be taken in patients with pancreatitis, shock or co-existent respiratory disease.

Urine tests

Perform a urinalysis (dipstick) on all patients presenting with abdominal pain. The following results give an indication of underlying pathology:

- urobilinogen/bilirubin – indicative of liver or biliary tract disease
- blood – may suggest a renal or urological cause of the pain (e.g. urinary tract infection or renal stone)
- ketones and glucose – indicate diabetic ketoacidosis

A urine pregnancy test should be requested in all women of child-bearing age presenting with abdominal pain. The results of such tests are confidential to the patient.

Electrocardiogram

Consider recording a 12-lead ECG in all patients as an acute myocardial infarction can present with abdominal pain. Atrial fibrillation can result in mesenteric embolic infarction.

Radiological investigations

An erect chest X-ray is required if a perforated viscus is suspected and should be considered in patients with co-existent chest pathology. The patient should be sitting up for at least 5 minutes before the X-ray is taken. If the patient is unable to sit or stand, an abdominal lateral decubitus film may show extraluminal gas.

A supine abdominal X-ray can be helpful if either intestinal obstruction or toxic megacolon are suspected. If either ureteric or renal colic is the differential diagnosis, a KUB (kidneys, ureter and bladder) film should be requested. An erect abdominal X-ray is rarely helpful and should not be requested 'routinely'.

Subsequent investigations may include the following.

Ultrasound scan. If a leaking abdominal aortic aneurysm is suspected, an ultrasound scan is required urgently. Suspected biliary tract or urinary tract obstruction is also an indication for urgent ultrasound scanning.

Intravenous urography. An IVU is often required in patients presenting with ureteric colic to illustrate a calculus and assess the extent of any obstruction of the ureter and kidney. In most hospitals this has been superseded by CT scanning.

CT scan. This is likely to provide more information than an ultrasound scan in the investigation of pancreatic abnormalities. It might be the preferred investigation for a patient presenting with an abdominal mass or suspected visceral perforation. It is prudent to discuss the appropriate radiological investigation in the acute setting with a radiologist.

Angiography. Mesenteric angiography may be used to establish the bleeding point in gastrointestinal haemorrhage. It has the advantage over a labelled red cell scan that therapeutic embolisation can be achieved at the time of angiography. A labelled red cell scan, however, is more sensitive in detecting the area of bleeding. Mesenteric angiography is also useful if mesenteric ischaemia is suspected.

Unprepared contrast enema. This might be required urgently to establish the cause of a suspected large bowel obstruction and to exclude a pseudo-obstruction.

Indications for referral

During the primary assessment, the patient may have been referred to the surgical team. Having completed the secondary assessment, it is worth reconsidering the indications for referral to the surgical team. These include, but are not limited to, suspected:

- hypovolaemic shock not responding to fluid resuscitation
- perforated viscus
- peritonitis, generalised or local
- bowel obstruction
- pancreatitis
- leaking abdominal aortic aneurysm
- bowel infarction or ischaemia
- upper gastrointestinal bleeding in a high-risk patient (see Box 9.3)
- lower gastrointestinal bleeding

Patients with ureteric colic should be referred to the urology team or general surgeon, dependent on local arrangements.

Gynaecological assessment is required if any of the following conditions are suspected:

- ectopic pregnancy
- miscarriage

- pelvic inflammatory disease
- complications of an ovarian cyst

Causes of abdominal pain and upper gastrointestinal bleeding

Of all patients presenting with a medical emergency, 13% will have an acute gastrointestinal condition. There are many causes of abdominal pain and upper gastrointestinal bleeding (see Box 9.4), with no specific diagnosis being made in one-third of patients presenting with acute abdominal pain.

In this section, the pathophysiology, assessment and management of three of the more common conditions will be discussed:

1 Acute upper gastrointestinal bleeding
2 Acute gastroenteritis
3 Inflammatory bowel disease

Features of some of the less common, but still important, conditions will be discussed briefly.

Acute upper gastrointestinal bleeding

Cause

Upper gastrointestinal bleeding is a common cause for acute medical admission and, overall, has a mortality of 5 to 14% (Rockall et al. 1995; Gralnek et al. 2008). Many conditions can cause acute upper gastrointestinal bleeding. Although in approximately 20% of cases no lesion is detected, the following conditions are most often found (in order of frequency):

- duodenal ulcer
- gastric ulcer
- gastric erosions
- Mallory–Weiss tear

Less common causes of upper gastrointestinal bleeding include:

- duodenitis
- oesophageal varices
- oesophagitis
- tumours

Pathophysiology

Duodenal ulcer

As many as 95% of duodenal ulcers are associated with the presence of *Helicobacter pylori* (McDonald et al. 1999) which causes an antritis, hypergastrinaemia and increased gastric acid secretion resulting in ulceration in the duodenal cap. Ingestion of NSAIDs can precipitate or exacerbate bleeding from a duodenal ulcer.

Gastric ulcer

Approximately 70% of gastric ulcers are associated with *Helicobacter pylori* (McDonald et al. 1999). Use of NSAIDs increases the risk of developing a gastric ulcer. Chronic, benign ulceration is associated with smoking. Additional proposed mechanisms include impairment of the mucus-bicarbonate barrier, acid-pepsin damage, deficient gastric mucosal blood flow and duodenogastric reflux. Benign gastric ulcers tend to occur on the lesser curve of the stomach. Ulcers on the greater curve, fundus and in the antrum are more commonly malignant.

Gastric erosions

Gastric erosions are small, shallow lesions, usually < 5 mm in diameter, which heal with no sign of scarring. They are commonly seen in an acute gastropathy associated with ingestion of NSAIDs or alcohol. Gastritis is a term that should be reserved for a histological diagnosis.

Mallory–Weiss tear

This is a mucosal tear at the oesophago-gastric junction caused by forceful vomiting.

Presenting features

Haematemesis and/or melaena are often, but not always, present. A patient who has had an upper gastrointestinal bleed may present with shock and few other clinical features; most however have no signs of shock. There may be a previous history of weight loss or dysphagia, which may be suggestive of underlying malignancy. Establish whether there is a history of gastrointestinal bleeding and, if so, its cause. Make a note of medications, particularly NSAIDs and warfarin, alcohol, liver disease and any other co-morbidities. Determine if the patient has had an aortic graft as, in these cases, an aortoenteric fistula can form which leads to upper gastrointestinal bleeding.

On presentation, if the patient shows signs of shock, initiate treatment as outlined in the primary assessment. During the examination in the secondary assessment, note the presence or absence of signs of chronic liver disease. If abdominal scars are present, establish their history. The presence or absence of melaena must be confirmed by a digital rectal examination.

Numerical scoring systems can be used after acute upper gastrointestinal haemorrhage e.g. Rockall and Glasgow-Blatchford scores (Rockall et al. 1996; Blatchford et al. 2000). These may be used to identify patients who are at low risk of re-bleeding and can be considered for early discharge or outpatient treatment.

Immediate management and investigations

The aims of managing patients presenting with acute upper gastrointestinal bleeding are to:

- resuscitate or stabilise the patient
- stop active bleeding
- prevent recurrent bleeding

The immediate management of a shocked patient has been described earlier in this chapter (and in Chapter 5 – Shock). Endoscopic therapy has an important role in stopping active bleeding and should be arranged as soon as possible. The surgical team should be involved before an operation is necessary rather than when it is inevitable. Ideally, the patient should be admitted to a designated high dependency unit.

Initial investigations include full blood count, coagulation studies (when liver disease is present or suspected), urea, electrolytes, creatinine and arterial blood gases (in those with respiratory disease). An urgent upper gastrointestinal endoscopy is essential. This will confirm the diagnosis and facilitate therapeutic intervention in active bleeding from, for example, peptic ulceration and oesophageal varices. The exact timing and place of endoscopy will depend on local arrangements, but should take place within 24 hours. Remember that measured haemoglobin is a poor indicator of transfusion requirement. Haemodynamic status is a better guide.

Ongoing assessment

The ongoing assessment in a patient who has had an upper gastrointestinal bleed is very important. Initially, monitor vital signs every 15 minutes. A rising pulse rate, rising diastolic blood pressure with reduction in pulse pressure, falling systolic blood pressure or decreasing urine output suggest continued bleeding or a re-bleed. The insertion of a central venous line to monitor the central venous pressure is appropriate in elderly patients and those with a history of cardiac disease or poor peripheral venous access.

A comprehensive review of this subject is beyond the scope of this chapter. A more detailed overview can be found in the additional reading list.

Acute gastroenteritis

Cause

Acute gastroenteritis is usually caused by the ingestion of bacteria, viruses and toxins (bacterial and chemical) from contaminated food or water. It can also have an airborne source, e.g. Noro virus.

Pathophysiology

There are three different pathophysiological mechanisms.

1. Inflammatory diarrhoea

Bacterial invasion of the mucosa of the distal small bowel and colon results in both impairment of the absorptive function of the intestine together with loss of blood protein and mucus leading to blood- and mucus-stained diarrhoea. Typical organisms causing inflammatory diarrhoea include *Salmonella enteritidis, Shigella, Campylobacter jejuni* and *Entamoeba histolytica. Clostridium difficile* and verotoxin-producing *Escherichia coli* (e.g. *E. coli* 0157) produce cytopathic toxins.

2. Secretory (non-inflammatory) diarrhoea

A toxin blocks the *passive* absorption of sodium (and water) and stimulates active sodium (and water) excretion in the small bowel, resulting in large amounts of isotonic fluid being secreted into the bowel lumen. This situation exceeds the absorptive capacity of the intestine with resulting profuse watery diarrhoea. *Active* sodium absorption by a glucose-dependent mechanism is not generally affected; therefore rehydration can be achieved by oral glucose solutions which contain both sodium and carbohydrate. Classically, the enterotoxin of *Vibrio cholerae* causes secretory diarrhoea, but *Giardia lamblia, Cryptosporidium, Bacillus cereus* (found in rice), enterotoxogenic *Escherichia coli* and rotavirus, among others, can do so.

3. Systemic infection

This occurs when infection penetrates the mucosa of the distal small bowel, invades lymphatovascular structures and causes a bacteraemia. Such invasive organisms include *Salmonella typhi, Salmonella paratyphi* and *Yersinia enterocolitica.*

Presenting features

Diarrhoea, abdominal pain, fever, nausea and/or vomiting can occur in various combinations with varying severity.

The presence of blood and pus in diarrhoea is indicative of an inflammatory origin. Inflammatory diarrhoea characteristically contains faecal leucocytes on microscopy. Severity varies from short-lived episodes of diarrhoea with spontaneous resolution to severe colitis complicated by toxic megacolon, perforation, septicaemia and death.

In cases of secretory (non-inflammatory) diarrhoea, there is profuse watery diarrhoea with vomiting. This can cause severe dehydration, leading to hypovolaemic shock and death.

With a systemic infection, about 50% of patients with typhoid fever develop constipation that precedes the diarrhoea and fever. Other features include malaise, headache, cough, relative bradycardia with high fever, myalgia, abdominal pain and splenomegaly. Complications include small bowel ulceration and occasionally perforation.

A history of overseas travel or of similar symptoms in family members or other contacts might be considered. Preceding antibiotic use or hospital admission might suggest *C. difficile* colitis. Key clinical features suggestive are:

- age > 65 years
- preceding antibiotic use
- neutrophil count > 15

Immediate management and investigations

Fluid replacement with monitoring of fluid balance and oral rehydration may be sufficient in most cases. Antibiotics are rarely required but should be considered in the following cases:

- *Clostridium difficile* toxin-related diarrhoea
- Severe *Salmonella* or *Campylobacter* infections, particularly in those who are immuno-compromised or who have co-existent medical problems
- Cholera
- Parasitic infections

These cases should be discussed with colleagues at the local Public Health Laboratory. Anti-diarrhoeal agents should be avoided but analgesia and anti-emetics can be given as required. If *Clostridium difficile* toxin-associated diarrhoea is suspected, pre-emptive oral antibiotic treatment is advocated, e.g. metronidazole 400 mg TDS or vancomycin 125 mg QDS according to local antibiotic guidelines.

Remember that the Consultant in Communicable Disease Control (CCDC) must be notified regarding the following diseases:

- Food poisoning (any)
- Dysentery (amoebic, typhoid/paratyphoid)
- Cholera

A stool specimen for microscopy (leucocytes, red blood cells, ova, cysts and parasites) and culture (*Salmonella, Shigella, Campylobacter* and *E. coli* 0157) and toxin detection (*C. difficile*) should be sent as soon as possible. If appropriate, a hot stool should be sent for examination for trophozoites of *Amoeba*. Relevant blood tests are likely to include full blood count, urea, creatinine, electrolytes and blood cultures.

Ongoing assessment

In the continuing assessment of patients with acute gastroenteritis, it is important to look for dehydration, shock and abdominal symptoms and signs of perforation.

Inflammatory bowel diseases (ulcerative colitis and Crohn's disease)

Cause

The cause of the inflammatory bowel diseases is not known. Ulcerative colitis is a recurrent inflammatory disease of the large bowel and virtually always involves the rectum and spreads in continuity proximally to involve a variable amount of the colon. Crohn's disease can affect any part of the gastrointestinal tract from the mouth to the anus with unaffected areas between the transmural inflammation. However, Crohn's disease usually affects the terminal ileum and ileo-caecal region.

Presenting features

Abdominal pain tends to be a more prominent feature in Crohn's disease than in ulcerative colitis. Patients with Crohn's disease may present with abdominal pain associated with vomiting, diarrhoea and weight loss. The site of the disease influences presentation. Crohn's disease involving the colon may present like ulcerative colitis. In ulcerative colitis, the principal symptoms are diarrhoea with rectal bleeding. Patients with ulcerative colitis often complain of abdominal discomfort with cramps, but severe, persistent pain suggests a complication or different diagnosis.

In those with severe ulcerative colitis, or less frequently, Crohn's colitis and other forms of colitis, toxic dilatation of the colon can occur. Features associated with toxic dilatation include fever, tachycardia, hypotension and abdominal tenderness. It is important to remember that patients can present with the features of toxaemia (listed above) without any evidence of colonic dilatation. In addition, those who have a previous history of inflammatory bowel disease can, and do, develop other conditions. For example, a patient, with a previous history of Crohn's disease who presents with right hypochondrial pain may have acute cholecystitis, not an exacerbation of Crohn's disease.

Immediate management and investigations

The immediate management of patients with inflammatory bowel disease will depend on the type, site, extent and severity of the disease. Attention should be given to analgesia, fluid balance, nutrition and the administration of steroids ± antibiotics. The patient should be reassessed regularly. Involvement of the surgical team should be considered early.

Remember that the clinical appearance can be deceptive if a patient is taking any form of immunosuppressant therapy, especially steroids. Despite impending perforation in toxic dilatation, the patient may have few symptom and signs.

The initial investigations in patients who are admitted with inflammatory bowel disease, or suspected inflammatory bowel disease, include blood tests (full blood count, urea, electrolytes, creatinine, glucose, albumin, inflammatory markers and blood cultures) and radiological investigations (abdominal X-ray±an erect chest X-ray). In severe colitis, consider abdominal X-ray on a daily basis to look for the colonic dilatation. Stool should be sent for microscopy and culture, with examination for *Clostridium difficile* toxin.

Serological investigation for *Yersinia* antibodies and titre is indicated when terminal ileal disease is diagnosed in the absence of a proven diagnosis of Crohn's disease. *Yersinia enterocolitica* is a Gram–negative bacillus and, in some countries, is a common cause of gastroenteritis. Subsequent investigations may include lower gastrointestinal endoscopy (with limited or no preparation), CT scanning and contrast radiological examination.

Ongoing assessment

Patients with toxic dilatation of the colon, and those who are at risk of developing it, need close, regular assessment. Symptoms, including the severity of abdominal pain and frequency of defaecation, need to be recorded. Temperature, pulse and blood pressure should be monitored at least 2-hourly in those with severe colitis along with daily checks of haemoglobin, platelet count, albumen and C-reactive protein.

Other causes of abdominal pain and upper gastrointestinal bleeding

A variety of other conditions can cause abdominal pain and/or upper gastrointestinal bleeding (see Box 9.4). There are too many to discuss in detail in this chapter but features of some important, albeit sometimes rare, conditions include:

- diabetic ketoacidosis
- hypercalcaemia
- adrenal insufficiency
- *Yersinia* infection
- acute intermittent porphyria
- lead poisoning

Diabetic ketoacidosis

(See Chapter 6 – Altered consciousness.)

Abdominal pain occurs in up to 46% of patients presenting with diabetic ketoacidosis (Umpierrez & Freire 2002). Acute pancreatitis must be excluded in these patients, but remember that a mildly elevated serum amylase can occur in diabetic ketoacidosis without associated acute pancreatitis.

Hypercalcaemia

Causes of hypercalcaemia include malignant disease (myeloma, bone metastases, production of parathyroid hormone related peptide – PTHrP) and primary hyperparathyroidism. Symptoms include abdominal pain, vomiting, constipation, confusion and renal failure. Rehydration with intravenous fluids is very important in the immediate management of hypercalcaemia.

Adrenal insufficiency

Patients with adrenal insufficiency can occasionally present with abdominal pain. Other symptoms include weight loss, myalgia and confusion. In acute adrenal insufficiency (Addisonian crisis) the patient may present with shock. Usually, the patient will be known to have Addison's disease but, alternatively, the patient may have been taking steroids long-term and suddenly stopped them. Hyperpigmentation may be seen on examination. Blood tests are likely to show hyponatraemia, hyperkalaemia and an elevated urea.

Yersinia infection

Yersinia infection can cause a variety of clinical syndromes. These include acute mesenteric adenitis and terminal ileitis. A mistaken diagnosis of appendicitis or Crohn's disease may be made initially. A serological test for antibodies (and titre) will confirm the diagnosis.

Acute intermittent porphyria

Abdominal pain, vomiting and constipation are features of acute intermittent porphyria. Usually there is a family history of porphyria but this is not always the case. Drugs such as phenobarbitone, sulphonamides, oestrogens and alcohol can precipitate attacks. Urine porphobilinogen is raised during attacks and often between them.

Lead poisoning

'Lead colic' was described first by Hippocrates. Severe lead poisoning causes abdominal pain (which is usually diffuse), constipation, vomiting and encephalopathy. The 'classic' sign of a fine blue line on the gums is rarely seen. Basophilic stippling of red blood cells occurs and may be observed on microscopy. The blood lead level can be measured.

In some hospitals, conditions such as pancreatitis and gastrointestinal haemorrhage are managed jointly by the medical and surgical units, on specialist units. In these cases, it is important that communication and referral arrangements are in place to ensure effective continuity of care for the patient and their family.

Summary

Abdominal pain and upper gastrointestinal bleeding are common presentations in acutely ill patients. This chapter has described how to assess these patients in a structured and accurate way. Three of the most common conditions (acute gastro-intestinal bleeding, acute gastroenteritis and inflammatory bowel disease) have been described with reference to cause, pathophysiology, presenting features, immediate management, diagnostic tests/investigations and ongoing assessment. Several other conditions which are not as common but nevertheless important have been discussed briefly.

References

Advanced Life Support Group (2010) *Acute Medical Emergencies: The Practical Approach* (2nd edition). Oxford: Wiley-Blackwell.

Blatchford O, Murray W & Blatchford M (2000) A risk score to predict need for treatment for upper gastrointestinal haemorrhage. *Lancet*, 9238(356), 1318–1321.

Gralnek IM, Barkun AN & Bardou M. (2008) Management of acute bleeding from a peptic ulcer. *New England Journal of Medicine*, (359), 928–937.

McDonald J, Burroughs A & Feagan B (eds) (1999) *Evidence-Based Gastroenterology and Hepatology*. London: BMJ Books.

Rockall T, Logan R, Devlin H & Northfield T (1995) Incidence of and mortality from acute upper gastrointestinal haemorrhage in the United Kingdom. *BMJ*, (311), 222–226.

Rockall T, Logan R, Devlin H & Northfield T (1996) Risk assessment after acute upper gastrointestinal haemorrhage. *Gut*, 38(3), 316–321.

Umpierrez G & Freire A (2002) Abdominal pain in patients with hyperglycaemic crises. *Journal of Critical Care*, 17, 63–67.

Further reading

Cotton P & Williams C (2008) *Practical Gastrointestinal Endoscopy* (6th edition). Oxford: Wiley Blackwell.

Kumar P & Clark M (2009) *Clinical Medicine* (7th edition). London: WB Saunders.

Munro J & Campbell I (2000) (eds) *MacLeod's Clinical Examination* (10th edition). London: Churchill Livingstone.

Scottish Intercollegiate Guidelines Network (2008) Management of Acute Upper and Lower Intestinal Bleeding: A national clinical guideline. Guidance 105. Edinburgh: SIGN.

Travis S, Taylor R & Misiewicz J (1998) *Gastroenterology* (2nd edition). Oxford: Blackwell Science Ltd.

Warrall D, Cox T & Firth J (eds) (2010) *Oxford Textbook of Medicine* (5th edition). Oxford: Oxford University Press.

10 Extremity Pain and Swelling
Ian Wood

Aims

This chapter will:

- describe the questions to ask when taking a history from a patient presenting with extremity pain and swelling
- discuss the causes, pathophysiology, investigation and treatment of patients with the following conditions:
  - deep vein thrombosis
  - thrombophlebitis
  - cellulitis

Immediate management – initial stabilising measures

An assumption has been made in this chapter that the patient has had an overall initial assessment and that any immediately life-threatening problems have been identified and treated.

Patients presenting with painful or swollen extremities can be nursed on a stretcher or couch, in a bed or in a chair. The principle of nursing care is that the patient will be in a position comfortable for them with their leg elevated and supported on a pillow. Elevation encourages venous drainage with the aim of reducing swelling.

The clinical features associated with disorders of the extremities are outlined in Box 10.1.

Initial assessment of painful and/or swollen limbs

Clinical assessment starts when the nurse first sees the patient and starts with a visual inspection and physical examination (see Box 10.2).

Verbal questioning to collect a history of the current problem supports this assessment (Box 10.3) including asking about possible predisposing factors outlined in Box 10.4.

Initial Management of Acute Medical Patients: A Guide for Nurses and Healthcare Practitioners, Second Edition. Edited by Ian Wood and Michelle Garner.
© 2012 John Wiley & Sons, Ltd. Published 2012 by John Wiley & Sons, Ltd.

Box 10.1   Common presenting features associated with extremity pain and swelling

- Oedema
- Calf pain
- Tenderness
- Swelling of calf or leg
- Increased skin temperature
- Slight fever
- Erythema
- Engorgement of superficial leg veins
- Positive Homan's sign

Box 10.2   Initial assessment by observation and examination

Observation
- Observe and record skin colour. Compare with unaffected side.
- Is the area swollen? Compare with unaffected side.
- Is oedema present?
- Is the area painful? Check for pain at rest or on movement.
- Is the area reddened? Compare with unaffected side.
- Are any wounds present? If so, how long have they been present? Have they been treated? By whom?

Physical examination
- Check and record presence of distal pulses on the affected limb and compare with the unaffected side.
- Check and record heart rate, respiratory rate and depth, blood pressure and temperature.
- Is the area hot? Compare with unaffected side.
- Palpate the area for pain or tenderness. Compare with the unaffected side.
- Check for range of movement of proximal and distal joints. Does this increase pain?
- Can the patient walk normally on the affected limb(s)?

Box 10.3   Information to be collected during history taking

Information to be collected verbally
- History of present problem:
  - How long has it been present?
  - When did it start?
  - Is it constant or intermittent?
  - Is it worse today than usual?
- Is there any previous history of same or similar problem?
- Is there any recent history of injury to the affected area?
- Has there been any recent long-distance travel (>4 hours), in last 4 weeks?
- Has there been any previous surgery especially orthopaedic, pelvic or abdominal?
- Is the area painful? If so, does anything relieve the pain or make it worse?
- Has any medication been taken to relieve the problem?

Box 10.4   Risk factors associated with the development of VTE

- Exponential increase in risk with age. In the general population:
  - <40 years – annual risk 1/10,000
  - 60–69 years – annual risk 1/1,000
  - >80 years – annual risk 1/100
- Obesity (3 × risk if obese: body mass index ≥ 30)
- Immobilisation longer than 3 days (plaster cast, paralysis, 10 × risk; increases with duration)
- Pregnancy and post-partum period (10 × risk)
- Plane or car journey >4 hours in previous 4 weeks (risk appears higher in patients with known risk factors and in flights >3000 miles)
- Hospitalisation (major surgery, acute trauma, acute illness 10 × risk)
- Previous VTE (DVT or PE) (Recurrence rate 5% per year, increased by surgery)
- Varicose veins (1.5 × risk after major general or orthopaedic surgery but low risk after varicose vein surgery)
- High-dose oestrogen therapy or oral contraceptives (oral combined contraceptives, HRT, raloxifene, tamoxifen 3 × risk, high-dose progestogens 6 × risk
- Malignancy (7 × risk in the general population)
- Recent myocardial infarction, cerebrovascular accident, heart failure, severe infection, inflammatory bowel disease, nephrotic syndrome, polycythaemia, paraproteinaemia, Bechet's disease, paroxysmal nocturnal haemoglobinuria
- Thrombophilias (low coagulation inhibitors (antithrombin, protein C or S), activated protein C resistance (e.g. factor V Leiden), high coagulation factors (I, II, VIII, IX, XI), antiphospholipid syndrome, high homocysteine)
- Anaesthesia (2 × general versus spinal or epidural)
- Injecting drug user

Source: SIGN (2002)

Conditions most commonly causing lower limb pain and swelling are:

1   Deep vein thrombosis
2   Thrombophlebitis
3   Cellulitis
4   Peripheral oedema due to heart failure (see Chapter 7 – Shortness of breath)

Deep vein thrombosis

Deep vein thrombosis (DVT) and its sequela pulmonary embolism (PE) are important and potentially preventable causes of mortality and morbidity in hospitalised patients; together they are referred to as venous thromboembolism (VTE). It is estimated that 25,000 people die each year from preventable hospital-acquired VTE (House of Commons Health Committee 2005) and that, in the general population, the incidence of VTE increases with age from about 2–3 per 10,000 person years at age 30–49 to 20 per 10,000 person years at age 70–79 (Fowkes et al. 2003). Incidence is similar in males and females and, according to SIGN, incidence of symptomatic DVT in the general population is approximately 1 in 1000 (SIGN 2002).

Causes

The causes of DVT centre on pathophysiological changes that occur most commonly in the veins of the lower leg. An individual patient's likelihood of developing a DVT increases when they possess one or more predisposing risk factors (Box 10.4).

Pathophysiology

A combination of factors is thought to lead to the development of DVTs. Known as Virchow's triad; these factors comprise venous stasis, vessel wall injury and hyper-coagulability of the blood. The relative importance of each of these factors is still not fully understood but the mechanism for the formation of DVTs is best summarised as the activation of coagulation factors in areas where blood flow is reduced (Patel et al. 2011).

DVT usually starts in the veins of the calf with coagulation originating around valve cusps. Calf DVTs are probably not dangerous if they remain isolated distally. However, between 5% and 20% of calf DVTs will progress proximally. In these cases, the primary thrombus extends within and between the deep and superficial veins of the leg and, as a result, can cause venous obstruction, valvular damage and, possible, thromboembolism (Gorman et al. 2000). Half of all proximal vein thromboses embolise to the lungs if left untreated (Moulton & Yates 2006). More rarely, cases of primary DVT can arise in the ileo-femoral veins, primarily after vessel wall damage from orthopaedic surgery or venous catheterisation.

Initial assessment

The classic presenting features of DVT include boring, unilateral calf pain with swelling, tenderness to touch/palpation, localised warmth and skin erythema. This 'textbook' presentation is, however, rare. In reality, the presenting features of DVT relate to the degree of venous obstruction and inflammation of the vessel wall. Many thrombi do not cause enough obstruction to significantly reduce blood flow, and collateral circulation can develop to ensure adequate venous return. Inflammation of vessel walls may not cause significant pain or swelling and, consequently, patients suffering from DVT can often be asymptomatic and the findings of a physical examination alone are often inconclusive. According to Jenkins and Braen (2005), clinical features of DVT are misleading, unreliable or absent in approximately 50% of patients. The clinical features that may be present are outlined in Box 10.5 and these, linked with the predisposing factors above, give a clearer indication of the likelihood of DVT being present.

The British Committee for Standards in Haematology (BCSH) (2004) recommend that all pregnant women (and those who are within the first 6 weeks postpartum) who are suspected of having a DVT should undergo diagnostic imaging.

On rare occasions, severe DVT can lead to arterial compromise with resultant severe pain, swelling, cyanosis and rapid development of tense oedema

---

Box 10.5   Possible presenting features of deep vein thrombosis

- Oedema, often unilaterally
- Calf pain (occurs in 50% of cases but is non-specific to DVT)
- Tenderness to touch (occurs in 75% of cases of DVT but is also found in 50% of patients without confirmed DVT)
- Purple or red discoloration of the skin
- Swelling below knee in distal DVTs and up to groin in proximal DVTs
- Increased skin temperature
- Engorgement of superficial leg veins (only in minority of cases)
- Slight fever
- Positive Homan's sign* (in less than 20% of cases and not a reliable indicator)

* Homan's sign: discomfort in calf muscles on forced dorsiflexion of the foot with the knee straight – not a reliable indicator of DVT

(phlegmasia cerulea dolens). In such cases, an urgent surgical referral is required along with elevation of the leg and fluids to replace extravasation (Bedside Clinical Guidelines Partnership 2009).

Immediate management and investigations

Patients with suspected DVT can be nursed on a stretcher, couch, in a bed or on a chair though ambulation should be encouraged if appropriate. If seated or lying down, elevate the affected leg with some flexion of the knee (to encourage venous drainage) and support it on a pillow in the position most comfortable for the patient. Take a history (Boxes 10.2 and 10.3), measure and record vital signs, gain intravenous access and take blood samples for full blood count, urea and electrolytes, D-dimer and clotting screen (FBC, INR & APTT). In addition, oxygen saturations may be measured and oxygen given if the patient is unusually short of breath. Prediction of probability for DVT should be undertaken using a clinical scoring model such as that outlined in Box 10.6. Measurement of calf circumferences to provide a baseline for further evaluation may be carried out 10 cm below the tibial tuberosity. A swelling of 3 cm greater than the asymptomatic side is a relative indicator of DVT but is not definitive.

Measurement of circulating D-dimer concentrations (a normal by-product of fibrin degradation) acts as an aid to diagnosis. A normal D-dimer level virtually rules out a DVT but a positive result on its own does not confirm DVT as raised levels can be caused by other pathology. When combined with ultrasound investigations, D-dimers have up to 98% sensitivity for proximal (thigh or pelvic) DVTs with a high negative predictive value (Bernardi et al. 1998; Gorman et al. 2000; Ofri 2000). However, D-dimer tests are less accurate when detecting calf vein thrombosis and have poor specificity as other conditions can cause raised levels (see Box 10.7).

In general terms, a low pre-test probability score combined with a normal D-dimer level indicates absence of DVT and no further investigations are required.

Box 10.6   The Wells clinical prediction guide for deep vein thrombosis

Clinical feature	Score
Active cancer (treatment on going or within 6 months or palliative)	1
Paralysis, paresis or POP on lower leg	1
Recently bedridden >3 days or major surgery within 4 weeks	1
Localised tenderness along distribution of deep vein system	1
Calf diameter >3 cm larger than the asymptomatic leg*	1
Pitting oedema	1
Entire swollen leg	1
Collateral superficial veins (non-varicose)	1
Alternative diagnosis (as likely or greater than that of DVT)	–2

* Measured 10 cm below tibial tuberosity

Adding the scores with a total as follows indicates probability of DVT:
0 = low probability	= 3% frequency of DVT
1–2 = medium probability	= 17% frequency of DVT
>3 = high probability	= 75% frequency of DVT

Source: Anand et al. (1998), Gorman et al. (2000) and Ofri (2000)

Box 10.7   Examples of conditions which may cause a D-dimer result to be raised

- Acute myocardial infarction (MI)
- Chronic subdural haematoma
- Disseminated intravascular coagulation
- Gram-negative bacteraemia
- Leukaemia
- Liver disease
- Metastatic malignancy
- Peripheral vascular disease
- Pregnancy
- Recent surgery
- Renal disease
- Rheumatoid disease
- Sickle cell crisis
- Subarachnoid haemorrhage
- Thrombolytic therapy
- Trauma with pathological thrombosis

Source: BCGP (2009)

All other cases should have a Doppler ultrasound carried out. This technique measures the velocity of moving objects such as red blood cells in comparison to other objects. Scanning time can be further reduced by the use of colour Duplex ultrasonography. In the case of venous thrombosis, colour Duplex scanning has a 90–100% accuracy for detecting proximal DVTs (from the common femoral vein to the popliteal vein) but is less reliable for diagnosing calf vein thrombosis (Donnelly et al. 2000). Impedance plethysmography (IPG) is a non-invasive investigation used in some centres. This procedure is based on recording changes in blood volume in a limb, which are directly related to venous outflow. IPG has been shown to be sensitive and specific for proximal vein thrombosis but it is insensitive for calf vein thrombosis, non-occluding proximal vein thrombus and ileo-femoral vein thrombosis above the inguinal ligament (Patel et al. 2011).

In summary, the combination of pre-test probability testing, D-dimer measurement and diagnostic imaging (ultrasonography) give better accuracy than any single approach when assessing the likelihood of distal as well as proximal DVTs.

Unless the patient has a condition other than DVT that requires admission to hospital, they should be treated as an outpatient (BCGP 2009). The principles in managing patients with a DVT are oral analgesia (e.g. co-codamol) and early initiation of effective anticoagulant therapy with the aim of preventing further progression of the thrombosis to the proximal veins and, thereby, pulmonary embolism. Given that diagnosis on the basis of clinical features is often inconclusive, management of suspected DVT is based on the results obtained from one or more objective diagnostic investigations. To support this, clinical risk factors (Box 10.4) are also assessed and taken into account as confirmation rates of DVT rise with the number of factors present. Identification of an underlying cause, if present, will also guide the treatment and prevention of further episodes (Gorman et al. 2000).

Treatment usually starts with subcutaneous low molecular weight heparin (LMWH) with the dose determined by platelet count and the patient's body weight (make sure you weigh them rather than relying on their own estimation). LWMH (e.g. dalteparin) has been shown to be at least as effective as the traditionally used unfractionated heparin in preventing recurrent venous thromboembolism. In addition, it significantly reduces the occurrence of major haemorrhage during initial treatment and reduces overall mortality at the end of the patient's follow-up period (van den Belt et al. 2000). It should continue for at least 5 days after warfarin treatment has been commenced (NHS Clinical Knowledge Summaries 2009). Oral warfarin is usually started on day one (except in pregnancy and other contra-indications) with the dose determined by algorithm. Application of graduated elastic compression stockings is recommended as they may reduce post-thrombotic syndrome by up to 50% (Brandjes et al. 1997). However, evidence as to whether these should extend to above or below the knee is inconclusive (NHS CKS 2009). Correctly fitting stockings should be worn for at least 2 years as the risk of post-thrombotic syndrome may last 8–10 years. According to BCGP (2009) absolute and relative contra-indications for the application of compression stockings include:

Absolute contra-indications

- advanced peripheral arterial disease – feel for foot pulses, but note that pulses may be impalpable because of oedema
- heart failure
- septic phlebitis
- phlegmasia caerulea dolens (see above)

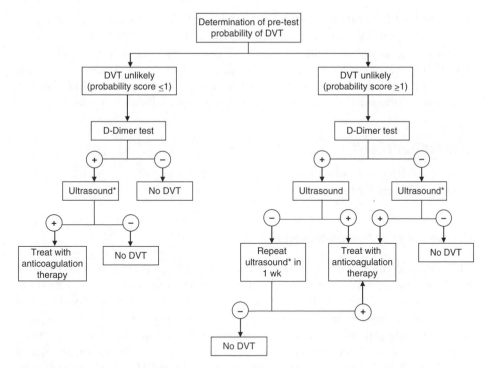

Figure 10.1 Example of a diagnostic algorithm using D-dimer testing and ultrasound imaging in patients with suspected deep vein thrombosis (from Scarvelis & Wells 2006). *Imaging done from proximal veins to calf trifurcation.

Relative contra-indications

- chronic arthritis of affected leg
- leg ulcers
- numbness or paralysis of affected leg
- suppurative dermatosis
- prognosis < 6 months
- intolerance of elastic stocking fabric

Based on the principles outlined above, local arrangements for assessing, investigating and treating suspected DVT will be available. An example of an assessment and treatment algorithm is shown in Figure 10.1.

Ongoing assessment and treatment

Gorman et al. (2000) suggest that the patient's activated partial thromboplastin time (APTT) is checked every 6 hours until the target of 1.5–2.5 is reached or according to the algorithm being used. Once reached, this should be checked daily to maintain this range. Platelet count should also be measured at the start of treatment and on day 5 to rule out thrombocytopenia. In cases of first DVT, warfarin is recommended for at least 3 months and prolonged treatment continues to reduce the risk of repeat DVT when compared with no treatment(NHS CKS 2009).

Many patients who are referred with DVT can be discharged once initial investigations and treatment have been completed. Deagle et al. (2005) give an example of how a nurse-led service that uses duplex ultrasound along with LMW heparin and compression for the assessment and treatment of ambulatory patients.

Thrombophlebitis

Thrombophlebitis is an inflammatory response that may affect superficial or deep veins of either the upper or lower limbs.

Causes and pathophysiology

Thrombophlebitis is characterised by pathophysiology that is similar to DVT, involving venous stasis, hypercoagulability and vessel wall injuries. It can occur spontaneously or as a result of invasive interventions such as venepuncture or intravenous administration of medication (either therapeutically or socially). Identifiable clinical risk factors associated with thrombophlebitis are a previous history of superficial phlebitis, DVT or pulmonary embolism; however, absence of risk factors is not a prognostic indicator (Kelver & Rosh 2010). In the lower limbs, it is associated with superficial varicosities, pregnant or postpartum women as well as recent surgery, prolonged immobilisation or underlying malignancy.

Initial assessment

Features of superficial thrombophlebitis include a gradual onset of tenderness, inflammation and swelling of the superficial veins. The area may be hot and erythema may be present along the path of the affected vein. A history of local trauma may be evident. Thrombophlebitis should be assumed to be DVT until proven otherwise as clinical examination cannot satisfactorily exclude deep vein involvement. As with DVT, visual examination is unreliable as the features present could be attributed to a number of conditions such as venous complications of liver disease, heart failure, renal disease, infection or trauma. Palpation usually indicates a painful or tender area and may reveal a firm, thickened and thrombosed vein (Kelver & Rosh 2010). Screening for meticillin-resistant *Staphylococcus aureus* (MRSA) is appropriate in accordance with local infection prevention and control policies.

Immediate management and investigations

Management of lower limb inflammation centres on resolving symptoms, prevention of extension to the deep veins and the exclusion of underlying DVT (see section above). Nurse the patient in the most comfortable position for them, ideally with their leg elevated, slightly flexed at the knee and elevated on a pillow. Record vital signs and take blood samples for full blood count, urea, electrolytes, D-dimer and clotting screen. Calf measurements may be recorded for comparison with the unaffected side. If the upper limb is affected, it should be elevated and supported in a position most comfortable to the patient. Once DVT has been excluded, superficial thrombophlebitis can be treated with a short course of an appropriate non-steroidal anti-inflammatory agent (Wyatt et al. 2005). Infective thrombophlebitis must be considered in patients who have a fever, raised white cell count, cellulitis or who have had recent venepuncture (including illicit drug use) or cannulation.

Ongoing assessment and treatment

If it is not possible to exclude infection, re-examination within 24–48 hours is recommended. If confirmed, patients with infective thrombophlebitis require admission for intravenous antibiotics.

Cellulitis

Causes and pathophysiology

Cellulitis literally means inflammation of cellular tissue. This common condition is caused when micro-organisms enter a break in the skin and lead to the spread of an acute infection usually caused by group A *Streptococcus* or *Staphylococcus aureus* (Jenkins & Braen 2005). It can occur anywhere on the body and may be associated with minor or unrecalled trauma or injecting drug use. The cellulitis disease cycle normally concludes with local infection or inflammation as the body's immune system responds. If, however, the body cannot compensate or if the infection becomes too overwhelming, this may lead to a more serious systemic infection. Patients with diabetes mellitus, immune deficiency disorders, chronic liver or kidney disease, peripheral arterial disease or systemic illness are prone to cellulitis (Herchline et al. 2011).

Initial assessment

Classic signs of cellulitis include a warm, reddened, swollen area that is tender to touch. Red 'track' marks may be visible on the skin proximal to the area of inflammation. These are characteristic of lymphangitis, an indication that infection is being carried through the lymph system.

Immediate management and investigations

Mild cellulitis can be treated with oral antibiotics on an outpatient basis. Systemic infection can be a sequela to undiagnosed or untreated cellulitis. Elevation of an affected limb can help to reduce swelling. Patients who fail to respond to oral antibiotics or who develop systemic signs including fever, dehydration, altered mental status, tachypnoea, tachycardia and hypotension may require intravenous antibiotics and management associated with a shocked patient (see Chapter 5 – Shock) (Herchline et al. 2011).

Ongoing assessment and treatment

Arrange follow-up either with the patient's GP or in the outpatient department 24–48 hours later to monitor the effectiveness of treatment. It is useful to mark the margins of the infection with a pen so that any changes are more obvious when the patient is reviewed. Give details of where to seek advice if the condition deteriorates. Patients who do not respond to oral antibiotics may require admission for intravenous antibiotics.

Less common conditions causing extremity pain and swelling

- Baker's cyst
- Torn gastrocnemius muscle
- Fracture
- Haematoma
- Acute arterial ischaemia
- Lymphoedema
- Hypoproteinaemia (e.g. cirrhosis, nephrotic syndrome)

Summary

This chapter has focused on the assessment and management of patients with painful and/or swollen lower limbs who may present in primary or secondary care settings. As a group of patients, these individuals can place considerable demands on the resources available within the acute admissions system. As new roles in nursing have developed, the care of these patients is an area in which nurses can have a positive impact on improving the service delivered and preventing hospital admission.

References

Anand S, Wells P & Hunt D (1998) Does this patient have deep vein thrombosis? *Journal of the American Medical Association*, 279,1094–1099.

Bedside Clinical Guidelines Partnership (BCGP) (2009) *Deep Vein Thrombosis*. West Mercia: BCGP.

Bernardi E, Prandoni P, Lensing A et al. (1998) D-dimer testing as an adjunct to ultrasonography in patients with clinically suspected deep vein thrombosis: prospective cohort study. *BMJ*, 317, 1037–1040.

Brandjes D, Buller H, Heijboer H et al. (1997) Randomised trial of effect of compression stockings in patients with symptomatic proximal-vein thrombosis. *Lancet* 349, 759–762.

British Committee for Standards in Haematology (BCSH) (2004) *Diagnosis of deep vein thrombosis in symptomatic outpatients and the potential for clinical assessment and D-dimer assays to reduce the need for diagnostic imaging.* London: BCSH.

Deagle J, Allen J & Rani R (2005) A nurse-led ambulatory care pathway for patients with deep venous thrombosis in an acute teaching hospital. *International Journal of Lower Extremity Wounds*, 4(2), 93–96.

Donnelly R, Hinwood D & London N (2000) Non-invasive arterial and venous assessment. *BMJ*, 320, 698 –701.

Fowkes F, Price J, & Fowkes F (2003) Incidence of diagnosed deep vein thrombosis in the general population: Systematic review. *European Journal of Vascular and Endovascular Surgery*, 25, 1–5.

Gorman W, Davis K & Donnelly R (2000) ABC of arterial and venous disease: Swollen lower limb 1: General assessment and deep vein thrombosis. *BMJ*, 320, 1453–1456.

Herchline T, Brenner B, Curtis D et al. (2011) Cellulitis. *Emedicine*.http://emedicine. medscape.com/article/781412-overview(accessed 15 April 2011).

House of Commons Health Committee (2005) *The prevention of venous thromboembolism in hospitalised patients.* London: Stationery Office.

Jenkins J & Braen G (eds) (2005) *Manual of Emergency Medicine* (5th edition). Philadelphia: Lippincott Williams & Wilkins.

Kelver R & Rosh J (2010) Superficial thrombophlebitis. *Emedicine*. http://emedicine. medscape.com/article/760563-overview (accessed 15 April 2011).

Moulton C & Yates D (2006) *Lecture Notes on Emergency Medicine* (3rd edition). Oxford: Blackwell Publishing.

NHS Clinical Knowledge Summaries (CKS) (2009) *Deep Vein Thrombosis Management*.www. cks.nhs.uk/deep_vein_thrombosis/management/scenario_deep_vein_thrombosis/follow_ up_for_dvt/basis_for_recommendation#-374373 (accessed 15 April 2011).

Ofri D (2000) Diagnosis and treatment of deep vein thrombosis.*Western Journal of Medicine*, 173, 194–197.

Patel K, Basson M, Borsa J et al. (2011) *Deep Vein Thrombosis and Thrombophlebitis.* Emedicine.http://emedicine.medscape.com/article/758140-overview (accessed 15 April 2011).

Scarvelis D & Wells P (2006) Diagnosis and treatment of deep-vein thrombosis. *Canadian Medical Association Journal*, 175, 1087–1092.

Scottish Intercollegiate Guidelines Network (SIGN) (2002) *Prophylaxis of Venous Thromboembolism.* Edinburgh: SIGN.www.sign.ac.uk/guidelines/fulltext/62/index.html (accessed 15 April 2011).

van den Belt A, Prins M, Lensing A et al. (2000) Fixed dose subcutaneous low molecular weight heparins versus adjusted dose unfractionated heparin for venous thrombo-embolism. *Cochrane Review* Vol.4. Oxford: Update Software.

Wyatt J, Illingworth R, Robertson C, Clancy M & Munro P (2005) *Oxford Handbook of Accident and Emergency Medicine* (2nd edition). Oxford: Oxford University Press.

Useful link and further reading

Advanced Life Support Group (ALSG) (2010) *Acute Medical Emergencies: The Practical Approach* (2nd edition). London: BMJ Books.

Emedicine.www.emedicine.com/emerg/contents.htm (requires free account login).

Index

Initial Management of Acute Medical Patients: A Guide for Nurses and Healthcare Practitioners,
Second Edition. Edited by Ian Wood and Michelle Garner.
© 2012 John Wiley & Sons, Ltd. Published 2012 by John Wiley & Sons, Ltd.